DISCARD

DATE DUE

Chicago Public Library

REFERENCE

Form 178 rev. 11-00

THE DEADLY TRUTH

The Deadly Truth

A HISTORY OF DISEASE IN AMERICA

Gerald N. Grob

HARVARD UNIVERSITY PRESS

CAMBRIDGE, MASSACHUSETTS,

AND LONDON, ENGLAND

2002

Library of Congress Cataloging-in-Publication Data

Grob, Gerald N., 1931–
The deadly truth : a history of disease in America / Gerald N. Grob.
p. cm.
Includes bibliographical references and index.
ISBN 0-674-00881-2 (alk. paper)
1. Diseases—America—History.   2. Medicine—America—History.   I. Title.

R150.G76 2002
616'.0097—dc21   2002017267

TO DAVID MECHANIC

Contents

Preface

This book is a product of nearly three decades of teaching and research. When I first became interested in the relationship between health and the environment in American history, I accepted many of the explanations about the etiology of disease and changing epidemiological patterns. Over time, however, I became more skeptical of contemporary theories that purportedly explained why people became sick and why they died. At present much of medical theory is based upon the belief that risk factors are responsible for cardiovascular diseases, cancer, and diabetes, and that behavioral and environmental changes provide the basis for their prevention. As will become clear in the following pages, I have serious doubts about the validity of these claims, which are seldom supported by empirical evidence. Indeed, we know very little about disease processes and mechanisms. This is not to disparage clinical medicine, which does yeoman work in managing and alleviating the symptoms of disease and thus contributes to the prolongation of life. Nevertheless the cure of most chronic or long-duration diseases, whether infectious or noninfectious in origin, remains only an ideal.

There are two ways of approaching the history of disease. The first (and dominant one) involves the study of the ways in which people have constructed and interpreted the meaning of disease. The second deals with the biological reality of disease. Both approaches are legitimate. The first (social construction) attempts to reconstruct past experiences, past meanings, and past perspectives. The second involves an effort to trace morbidity and mortality trends over time and to relate them to changing social, environmental, and behavioral factors. I have opted to focus upon the reality of disease rather than the manner in which different generations interpreted them.

My effort to understand past disease processes admittedly relies heavily on contemporary theories, which are themselves subject to change. Hence throughout the book I emphasize the limitations of our knowledge about the etiology and physiology of disease, and my delineation of past trends is stated in very tentative and probabilistic ways. I believe that it is better to admit what we do not know than to attempt overarching interpretations that rest on a slippery empirical foundation.

Throughout the book I present statistics dealing with life expectancy, morbidity, and mortality. These statistics represent at best an approximation of reality. Nor have I attempted to deal with all diseases, which would be an impossible task. Instead I have emphasized those disease categories which have been the major contributors to morbidity and mortality. Though touching upon gender, class, and racial differences in health and sickness, I have not made them central to my analysis. Finally, because of the methodological problems of translating past descriptions of diseases into modern diagnostic categories (which are themselves subject to change), many of my interpretations and generalizations are presented as probabilities rather than as certainties.

▼   ▼   ▼

In writing this book I have incurred many debts. The notes indicate the degree to which scholarship is a collaborative effort. A number of friends and colleagues not only engaged me in a fascinating dialogue but also read the entire manuscript, caught errors, and offered suggestions that have helped in numerous ways. I owe a particular debt of gratitude to George A. Billias, Lawrence J. Friedman, Allan V. Horwitz, Robert J. T. Joy, David Mechanic, Jay Neugeboren, Philip Pauly, and Joyce Seltzer. Each brought a different but illuminating perspective to the reading of the manuscript. Their comments and criticisms—always offered in a spirit of friendship and collegiality—made this book much better than it would have been. I must also thank Lila K. Grob—my wife and best friend—for her unwavering support and love during nearly fifty years of marriage.

Rutgers University
New Brunswick, New Jersey

THE DEADLY TRUTH

Prologue

"It is seldom recognized," wrote the distinguished biologist René Dubos in 1961, "that each type of society has diseases peculiar to itself–indeed, that each civilization creates its own diseases. Furthermore, there is no evidence that the techniques developed for dealing with the disease problems of one generation can cope with the problems of another." Conceding that new chapters in the history of medicine were likely, Dubos nevertheless argued that such chapters are "likely to be as full of diseases as its predecessors; [although] the diseases will only be different from those of the past."[1] To many Dubos's observations appear unduly pessimistic and obsolete, particularly in view of the advances in medical science since World War II. Before 1940, to be sure, the major function of medicine had been the diagnosis of disease; the therapeutic armamentarium was hardly impressive. With the exception of a limited number of medications (digoxin, thyroxine, insulin), immunization for a few infectious diseases, and surgical procedures, physicians had few means of coping with most infections, cardiovascular diseases, cancer, and many other illnesses of long duration. In an analysis of a classic medical textbook published in 1927, Paul B. Beeson found that most of the recommended treatments of the pre–World War II era had disappeared by 1975. Indeed, some of the therapies deployed before 1940 probably did more harm than good. The prevention of disease, however attractive, remained a utopian goal.[2]

After World War II medical practice underwent fundamental changes. The development of antibiotic drugs and vaccines seemed to

diminish the threat of infectious diseases. The introduction of the ste-
roids (cortisone and its derivatives) transformed a number of medical
specialties, made possible the treatment of childhood cancers, and facilitated organ transplantation. New medications and surgical interventions dramatically increased the ability to manage cardiovascular
disease. Technological innovations in laboratory analysis, imaging,
and instrumentation also played major roles in enhancing the capacity to manage many diseases that had previously proved fatal.[3] Potential advances in molecular biology and genetics offered the promise of
even greater progress. "[If] developments in research maintain their
current pace," according to William B. Schwartz, "it seems likely that
a combination of improved attention to dietary and environmental
factors along with advances in gene therapy and protein-targeted
drugs will have virtually eliminated most major classes of disease."[4]

That medical science alleviated many of the burdens of disease and
disability is incontrovertible. If its contributions to increasing longevity were more modest, the ability to manage disease clearly contributed to a better quality of life. To assume that continued progress will
eventually lead to the elimination of disease and presumably the
indefinite prolongation of human life, however, is more problematic.
Such a proposition rests on a fundamental misunderstanding of the
biological world and the nature of life itself. Taken to its extreme, the
belief that the conquest of disease is possible is but a modern version
of humanity's perennial quest to postpone death and to achieve a
form of immortality.

Modern humans no longer search—as Ponce de León once did—for a
"Fountain of Youth." Yet they still view the conquest of disease as a
realistic goal. Some insist that medical science can develop appropriate therapies for virtually all diseases; some believe that environmental and behavioral changes can eliminate many diseases; and still others turn to alternative medicine as a panacea. However dissimilar
their views, all assume that disease is "unnatural" and that its virtual
elimination is a distinct possibility. Based on this supposition, a variety of specific disease lobbies compete for funding on the grounds
that research can result in the discovery of cures.

The belief that disease can be conquered reflects a fundamental
conviction that all things are possible, and that human beings have it
within their power to control completely their own destiny. Disease is
perceived as the "enemy" of humanity, and only a war can vanquish

it. As Susan Sontag brilliantly noted in her classic *Illness as Metaphor*, descriptions of cancer resort to the terminology of warfare. Cancer cells "do not simply multiply; they are 'invasive.'" They "'colonize' from the original tumor to far sites in the body, first setting up tiny outposts ('micrometastases')." Medical treatment also employs military language. Radiotherapy resembles aerial warfare; patients are "bombarded" with toxic rays. Chemotherapy is akin to "chemical warfare, using poisons." That healthy cells are damaged or destroyed is but the collateral cost of conflict. The "war on cancer" must be fought to the finish, and the only acceptable outcome is unconditional surrender.[5]

The faith that disease is unnatural and can be conquered rests on a fundamental misunderstanding of the biological world. If cancer is the enemy, then we ourselves are the enemy. Malignant cells, after all, are hardly aliens who invade our bodies; they grow from our own normal cells. The biological world, moreover, includes millions of microorganisms. Some are harmless, while some are parasitic and have the potential to cause infection. Others play vital symbiotic roles that nourish and maintain organic life. Indeed, in the world of nature there is little clarity. Some microorganisms contribute to soil fertility by converting plant debris into humus, while others destroy crops. Some microorganisms cause disease in humans, but others that reside in the gastrointestinal tract play constructive and vital roles. Efforts to destroy pathogenic microorganisms through a variety of drugs seem doomed to failure, if only because of the ability of these microorganisms to develop resistant properties, which pose even greater dangers.

Environmental changes, moreover, can enhance the virulence of microorganisms or magnify other health risks. "Threats to health," Dubos observed in words that are still relevant as they were more than forty years ago, "are inescapable accompaniments of life." Conceding the ability to find methods of control for any given pathological state, he nevertheless insisted that "disease will change its manifestations according to social circumstances." Medical science traditionally sought "methods of control for the problems inherited from past generations," but it could not "prepare solutions for the specific problems of tomorrow because it does not know what these problems will be." Physicians–like soldiers–are always "equipped to fight the last war."[6]

Besides its inability to predict future threats to health, contemporary medical science for the most part can neither cure nor prevent most of the long-duration illnesses that account for the bulk of mortality. Its importance derives from its capability to manage and alleviate the symptoms of disease and thus to prolong life. Inflated rhetorical claims to the contrary, the etiology of most of the diseases of our age–notably cardiovascular disease, cancer, diabetes, mental illnesses—still remains a mystery. These intractable diseases reflect, as David Weatherall (Regius Professor of Medicine at Oxford) has written, "an extremely complex mixture of nature and nurture, set against the background of aging, which itself may be modified by both genes and environment. They are likely to have multiple causes, and there may be many different routes to their pathology."[7]

As our knowledge of specific diseases expands, their etiology and mechanisms grow more elusive. Diabetes offers an instructive illustration. Insulin-dependent (Type I) diabetes results from the self-destruction of the pancreatic islet cells. What causes this remains unknown. Though partially controllable by insulin, this disease still results in major complications, including blindness, coronary artery disease, circulatory problems in the lower limbs, and kidney failure. Nor does accurate control of the sugar level in the blood necessarily prevent these complications. Non-insulin-dependent diabetes (Type II) occurs in later life and results in disease of blood vessels. The causes of the complications that follow both forms of the disease remain unclear. "The more we have learned about this disease," Weatherall noted, "the more complex it has turned out to be." Much the same holds true for many other diseases.[8]

Nor are the benefits of medical treatment without risk. As a result of the introduction of chemotherapy in the treatment of cancer in the latter part of the twentieth century, a variety of new infections–some of which were previously virtually unknown–appeared. The microorganisms responsible for these infections were particularly dangerous to individuals whose immune system had been compromised by cancer treatment. The same phenomenon was evident among those undergoing organ transplantation, which required immunosuppressive drugs in order to prevent rejection.[9] Equally significant, many microorganisms developed resistance to antibiotics and were capable of causing life-threatening infections for which no therapies were available. Anesthesia, surgery, and sophisticated diagnostic procedures, even when competently undertaken, had the potential to induce iatrogenic illnesses. The rapidly expanding drug armamentarium was often accompanied by serious side effects. Finally, medical errors often resulted in both morbidity and mortality. A study by the Institute of Medicine of the National Academy of Sciences concluded that at least 44,000 and perhaps as many as 98,000 Americans died each year as a result of medical errors. One study of 815 consecutive patients on a general medical service of a university hospital found that 36 percent had a iatrogenic illness (defined as "any illness resulting from a diagnostic procedure, from any form of therapy, or from a harmful occurrence that was not a natural consequence of the patient's disease"). Medication errors in both hospitals and community settings were not uncommon.[10]

The generalizations offered by Dubos, Weatherall, and others clearly run counter to the contemporary myth that medical science has the capacity to uncover the precise etiology and mechanisms of all diseases and to develop appropriate cures. It is much easier, after all, to believe that disease can be eradicated than it is to accept the view that disease is an inevitable concomitant of the biological and natural environment. The world in which we live undergoes constant changes, which in turn create novel risks to human health and life. In this sense there can be no final victory over disease. The challenge facing medical science will be to minimize and control the health risks that accompany unforeseen environmental changes.

Nowhere is the validity of these generalizations better illustrated than in the history of sickness and death in America (as well as elsewhere). From the first settlements in the Americas to the end of the nineteenth century infectious diseases were the most important factor in mortality. This is not to imply that chronic degenerative or long-term diseases were absent; but the overwhelming presence of acute infectious diseases, which resulted in extraordinarily high mortality rates among infants and children, tended to conceal the presence of other categories of disease. The decline in acute infectious diseases as the major cause of mortality after 1900 led to shifts in the pattern of mortality and recognition of the presence of other long-duration illnesses that in the past had appeared less important because of the fact that fewer people survived to adulthood and old age.[11] What is most

impressive is that the decline of particular diseases was invariably followed by increases in the prevalence of other diseases. There is little
reason to assume that such trends will not continue.

The "lessons" of history are admittedly ambiguous. Nevertheless,
the discipline offers a perspective that illuminates many of the forces
that shape morbidity and mortality patterns in an ever-changing
world. It may offer little support to the utopian dream of a disease-
free society and a life span without well-defined limits, but at the very
least it provides the basis for a more realistic appreciation of the individual, social, and biological determinants of human health. To offer
such a sober view of the past is not synonymous with a paralyzing
pessimism. On the contrary, the very uncertainty of the future gives
meaning to our lives and forces us to think of a variety of possibilities
to deal with the challenges posed by ever-changing circumstances.

CHAPTER 1

The Pre-Columbians

The oldest known Chinese medical treatise, published between two and three thousand years ago, alluded to a legendary era of health and happiness in the remote past. "In ancient times," wrote the Yellow Emperor in his *Classic of Internal Medicine,* "people lived . . . to be over a hundred years, and yet they remained active and did not become decrepit in their activities." Nowadays, he added, "people reach only half of that age and yet become decrepit and failing." What accounted for this shift? The answer to this question, according to one of the sages, lay in behavioral changes. In the past

> those people who understood Tao [the way of self-cultivation] patterned themselves upon the Yin and the Yang [the two principles in nature] and they lived in harmony with the arts of divination.
>
> There was temperance in eating and drinking. Their hours of rising and retiring were regular and not disorderly and wild. By these means the ancients kept their bodies united with their souls, so as to fulfill their allotted span completely, measuring unto a hundred years before they passed away.
>
> Nowadays people are not like this; they use wine as beverage and they adopt recklessness as usual behavior. They enter the chamber (of love) in an intoxicated condition; their passions exhaust their vital forces; their cravings dissipate their true (essence); they do not know how to find contentment within themselves; they are not skilled in the control of their spirits. They devote all their attention to the amusement of their minds, thus cutting themselves off from

the joys of long (life). Their rising and retiring is without regularity. For these reasons they reach only one half of the hundred years and then they degenerate.[1]

The Yellow Emperor's vision of a utopian and harmonious past has been widely shared. Indeed, many assume that the ideal environment is one that has remained in a natural state unchanged by human intervention. Yet in the world of nature change is the rule rather than the exception; weather patterns and the physical surface of the Earth have undergone cataclysmic alterations, and there have been radical transformations in vegetation and animal populations.[2] The same is true of humankind; behavior and social organization over many millennia have rarely remained static.

▾   ▾   ▾

The notion that a pristine environment in the remote past was synonymous with health is a romantic dream. Though inhabiting a very different world, our prehistoric ancestors also confronted the reality of disease.

The data on prehistory are extraordinarily scanty; nearly all the "facts" are speculative or extrapolated from tiny samples. Hence generalizations are at best contingent and provisional. Yet it is clear that our remote ancestors, like ourselves, faced a variety of threats to health and life that reflected the world they inhabited.

For several million years humans survived by hunting and gathering food from whatever sources were available. They lived in small groups and tended to be nomadic because of the need to find adequate food supplies. Generally speaking, they neither cultivated crops nor kept domestic livestock, and their daily existence was shaped largely by the physical environment. Life was harsh, accommodation to natural forces necessary, and survival fragile.

Such groups faced very different threats to health and life from those confronting their modern successors. Their low population density and nomadic way of life allowed only limited opportunities for infectious diseases to strike or spread. The very small size of these groups did not generally allow microbial parasites to maintain a presence in human hosts. Low population density invariably broke the chain of transmission; the lack of a sufficient number of susceptible individuals (those not previously exposed and hence lacking protective antibodies) precluded the continuous presence of the pathogen. Hence many of the endemic and epidemic infectious diseases that would play such a prominent role in later periods were of minor importance in the remote past.[3]

The small nomadic bands of prehistoric times, however, did not enjoy an idyllic and healthy life. Their members were exposed to a variety of parasites found in vegetation, animals, or the soil. Zoonoses or zoonotic infections (animal diseases capable of being transmitted to humans) were caused by organisms that survived in animal hosts. Their transmission to humans was usually the result of chance contacts with wild animals. Such zoonotic diseases as rabies, hemorrhagic fevers, and anthrax—to cite but a few—were significant causes of disease among prehistoric populations. Though common, zoonotic diseases tended to be self-limiting because they were not transmitted by human contact. Such infections often resulted in death, however, because any immunity prior to exposure was lacking.

The conditions of prehistoric life also enhanced the risks of other diseases. The anaerobic bacteria that cause gangrene and tetanus were present in the soil and animal intestines, and humans were exposed to them while traveling in the wilds or butchering carcasses. Worms and tapeworms survived in the soil and water and could easily infect humans. Eating animal flesh posed additional risks, since many food animals harbored a variety of worms or tapeworms. Animal populations carried fleas and ticks that caused bubonic plague as well as such rickettsial diseases as Rocky Mountain spotted fever and Lyme disease. Mosquitoes transmitted various pathogens from animal and bird hosts to humans.

Prehistoric populations also carried organisms that survived for extended periods, causing mild chronic infections. Such organisms passed from one human to another by personal contact or food, or through atmospheric droplets from infected family members. Many bacteria, including staphylococcus, streptococcus, various forms of salmonella, and intestinal protozoa, were of ancient lineage; they survived in humans sometimes without producing symptoms. Yet they were capable of causing mild or even fatal infections. These and other pathogens possessed the ability to survive in small groups of humans, maintaining a presence in successive generations.[4]

The distribution of infectious diseases among prehistoric humans was by no means constant. Migration to new areas with different environments produced new patterns. Indeed, as prehistoric groups left Africa (where humankind probably originated), they left behind many of the parasites and microorganisms found primarily in tropical climates. In more temperate zones, conditions less hospitable to bacterial life diminished their diversity. In the Americas, moreover, perhaps 80 percent of large wild mammals became extinct during the last Ice Age, around 13,000 years ago. Their inhabitants—unlike their counterparts in Eurasia—thus had far fewer herd animals to domesticate as a result of the decline of animal species. Consequently, animal-derived diseases played a much less significant role in the Americas than in Eurasia.[5]

Zoonotic and soil diseases were by no means the only or even the major threats to prehistoric humans. Fluctuations in climate—floods, droughts, temperature changes—diminished the food supply and increased human vulnerability through starvation or lack of necessary nutrients. Accidents and violence between groups took a high toll as well. Mothers and infants undoubtedly experienced high mortality rates. The migratory style of life also made it difficult or impossible to provide care for sick persons or to nurse them back to health. Although data on average duration of life are extraordinarily sketchy, surviving skeletal evidence suggests that considerably more than half of all people died before the age of 20, and few lived beyond 50.[6]

Nomadic hunting groups depended for their survival on the presence of large-bodied animals. Over time, however, many animal species serving as sources of food became extinct. Whether as a result of excessive hunting or natural disasters (e.g., fires, floods, earthquakes) that destroyed indigenous habitats, the decline in the animal population posed a dire threat to humans. In response to a variable and diminishing food supply, humans began to alter their living pattern. Between 10,000 and 2,000 years ago a sedentary lifestyle slowly replaced nomadism as humans turned to agriculture to ensure a more stable food supply.

The transition from hunting to agriculture had profound consequences. Nomadic groups had relatively little capacity to alter the environment. Sedentary populations, on the other hand, transformed the landscape in many ways. As archaeological excavations demonstrate, humans cleared the land, built drainage and water systems, and kept domesticated animals. As the food supply became more dependable, populations began to grow in both size and density. Humans increasingly lived in villages, towns, and subsequently cities, where more crowded conditions prevailed. Additional contacts between groups followed the inevitable rise of trade and commerce.

Sedentary communal patterns led to the first epidemiological transition. By altering the material conditions of their lives, humans changed the intricate relationships between themselves and the many microorganisms inhabiting the Earth. The development of agriculture inhibited natural ecosystems and created favorable conditions for the transmission of a variety of disease parasites that flourished in shallow water. Human beings, as well as their animals and crops, began to experience the consequences. Sedentary patterns and agriculture created circumstances propitious to the emergence of infectious endemic and epidemic diseases, which became the major determinants of morbidity and mortality.

Sedentary modes, to be sure, conferred certain benefits. The environmental modifications that followed the adoption of an agricultural way of life reduced the number and variety of pathogens and enabled humans to create a host-parasite relationship benign to both. The emergence of a sedentary society also improved the ways in which sick people received care, and thus their chances of survival. The benefits of sedentary patterns, however, may well have been outweighed by disadvantages. Better and permanent housing, for example, attracted insects and rats, thus increasing the potential for such diseases as malaria and plague in endemic form. Housing also promoted the transmission of disease from one person to another either by actual contact or by airborne droplets from the secretions of sick individuals. Sanitation likewise became a greater problem, for concentration of the wastes of humans and animals promoted fecal-oral transmission of diseases.

The creation of stable communities permitted microorganisms to establish themselves in environments that had previously been inhospitable. Irrigation practices, for example, created stagnant bodies of water, thereby providing better conditions for snails carrying schistosomiasis or mosquitoes serving as vectors for malaria and yellow fever. Domestication of animals, however beneficial, placed humans in close contact with them, thus facilitating the transmission of zoonotic diseases or, as in the case of influenza, permitting the mixing of animal and human strains of the virus that from time to time mutated

into more virulent forms. The increase in population density promoted infectious diseases, particularly when the number of susceptible persons reached a critical mass. The expansion of trade and commerce moved pathogens over long distances, enabling them to find
new host populations, often with catastrophic consequences. The
opening of areas previously uninhabited by humans and the transformation of established environments disseminated new viruses and
microorganisms that led to devastating epidemics among those lacking immunologic defenses. Prevailing mortality patterns ensured that
the proportion of aged persons in the general population remained
low. Consequently, long-duration diseases—the primary causes of
mortality among the aged—were not and would not be of major
significance until the twentieth century.[7]

Infectious diseases were established in human hosts relatively early,
as Egyptian mummies and papyri reveal. Descriptions from the latter
indicate the presence of intestinal infections and urinary disorders, including schistosomiasis (a parasitic disease often spread by freshwa-
ter snails) and such treponemal diseases as yaws, pinta, and bejel.
Worm and tapeworm infections were also common. The Egyptian Pa-
pyrus Ebers includes a passage describing symptoms compatible with
tuberculosis: "If thou examinest a man for advanced illness in his
chest, whose body shrinks, being altogether bewitched; if thou
examinest him and dost not find any disease in his belly, but the
'hnwt' of his body is like 'pjt,' then shalt thou say to him: It is a decay
of thy inside."[8]

Ancient Near Eastern texts often refer to periods of pestilence. A
Hittite prayer written in the late fourteenth century B.C.E. notes the
presence of a devastating plague:

> The Hatti land has been cruelly afflicted by plague. For twenty years
> now men have been dying in my father's days, in my brother's days,
> and in mine own since I have become the priest of the gods. When
> men are dying in the Hatti land like this, the plague is in no wise
> over. As for me, the agony of my heart and the anguish of my soul I
> cannot ensure any more . . . Because I humble myself and cry for
> mercy, hearken to me, Hattian Storm-god, my lord! Let the plague
> stop in the Hatti land![9]

The Hebrew Bible frequently alludes to sudden outbreaks of lethal
diseases, which Jews interpreted as the work of God. The book of Ex-

odus describes the lethal visitation upon Egypt's firstborn that left "not a house where there was not one dead." Other passages detail a variety of epidemics visited upon enemies of Israel as well as the Israelites themselves. When David sinned, God "sent a pestilence upon Israel . . . and there died of the people from Dan even to Beer-sheba seventy thousand men."[10]

Greek texts from the classical era echo these descriptions. Thucydides' *History of the Peloponnesian War* includes a sketch of the plague that devastated Athens about 430 B.C.E. "The disease began with a strong fever in the head, and reddening and burning heat in the eyes; the first internal symptoms were that the throat and tongue became bloody and the breath unnatural and malodorous." Many perished within a week from the "internal burning" even though they retained some strength. Those who escaped the first symptoms found that the "disease descended to the belly; there violent ulceration and totally fluid diarrhoea occurred, and most people then died from the weakness caused by that." The magnitude of the plague was such that the "bodies of the dead and dying were piled on one another." Thirty-five years later the Carthaginian army besieging Syracuse was struck by a plague. Its symptoms included sore throats, dysentery, pain, pustules covering the entire body, and disorientation. Death, according to Diodorus Siculus in his *History,* "came on the fifth day, or the sixth at the latest, amidst such terrible tortures that all looked upon those who had fallen in the war as blessed." The writings of Hippocrates confirm the importance of numerous infectious diseases in the ancient world, including malaria, dysentery, and respiratory disorders of one sort or another.[11]

▼   ▼   ▼

In a classic study William H. McNeill emphasized the confluence of disease pools in Eurasia between 500 B.C.E. and 1200 A.D. Ancient societies—whether in the Middle East, continental Europe, the British Isles, the Mediterranean littoral, or Asia—experienced periodic epidemics as increased commercial contacts moved pathogens between them. By 900 A.D., however, an uneasy epidemiological equilibrium, which allowed for significant population growth, had been established in Eurasia between human hosts and pathogens. It was upset only occasionally when the number of susceptible persons reached a point that permitted the outbreak of epidemic diseases.[12]

Despite the presence of infectious diseases, European population grew rapidly from the eleventh to the fourteenth centuries. Although precise figures are lacking, it is clear that the continent was densely populated by the beginning of the fourteenth century. At its peak, for example, the Italian region of Tuscany may have had as many as 2 million inhabitants—a figure that would not be matched until the middle of the nineteenth century. To be sure, infectious diseases persisted in endemic and epidemic form. Yet many existed in nonlethal and mild forms—smallpox being an example—and resulted in relatively low mortality.[13]

The circumstances that promoted European population growth for nearly three centuries came to an abrupt halt about 1347 with the advent of the Black Death, or bubonic plague. Persisting sporadically for more than three centuries, this disease was responsible for a massive decline in the populations of Europe and the British Isles as well as the Middle East and Asia. By 1420 Europe may have had only a little more than a third of the population it had a century earlier. In some areas the population fell 80 percent. The experiences of London were by no means atypical. In 1563 more than 17,000 died, perhaps a fifth of the population. Before the end of the century three additional outbreaks took heavy tolls. In 1603 and 1625 the total deaths from plague were 30,000 and 40,000, respectively. The final epidemic in 1665 resulted in perhaps 100,000 fatalities, or one-sixth of the city's population. "We are in good hopes," wrote an official of St. Paul's Cathedral,

> that God in his mercy will put a stop to this sad calamity of sickness. But the desolation of the City is very great; that heart is either steel or stone that will not lament for this sad visitation, and will not bleed for those unutterable sorrows . . . What eye would not weep to see so many habitations uninhabited, the poor sick not visited, the hungry not fed, the grave not satisfied? Death stares us continuously in the face of every infected person that passes by us, in every coffin which is daily and hourly carried along the streets. The bells never cease to put us in mind of our mortality.[14]

Bubonic plague in its origins was a disease of small animals, including rodents, prairie dogs, and other wildlife living far from human habitats. The primary organism was a bacillus (*Yersina pestis*).

Patterns of settlement and trade moved an enzootic disease westward
from Mongolia through central Asia and eastern Europe. The presence of a large rodent population and rat fleas in populated regions
created conditions conducive to the spread of the disease to human
hosts. When infected rodents perished, the rat flea sought other hosts.
Though preferring a rodent host, fleas were able to infect humans
with the bacillus. The result was a plague that took three forms—bubonic, septicemic, and pneumonic. In the bubonic form (in which
lymph involvement is characteristic) the mortality rate can approach
60 percent. The other two forms had mortality rates of nearly 100
percent and were spread among humans by droplet infection. Not all
scholars concede that bubonic plague was solely responsible for the
depopulation that occurred after 1347. Indeed, it may be that such
high mortality rates were caused by a combination of infectious diseases working in tandem. Whatever the case, there is little doubt that
Europe, as well as the Middle East and Asia, suffered a human catastrophe lasting for several centuries. Paradoxically, the expansion of
Europe beyond the continent occurred at precisely the time that inhabitants were experiencing a mortality crisis that seemed to endanger their very survival.

▼   ▼   ▼

Although humankind may have had a common biological origin, the
inhabitants and environment of the Americas differed in important
ways from those of other continents. Admittedly sketchy and inconclusive evidence suggests that its peoples had Asiatic origins and originally migrated across Beringia, a land bridge linking Alaska and Siberia during perhaps three or four successive ice ages over the past
70,000 years. Indeed, there may have been as many as four distinct
migrations separated by thousands of years. Recent scholars have
speculated—on the basis of limited archaeological evidence—that the
first migration possibly occurred more than 25,000 years ago and involved people from the Bakai region of Siberia. Their migration from
Alaska to South America may have involved sea travel, since North
America was covered by massive icecaps at the time. The second and
third migrations came from Eurasia and possibly from coastal eastern
Asia. When the ice age passed, an interior corridor opened up that facilitated the movement of peoples along the Pacific coast and into the

interior, and southward to Central and South America. The final migration from Siberia involved Eskimo-Aleut peoples, whose descendants remained in northern Canada and Alaska.[15]

Whatever the origins of human beings in the Americas, contacts—human as well as biological—between the Americas and Eurasia ceased when Beringia disappeared about 10,000 years ago. The population of the Americas therefore developed in cultural, physical, and biological isolation from the rest of humanity. Taken as a group, they were remarkably homogeneous from a biological point of view. The distribution of blood types in the Americas lacked the variability found everywhere else (except among Australian aborigines). Its peoples had far less heterogeneity in the polymorphic loci that control the immune system. Recent studies have shown that individuals in the Americas who are unrelated have a more restricted gene pool and many more lines of common descent than siblings from other parts of the world. The genetic homogeneity of the peoples of the Americas, therefore, was not only a consequence of their biological isolation, but may also have been an adaptive response to the environment in which they lived.[16]

The biological isolation of the Americas was reflected in the absence of many of the pathogens that played an important role elsewhere. The slow passage across Beringia and the harsh climate experienced by the migrants probably eliminated many pathogens. Those whose life cycles occurred outside the bodies of their hosts (e.g., hookworm) could not survive the low temperatures. Similarly, diseases such as malaria and yellow fever—both of which require both an insect vector and infected persons—were never able to gain a foothold because of the absence of active cases. The lack of a variegated domesticated animal population tended to minimize the risk of many zoonotic diseases. The relatively small number of migrants inhibited the continued existence of many viral diseases that required a large human reservoir to persist. The migratory lifestyle and small numbers of the early indigenous population who were hunters and food gatherers further diminished the possibility that many pathogens that existed elsewhere could survive without a sufficiently large number of susceptible hosts.[17]

The lack of a diverse animal population shaped the disease pool in the Americas. Most of North and South America's wild mammal population had become extinct during the Pleistocene period, when glaciers covered much of the region. Consequently, the possibility of domesticating animals was minimal. The absence of a domesticated animal population had a profound influence. In Eurasia many of the pathogens responsible for the infectious diseases that periodically ravaged residents probably evolved from ancestral microbes that originally preyed on animals. That people and a large variety of domesticated animals lived in close proximity ensured the continued presence of many infectious diseases. The inhabitants of the Americas, by contrast, had few, if any, domesticated animals, and thus the crowd diseases that played such a significant role in other parts of the world were largely unknown.[18]

These and other factors combined to give pre-Columbian America a disease environment somewhat different from the rest of the world. Many of the bacterial and viral diseases that had played such a critical role elsewhere—smallpox, yellow fever, measles, malaria—were unknown in the Americas. This is not to argue that its peoples led a disease-free existence. It is merely to suggest that threats to life and health diverged from patterns elsewhere, largely because environment, lifestyle, and genetic endowment were dissimilar.

To reconstruct the pattern of disease in the Americas before 1492 is extraordinarily difficult. Although human remains at pre-Columbian archaeological sites provide some data, they shed little light on acute viral and bacterial infectious diseases that left no lesions on the skeletal structure. Certain chronic bacterial infections left lesions but probably were not fatal because the immune response neither eliminated nor was overwhelmed by the bacterium. Early descriptions by Europeans of native diseases are equally problematic, nor do they correspond to contemporary diagnostic categories (which are themselves subject to change). Finally, there are numerous methodological problems in drawing inferences from skeletal remains; as a result there is as much disagreement as there is agreement among scholars who have attempted to employ skeletons to understand health and disease patterns of the pre-Columbian Americas.[19]

Within broad limits, however, it is possible to identify the patterns of morbidity and mortality while conceding that definitive statements are not possible.[20] Those patterns in the Americas generally reflected the ecological framework within which individuals and groups lived. The experiences of sedentary groups in the Americas paralleled those in other parts of the world, even if there were differences in terms of specific pathogens and magnitudes of health crises. Before the first contacts with Europeans, for example, the Ontario Iroquois already lived in densely populated communities with complex social structures. Crowded conditions, contamination of water supplies by human and organic wastes, and increased contacts with migrants created conditions in which endemic and epidemic infectious diseases persisted.[21] Before contact with Europeans, natives had not experienced the demographic disaster that occurred in Eurasia and elsewhere in the fourteenth and fifteenth centuries. But like their Eurasian brethren, they had to contend with dysentery and various bacterial and viral respiratory infections—all of which took a heavy toll, especially among infants and children.[22]

Differences notwithstanding, the populations of the Americas and Eurasia shared some infectious pathogens that had existed long before the appearance of human beings. Among these were the cocci group of bacteria that have had a long and generally intimate relationship with their human hosts. The most familiar are the varieties of staphylococcus and streptococcus, many of which are relatively harmless. The staphylococci, for example, are found on the skin of virtually all human beings and either are innocuous or else cause localized infections marked by pimples and boils. The streptococci can also cause annoying but not especially serious infections in the tonsils and sinuses. But some varieties of both can lead to life-threatening diseases such as meningitis, endocarditis, and infections that become systemic and are often fatal. There is no reason to believe that peoples in the Americas were exempt from cocci infections. Similarly, rheumatoid arthritis—a disease that may have very different etiologies—existed both in the Americas and elsewhere.[23]

Tuberculosis—a disease well known in Eurasia before 1492— was also present in the Americas. Tuberculosis is a chronic, or long-duration, disease caused by the *Mycobacterium tuberculosis* and exists in both human and bovine form. Though often identified as a pulmonary disease, it can affect all parts of the body, including the skeleton. Its history is marked by peaks and valleys because its virulence varied. Individuals were often infected in early childhood by inhaling droplets exhaled by those with the pulmonary form of the disease. Many never manifested clinical symptoms of tuberculosis. Some developed lesions as a result of other infections, inadequate nutrition, stress, and cofactors that are as yet unclear. But all these forms of the disease can compromise the immune system and lead to clinical cases and high mortality rates. Domestic herd animals as well as humans serve as a reservoir for the tubercle bacillus.

In recent decades the recovery of skeletal remains in both North and South America has provided evidence of the presence of tuberculosis. In one Illinois excavation, for example, there were 27 cases with clear and 5 with probable lesions associated with tuberculosis out of a population sample of 264. The remains in this agricultural community suggested that a sedentary lifestyle and a restricted food supply as a result of violent confrontations with neighboring groups created conditions in which opportunistic infections like tuberculosis could flourish.[24]

The distribution of tuberculosis in prehistoric America probably differed substantially from that in other parts of the world. Tuberculosis in the Americas was somewhat less virulent. Natives may have adapted to the particular strain of the tubercle bacillus they encountered. Moreover, ecological and environmental factors combined to prevent epidemics with high mortality rates. In many Eurasian settings high population density and the presence of domesticated herds played a more significant role in the ecology of the disease. In the Americas, by contrast, the persistence of hunting and gathering among mobile groups tended to limit the spread of the disease. But the existence of more sedentary populations that employed agriculture as their source of food and therefore had higher population densities provided conditions in which the disease could exist. The absence of domesticated herds may not have been a limiting factor, for other animal populations may have served as natural reservoirs.[25]

Treponematosis was another chronic infectious disease endemic in the Americas. A multifaceted disease that may have originated in the tropical or temperate zones of the Americas, it has appeared in no less than four distinct clinical forms: pinta, yaws, nonvenereal syphilis, and venereal syphilis. Whether it was caused by the spirochete *Treponema pallidum* or by different subspecies remains unknown. The organisms recovered from all clinical forms are morphologically and serologically indistinguishable. The first three forms were generally contracted in childhood by direct contact with skin lesions. Venereal syphilis can affect all tissues and organs, especially the central nervous system and brain. In the later stages the disease has a devastating impact on the body as well as a high mortality rate. Archaeological evidence indicates that treponematosis in the Americas was not a venereal disease, but rather was spread by external contact. Environmental conditions probably played an important role in determining the form of the disease. The fact that it was contracted in early childhood may have triggered an immune response that limited the disease to its nonvenereal forms. Rarely fatal, treponematosis was an annoying fact of life in the Americas. In fifteenth-century Europe, by contrast, different social and environmental conditions promoted venereal dissemination of the disease in a virulent form, especially among urbanized populations.

Skeletal excavations have provided data on the presence of tuberculosis and treponematosis among native peoples of the Americas. But it is highly probable that a variety of other infectious diseases that left no mark on skeletal remains were far more important in shaping morbidity and mortality patterns. Given the fact that few pre-Columbian peoples created an urbanized society that transformed the natural landscape, they remained vulnerable to diseases of nature. Pathogens responsible for these diseases generally inhabit ticks, fleas, rodents, and a variety of wild animals. The transmission of such pathogens to human hosts generally occur as a result of accidental contact, and the ensuing infections often had a devastating impact.

There are, of course, many diseases of nature. Some are specific to particular geographic regions; others tend to be more dispersed. The precise pattern of such diseases in pre-Columbian America may never be known. There is reason to believe, however, that the environment in which an indigenous population lived and their unique customs rendered them susceptible to certain of these diseases. As they traveled through wooded areas in the late spring and summer, for example, they became vulnerable to pathogens transmitted by ticks. A prominent example is Rocky Mountain spotted fever. It is caused by a rod-shaped extremely small bacterium (*Rickettsia rickettsii*) that is part of the rickettsial group. These bacteria—like viruses—conduct their life processes inside the cells of their hosts, often with devastating results. The pathogen responsible for Rocky Mountain spotted fever is found only in the Americas, and we can assume that it struck indigenous inhabitants. First identified in Montana in the early twentieth century, it was even more prevalent in such southern states as Maryland, Virginia, North and South Carolina, and Georgia. Depending on location, the disease has a mortality rate that can reach as high as 70 percent, but on average it kills about 20 percent of its victims. Those who survived, however, were often left with impaired organs that rendered them vulnerable to other diseases.

Nor was Rocky Mountain spotted fever unique. Present in western America was an orbivirus that caused Colorado tick fever. Throughout the Americas arboviruses that caused St. Louis encephalitis, Western equine encephalitis, and Eastern equine encephalitis survived in a large reservoir of reptiles, birds, and mammals and were in turn transmitted to human hosts by mosquito vectors. The ensuing inflammation of the brain resulted in high mortality rates. Undoubtedly mosquitoes, flies, fleas, bugs, and ticks that lived in proximity to human beings conveyed many other bacterial and viral infections. Because the pathogens and the vectors differed from region to region, the specific pattern of infectious diseases varied, depending in part upon climate, vegetation, and population density.[26]

Many of the pathogens that employed animals as hosts were equally capable of parasitizing human beings on their own. People who relied upon hunting as a source of food came into contact with animals that harbored a variety of pathogens. Eating meat from infected animals resulted in such diseases as anthrax. Other organisms were part of the indigenous environment. Both domesticated and wild animals harbored tapeworms that could infect human hosts. In the southeastern United States common intestinal roundworms were found among inhabitants.[27] The probability is high that Indians encountered viral infections of one sort or another in their daily life. Some proved innocuous, while others could lead to chronic diseases or even prove fatal.

The environment in which the indigenous population lived was also conducive to the transmission of mycotic infections. These infections were caused by fungi, including mushrooms, molds, mildew, and other life forms that lack chlorophyll and subsist upon dead or living organic matter. Most fungal infections have a specific geographic distribution. In the contiguous United States coccidioidomycosis was generally confined to the Southwest, while histoplasmosis was found in the East and Midwest. In both instances the infection was spread by spore-laden dust. The acute form of both infections is generally benign, and resembles more common respiratory infections. But if the organisms disseminate in the individual, mortality rates can be as high as 60 percent. Skeletal remains in the Americas indicate that mycotic infections were fairly widespread even though the majority were relatively benign.[28]

Levels of health among pre-Columbian populations were not simply a function of the presence or absence of specific pathogens. A variety of other factors shaped morbidity and mortality patterns. In the Southwest skeletal excavations at several sites reveal high rates of fetal and infant mortality from congenital malformations, trauma, malnutrition, and infection. The process of giving birth, the presence of maternal health problems, and the youth of mothers all played a role as well. Common respiratory and intestinal disorders took a very heavy toll during the first 8 years of life. The pattern among prehistoric California Indians was similar. Skeletal remains reveal that individuals under the age of 20 accounted for one-quarter to nearly a third of all deaths. Given the fact that infant and child skeletal bones are less likely to be recovered, the actual figure may be considerably higher. Indeed, surviving evidence suggests that infant and maternal mortality may have been much higher in the Americas than in Europe, and that differing patterns of care contributed to the increased risk of death among infants and children.[29]

Violence within and between groups and accidents were also significant causes of mortality. Nor was the food supply always adequate. On occasion climatic changes had adverse effects on both vegetation and animal life, which in turn led to malnutrition and the complications that followed. In some cases the absence of vital nutrients led to such diseases as goiter (caused by iodine deficiency). Skeletal remains offer substantial evidence of both trauma and malnutrition. Individual and group interactions, social and cultural patterns, and environmental forces beyond human control, together with existing infectious organisms, shaped the lives of pre-Columbian Americans in ways not fundamentally dissimilar from Eurasian populations.

▼   ▼   ▼

In Europe the major causes of mortality were epidemic and endemic infectious diseases associated with high-density populations and established patterns of trade and commerce. The absence of many of these "crowd" diseases fostered the belief that the Americas provided a healthier and less risky habitat. In part such beliefs reflected the attitude that America was an Eden, utopia, and a place for humanity to start over anew. Even the native population made distinctions between European and indigenous diseases. A Mayan noted that before the coming of the Spanish there was "no sickness; they had then no aching bones; they had then no high fever; they had then no smallpox; they had then no burning chest; they had then no abdominal pain; they had then no consumption; they had then no headache."[30]

Such images notwithstanding, the reality was quite different. Although the indigenous inhabitants did not experience the catastrophic epidemics that ravaged Europe and Asia in the fourteenth and fifteenth centuries, they faced equally serious threats to health and life. Mortality data from precontact populations indicate that European perceptions of health and disease patterns in the Americas were largely erroneous. Skeletal remains indicate that the mean life span of nonagricultural and nomadic Texas Indians between 850 and 1700 was about 30. But when account is taken of the fact that infant skeletons are often unrecoverable, the average age at death was perhaps closer to 24. A large percentage of deaths occurred between the ages of 20 and 34, and only 14 percent (or less) lived beyond 55. The mean age at death of an agricultural community at Pecos Pueblo in New Mexico during the same period was also 25 years or less. Two excavations in the tidewater Potomac region of Maryland provided comparable findings. At the first site life expectancy at birth was 21 years, and a child surviving to age 5 lived on average another 24 years, while at the second site the figures were 24 and 27 years, respectively.[31]

Time, place, and circumstances resulted in significantly different mortality patterns. Excavations at two Illinois sites for different periods (1050–1200 and 1200–1300) are illustrative. At the earlier one inhabitants lived largely by hunting and gathering, although evidence of some agricultural activity was present. At the latter site the community relied on maize. Its population was both sedentary and larger, and trade and contacts with other groups more extensive. Life expectancy at the later site was 24, as compared with 33 at the older. Sixty percent of those at the later site failed to reach adulthood (i.e., age 20), as compared with 43 percent at the earlier site. At the younger site infectious disease and dietary problems played a more prominent role. Reliance on maize resulted in a deficient diet. At the same time population growth and sedentary lifestyles promoted more permanent host-pathogen relationships. The result was an increase in chronic and endemic infectious disease, and a decrease in life expectancy. Other excavations have revealed similar patterns.[32]

Skeletal remains suggest both phenomenal variability in the pre-Columbian Americas and a long-term deterioration in health as people shifted from reliance on hunting and gathering to agriculture. The food supply became less varied; the quality of protein decreased; the lower demands of work led to reduced muscle and bone growth; and the increase in population and decline in mobility heightened the importance of infectious pathogens. Political upheavals, warfare, and resource depletion may also have contributed to declining health. At two Kentucky sites the hunting and gathering group at Indian Noll had significant advantages over a maize-growing community at Hardin Village. At the latter infant and child mortality was higher and life expectancy at all ages was lower. Life expectancy at birth at Indian Noll was 22 for males and 18 for females; at Hardin the comparable figures were 16 and 17. The advantage persisted even among those who survived to adulthood. At age 35 life expectancy at the former was 13 for males and 12 for females; at the latter, 7 and 10, respectively.[33]

European demographic data exhibit comparable patterns. Aside from the spikes that accompanied crop failures or plague years, life expectancy and mortality rates in England and on the Continent were not fundamentally different. In four preindustrial London parishes between 1580 and 1650, life expectancy ranged from a low of 21 to a high of 36. Well-to-do groups tended to do better than others, but the differences were not stark. Between 1550 and 1574 life expectancy at birth for members of the British peerage was about 38. As in the precontact Americas, less populated areas in Europe proved more conducive to health and longevity.[34]

The similarities in life expectancy conceal some significant differences between the two continents. By the beginning of the fifteenth century Europe's population (excluding Russia) was perhaps 60 to 70 million, and its more concentrated population thus permitted "crowd" infectious diseases to play a much more significant role in shaping morbidity and mortality patterns. The Americas, by contrast, contained a large number of inhabitants, but they were (with some notable exceptions) dispersed over a very large land mass. Population estimates for the Americas around 1500 range from a low of 8.4 million to a high of 100 million. The estimates for North America are equally broad, ranging from 900,000 to 18 million. Given the paucity of evidence and the numerous if inconclusive methodologies employed to determine population levels, it is doubtful that we will ever know the size of the population of the Americas before 1492. Whatever the number, it is evident that the Western Hemisphere, including the contiguous United States, contained a substantial indigenous population.[35]

In 1492 the Americas were peopled by a multiplicity of groups whose economies, cultures, languages, social structures, and genetic endowment diverged from those found in Europe and Asia. Although life spans were not greatly dissimilar, the diseases and causes of mortality were quite different. In Eurasia "crowd" infectious diseases played the most important part in shaping mortality patterns. In the Americas (which harbored some of the same pathogens) the circumstances of life were quite different, and mortality patterns were therefore more variegated. When the first contacts took place between the residents of the Americas and Europe, a variety of unforeseen consequences followed that would change forever the lives of both peoples and transform the environment in profound ways.

CHAPTER 2

New Diseases in
the Americas

"Great was the stench of the dead," according to a text written by the Cakchiquel Mayas recalling the events that followed the arrival of the Spanish. "After our fathers and grandfathers succumbed, half of the people fled to the fields. The dogs and vultures devoured the bodies. The mortality was terrible. Your grandfathers died, and with them died the son of the king and his brothers and kinsmen. So it was that we became orphans, oh, my sons! So we became when we were young. All of us were thus. We were born to die!"[1]

When Christopher Columbus set sail from Spain in August 1492, neither he nor his contemporaries anticipated the tragic consequences for the indigenous inhabitants of the Americas. The Europe he left had experienced more than a century of plague and other infectious diseases, along with periodic famine, wars, and violence within and between groups and nations. Indeed, the very future of the Continent appeared threatened by forces seemingly beyond human control. In 1492 it would have been difficult to predict that within a relatively brief period, Europeans would not only transform the environment of the planet in unimaginable ways, but also create a hegemonic relationship with much of the rest of the world.

Reflecting upon the events set in motion by Columbus and his successors, the redoubtable Adam Smith wrote in 1776 that the "discovery" of the Americas and the passage to the East Indies by way of the Cape of Good Hope were "the two greatest and most important events recorded in the history of mankind" even though their full consequences were as yet unknown. By uniting distant parts of the world, facilitating the exchange of goods, and encouraging the growth of industries, these two "discoveries" appeared "to be beneficial" to Europe. To the inhabitants of the Americas, however, "all the commercial benefits which can have resulted from those events have been sunk and lost in the dreadful misfortunes which they have occasioned."[2]

Smith's use of hyperbole notwithstanding, there is little doubt that he had grasped the significance of the juncture of these two different worlds: Europeans were the beneficiaries, and the inhabitants of the Americas clearly the losers. The former brought with them not only a novel culture but, more important, diseases with which the latter were biologically and culturally unprepared to cope. The result was a catastrophe of monumental proportions that resulted in the destruction of a large majority of the indigenous population and facilitated European domination of the Americas.

▼ ▼ ▼

The expansion of Europe that began in the fifteenth century set into motion complex social, economic, biological, ecological, and technological processes. Before that time human habitats and environments tended to be locally oriented and therefore retained some unique features. The distribution of plant and animal species, including many pathogens, reflected different indigenous ecologies. As Europeans migrated to other regions of the world they brought with them not only their cultures and traditions but also their plants, animals, and pathogens. In so doing they profoundly transformed the areas into which they moved.

The commercial outlook so characteristic of early modern capitalism—an outlook that promoted the movement of people and goods—also tended to alter local ecologies. Trade and commerce changed the ways in which land and resources were exploited, promoted agricultural development for markets, and hastened the emergence of more densely populated cities. To be sure, the process was by no means one-sided; inhabitants of the Americas contributed crops, animals, and pathogens to Europe, which led to greater biodiversity. The expansion of the food supply in the Americas helped fuel the phenomenal growth of world population that began in the eighteenth century. The driving force behind these environmental changes, however, was derived largely from European sources.[3]

In the years following Columbus' voyages Spain pursued an active policy of exploration and colonization in Central and South America, the southeastern and southwestern regions of the United States, and ultimately California. In these geographically separated regions they encountered a bewildering variety of native peoples. Despite common biological origins, the indigenous inhabitants of the Americas had created over many millennia very diverse societies with unique languages, economies, cultures, and social structures. Heterogeneity most accurately describes the inhabitants of the Americas at the time of the first contact with Europeans. Whereas Europe had relatively homogeneous nation-states, the Americas included distinctly dissimilar societies and cultures. Hunting and gathering groups existed alongside more sedentary populations that subsisted by a combination of hunting, gathering, and agriculture. But the Americas also included complex and densely populated societies in such different regions as Mexico and Peru. Similarly, health patterns varied in the extreme. "The Western Hemisphere before the arrival of Europeans," according to three scholars, "was so diverse that parts of it, at certain times, were like a Garden of Eden or an impoverished wasteland of health by standards of world history prior to the twentieth century."[4]

Nineteenth-century Romantic writers and painters were prone to portray the Americas in terms of a pristine and virgin environment in which nature reigned supreme. Such a portrait, however, had little to do with reality. The landscape of the Americas at the end of the fifteenth century was a thoroughly humanized one. By 1492, William M. Denevan has written, "Indian activity throughout the Americas had modified forest extent and composition, created and expanded grasslands, and rearranged microrelief via countless artificial earthworks. Agricultural fields were common, as were houses and towns and roads and trails. All of these had local impacts on soil, microclimate, hydrology, and wildlife."[5]

From the sixteenth through the eighteenth centuries the indigenous inhabitants of what became known as Spanish America were devastated by the introduction of certain European infectious diseases. The first such recorded example occurred on the Island of Hispaniola (Santo Domingo) during Columbus' second voyage to the Americas, in 1493. The exact population of Hispaniola at the time remains in doubt; estimates range from a low of 60,000 to a high of nearly a million. Shortly after the arrival of the Spanish, an epidemic broke out among members of the expedition. Contemporary observers noted that the outbreak was an acute, highly contagious infectious disease with a very brief incubation period. Its symptoms included a high fever, prostration, body aches, and respiratory involvement. Mortality even among the Spanish was high. But among the native population the epidemic proved catastrophic. By 1517 (a year before the introduction of smallpox into the Antilles), perhaps only 10,000 to 18,000 of the indigenous residents survived.[6]

Contemporary descriptions by Columbus and subsequent accounts by Bartolomé de Las Casas suggest that the epidemic that began in 1493 and persisted until 1517 was a form of influenza, a viral disease that may have not been present in the New World before 1493. Influenza is a disease of humans, pigs, and several other mammals, as well as of some avian species. Although there are three types of influenza viruses (A, B, and C), the most common form is Type A. The influenza virus undergoes genetic change from time to time. Under ordinary circumstances the changes in the virus from year to year are relatively minor (antigenic drift), and hence a form of herd immunity in the population limits the risks from the disease. On occasion, however, an antigenic shift takes place; the human form of the virus captures an antigen from avian influenza viruses. Under such circumstances influenza can emerge in a more virulent form.[7]

Normally influenza is a relatively mild disease. Two elements, however, may have played a role in the elevated virulence of the Hispaniola outbreak. First, the genetic homogeneity of the native population as well as of their immune systems, and the introduction of a disease for which prior immunity was nonexistent, led to high mortality levels. Equally important, the particular form of the virus may have played a role. After leaving Cadiz in September, Columbus' expedition stopped for provisions at the Canary Isles. Aside from food and water, the ships took on a number of domestic animals, including sows. The epidemic began the day after the fleet reached Hispaniola and quickly assumed a lethal character. There is a distinct possibility that an antigenic shift took place as the swine served as a mixing reservoir for the reassortment of human and avian forms of the influenza virus. Indeed, at least fourteen influenza Type A subtypes persist in avian hosts. The combination of avian and human viruses can lead to viruses with novel surface antigens that spread rapidly in human populations and give rise to epidemics with high mortality rates.

The swift proliferation of the swine population on Hispaniola created conditions conducive to such a continued reassortment. Influenza may have assumed an endemic character, and thus contributed to the decline of the population in succeeding years. Moreover, the introduction of a new disease left the indigenous population little time to develop appropriate systems of care, which in turn may have magnified its lethal effects. The Spanish suffered as well, but their mortality level remained far below that of the native population.[8]

The high native mortality in Hispaniola from 1493 to 1517 was but a portent of things to come. The arrival of the Spanish was invariably followed by devastating epidemics that resulted in a massive depopulation among the indigenous inhabitants. From the very beginning of the fifteenth through the nineteenth centuries infectious diseases shaped the destinies of the Americas in profound and tragic ways. To be sure, infectious diseases had taken heavy tolls in Europe, Asia, and Africa since biblical times. Yet none of these outbreaks—whatever their causes—equaled in devastation and loss of lives those that occurred in the Americas after 1500. An overwhelming majority of inhabitants succumbed to the ravages of infectious diseases. The social dislocations associated with such high mortality rates merely rendered them more vulnerable to foreign colonizers. The European conquest of the Americas had relatively little to do with military prowess or superior technology; it was largely the result of the ravages of disease.

Smallpox undoubtedly had the greatest impact on the native inhabitants of the Americas. It is a viral disease spread by human contact either through droplet infection from the nose or throat or through direct contact with pustules on the skin. The virus is an oddity in that it survives only in human tissue (a condition that made its eradication possible after World War II). The disease occurs in two major forms: *variola major* and *variola minor*. The former has been subdivided into five categories, the most virulent having a mortality rate approaching 100 percent and at the very least about 10 percent. *Variola minor* rarely has a mortality rate of more than 1 or 2 percent.[9] Oddly enough, smallpox in Europe before the end of the sixteenth century existed in a relatively mild and nonlethal form. London Bills of Mortality before 1630 indicate that the disease killed fewer than 1 percent of its victims. Only after 1632 did smallpox become a virulent disease.[10]

When smallpox reached the Americas around 1518 (if not earlier), its effects were devastating. In 1520 a Spanish expedition arrived in Mexico probably carrying an African slave who had smallpox. The disease quickly spread. Unlike the relatively benign form that existed in Europe, smallpox in the Americas seems to have been a virulent disease with an extraordinarily high mortality rate. Toribio Motolinía, a Spanish friar who arrived in Mexico in 1524, offered a dramatic portrait. "In most provinces," he noted,

> more than half the population died; in others the proportion was little less. For as the Indians did not know the remedy for the disease and were very much in the habit of bathing frequently, whether well or ill, and continued to do so even when suffering from smallpox, they died in heaps, like bedbugs. Many others died of starvation, because, as they were all taken sick at once, they could not care for each other, nor was there anyone to give them bread or anything else. In many places it happened that everyone in a house died, and, as it was impossible to bury the great number of dead, they pulled down the houses over them in order to check the stench that rose from the dead bodies so that their homes became their tombs.[11]

The devastation wrought by smallpox facilitated the Spanish conquest of the Aztecs. The social fabric of a sophisticated Aztec society came apart as the disease ravaged their leadership. Shortly before the fall of the capital of Tenochtitlán, a native text reported that

> a great plague broke out . . . and lasted for seventy days, striking everywhere in the city and killing a vast number of our people. Sores erupted on our faces, our breasts, our bellies; we were covered with agonizing sores from head to foot.
> The illness was so dreadful that no one could walk or move. The sick were so utterly helpless that they could only lie on their beds like corpses, unable to move their limbs or even their heads . . . If they did move their bodies, they screamed with pain.
> A great many died from this plague, and many others died of hunger. They could not get up to search for food, and everyone else was too sick to care for them, so they starved to death in their beds.

The Spanish, by contrast, seemed immune (largely because they had been infected during childhood). Some scholars have estimated that the population of central Mexico fell from 25.2 million in 1518 to

2.65 million in 1568. Although these numbers are probably grossly exaggerated because of the ideological assumptions of scholars, it is clear that the catastrophic effects of smallpox were replicated time and time again in Central and South America. In the century following the arrival of the Spanish in Peru, the once dense native population virtually disappeared.[12]

Though taking the highest toll, smallpox was by no means the only disease ravaging the indigenous populations of Central and South America; measles occupied second place in terms of mortality. An acute viral infection of short duration, its characteristic symptoms include fever, a spotted rash, and a cough. Highly contagious, it is generally disseminated by droplet infection. It is generally regarded as a disease of childhood, if only because the loss of temporary immunity from the mother renders the infant susceptible at an early age. The disease tends to follow a cyclical pattern. After an epidemic the number of immune persons reaches a peak. For another epidemic to occur, several years have to pass before the number of susceptible individuals reaches a critical mass. Although mortality rates varied, it was not regarded as a particularly lethal disease in Europe.

Measles was endemic in Spanish urban areas in the sixteenth century. Nevertheless, it arrived in the Americas somewhat later than smallpox, if only because its characteristic mode of transmission involved young children. The earliest Spanish arrivals in the Americas were adult males, most of whom had had the disease in infancy or childhood. By 1530, however, migration patterns had changed, and either alone or in conjunction with smallpox, periodic outbreaks of measles were accompanied by high mortality rates. The devastating outbreak of smallpox in Mexico was succeeded a decade later by a measles epidemic. "If great care had not been taken to prevent their bathing, and to use other remedies," noted Motolinía, "this would have been as terrible a plague and pestilence as [smallpox] . . . Even with all these precautions many died. They called this the year of the 'little leprosy.'"[13]

The path of diseases in Spanish America followed a regular pattern. Expeditions from Spain or intermediate points carried infectious diseases to the indigenous natives, and virulent epidemics followed. Even those who survived were left in a weakened state and hence rendered vulnerable to other diseases. Smallpox and measles may have taken the highest toll, but other infectious diseases also played roles in the depopulation of Spanish America. European expeditions transported not only goods but pathogens. After 1518 smallpox spread west and north from Hispaniola to Cuba, Guatemala, Mexico, and the American Southwest, and south to Panama, Venezuela, Columbia, Ecuador, and Bolivia. From 1601 to 1653 northwestern Mexico was battered by successive outbreaks of smallpox, measles, pneumonia, yellow fever, and other unidentified diseases. Nor were these epidemics sufficiently separated in time to permit any degree of recovery. Only twenty-nine of these fifty-three years remained free from epidemics. The experience of Mexico was not atypical; Brazil, Andean America, and Central America experienced comparable epidemics for much of the sixteenth century. By the time infectious diseases had run their course, perhaps 90 percent of the indigenous population had perished. "The century and a half after 1492," to quote Noble D. Cook, "witnessed, in terms of the number of people who died, the greatest human catastrophe in history, far exceeding even the disaster of the Black Death of medieval Europe."[14]

▼   ▼   ▼

As the Spanish were extending their hegemony over Central and South America (excluding Brazil), they were also exploring what became known as the Spanish Borderlands—the territory between Florida and California. Juan Ponce de León, who arrived on the mainland about 1513, gave to the lands whose coasts he explored the name La Florida—a region that eventually included the entire southeastern United States. This area exhibited striking differences in climate, elevation, and vegetation. The Indians who inhabited these lands were equally diverse in terms of lifestyle and social organization. Ponce de León was only the first of many Spanish adventurers; in succeeding years others would explore this region as well. Hernando de Soto began his famous journey in 1539, which ended with his death in 1542. He and his army commenced their travels in Florida and eventually marched through Georgia, the Carolinas, Tennessee, Alabama, and Mississippi.

Florida was one of the first regions within the contiguous United States to experience the impact of European infections. For several centuries before the European contacts the native population of Florida had been growing at a rapid rate as a result of the shift to agriculture and a more sedentary lifestyle. Archaeological excavations of skeletal remains reveal a higher incidence of dental caries, enamel defects, and porotic hyperostosis (iron deficiency anemia). Comparisons of the preagricultural and agricultural population reveal that the latter had a younger mortality peak and an earlier mean age at death. The decline in the quality of life in the precontact period may very well have enhanced the vulnerability of the indigenous inhabitants of Florida.[15]

As early as 1513 an epidemic swept through Florida, transmitted possibly by Cubans fleeing Spanish exploitation. Six years later smallpox arrived in the region and was followed by other epidemics in succeeding decades. All of these outbreaks had the same devastating impact as they had in other parts of Spanish America. One scholar has estimated that from 1517 through 1519 perhaps 50 percent of the indigenous residents died; in 1528 half of those who survived perished. By 1617 the Amerindian population of Florida was perhaps 5 percent of the total alive a century earlier. Although the precise character of the infectious diseases that decimated the inhabitants of the region cannot always be determined, they included gastrointestinal infections, measles, smallpox, plague and/or typhus, mumps, and influenza. By the seventeenth century yellow fever—a viral disease transmitted by a mosquito vector—had also been imported and added to the toll in human life.[16]

Surprisingly, the depopulation of Florida did not follow a straight line, nor were all groups equally affected. The Calusa, who lived along the southwestern coast of Florida on the Gulf of Mexico, survived for nearly one hundred fifty years following the first contacts. The Spanish were unable to establish long-term missions or settlements among this group. The Calusa had a nonagricultural economy and subsisted primarily on fishing, hunting, and gathering. Most important, they did not live in villages with high population densities, and hence were less susceptible to the spread of infectious diseases. But even where the Spanish were successful in establishing missions, some groups—despite experiencing epidemics that resulted in elevated mortality levels—were able to adjust. The Apalachee, for example, suffered a population decline during the seventeenth century but managed to adapt and by 1675 had reached an equilibrium that was not upset until the English raids in the early eighteenth century destroyed the Spanish missions.[17]

Epidemics were not confined to Florida; Spanish explorers transported diseases into Georgia, South Carolina, and Texas during the sixteenth and seventeenth centuries. Nevertheless, the depopulation of the Southeast was somewhat protracted and probably followed irregular patterns. The pandemics that resulted in high mortality rates sometimes came to an abrupt end when they reached cultural or natural limits. Moreover, high mortality rates in some areas reflected violent confrontations with would-be conquerors. De Soto, for example, had a penchant for enslaving young women, who were used for sexual pleasure, and middle-aged persons who were employed as burden bearers. A revolt among those enslaved in 1540 resulted in numerous fatalities; skeletal remains attest to the fierce struggles that took place between the Spaniards and natives.[18]

That disease was the crucial element in the depopulation of the American Southeast is obvious.[19] Yet recent case studies suggest that the relative inability of Amerindians to mount an adequate immune response to infectious epidemic diseases was not the sole factor. The examples of northwest Mexico and California suggest that social and environmental forces often magnified the impact of diseases. The extraordinary mortality levels in Spanish America, in other words, had complex origins that transcended their biological and genetic origins, and could differ both spatially and temporally.

The Spanish colonial policy of *congregación* was a distinctive factor in the spread of disease. Under this policy the indigenous inhabitants were resettled into compact communities, many of them established by Jesuit and Franciscan missionaries. These settlements had diverse objectives: the conversion of the native inhabitants to Christianity, their acculturation to European values, and the creation of a more hierarchical society stratified along racial lines. Indians were located at the bottom of the social structure. They were to supply the inexpensive labor required for economic development, pay tribute in the form of a poll tax to support the state, and serve as a market for goods. By the end of the seventeenth century the mission frontier had reached northern Sonora in Baja California, and after the 1760s had been extended to Alta California (the area north of San Diego).[20]

All these regions experienced a demographic collapse of the mission population because their compact communities facilitated the spread of pathogens. In northern Sonora and Baja California—

regions that had commercial contacts—periodic epidemics of infectious diseases took a high toll. During a measles epidemic in 1769 and a smallpox epidemic in 1781–82 about 10 percent of the inhabitants of Baja California perished. Mortality rates during these and other episodes were often double or triple those in normal years. Indeed, epidemics accounted for at least 50 percent of total deaths, and many were among young adults, thus inhibiting reproduction. Since mortality rates in nonepidemic years were higher than birthrates, the population was unable to recover.[21]

The experiences of the Alta California missions were somewhat different. Geographically isolated, Alta California natives were largely spared from the periodic epidemics spread by commercial contacts. Yet chronically high mortality rates were characteristic, and in nonepidemic years even exceeded those of Baja California. In the end the outcome was the same even though the process was different.

What other factors proved most important in the depopulation of native peoples? The answer may be found in the social environment of Alta California. In this region young women, infants, and children had disproportionately high death rates. Prenatal care was nonexistent. Moreover, missionaries required women to work, thus magnifying the risks associated with pregnancy. The destruction of indigenous childrearing practices may also have had an adverse impact on infants. Many of them perished from the complications of birth, congenital infections, and dehydration from enteric diseases. The Franciscans imposed a harsh disciplinary system that may have undermined native morale, while unsanitary and damp housing exacerbated environmental dangers. Young girls, unmarried females, and wives of absent or fugitive males were kept in dormitories to control presumably promiscuous sexual behavior. Its effect, however, was to disrupt normal living patterns, and to magnify health risks because of inadequate sanitation and overcrowding. The use of coerced labor and corporal punishment was also common. Above all, missionaries attempted to destroy the beliefs, traditions, and culture of the Indians in order to Christianize them. Many natives attempted to escape from the missions, only to be pursued into the interior and forcibly repatriated. Missionaries believed that their harsh actions ensured the eternal salvation of their converts, and Spanish officials insisted that the needs of the state mandated the policy of *congregación*. Whatever their intentions, such policies probably contributed to a complete de-mographic collapse of the mission population. By the early nine-teenth century the depopulation of the missions forced Spain to aban-don its *congregación* policy.[22]

▼ ▼ ▼

By the late sixteenth century England, France, and Holland were at-tempting to emulate the Spanish by creating their own overseas em-pires. The initial English settlement in 1585 at Roanoke, Virginia, disappeared within a few years, and the fate of its people remains a mystery. The first permanent settlement, at Jamestown in 1607, had an equally troubling if different history. Mortality among the settlers remained at such high levels that the very survival of the colony re-mained problematic for years. Upon arriving in Jamestown, the Eng-lish found a large native population. The Powhatan Confederacy, as it was known, included between twenty-six and thirty-two tribes. Its members occupied about one-fifth of the territory of present-day Vir-ginia and numbered, according to one authority, about 8,500 out of the state's total indigenous population of 17,000 (more recent esti-mates put the figures at 12,000 and 20,000–25,000, respectively).

From the very outset relations between the English and the natives were tense. Lacking provisions from the homeland, English settlers took over significant tracts of land for agriculture. By 1622 open warfare erupted. Casualties were high on both sides, but the native population suffered the most. Hostilities persisted for decades, and by the end of the seventeenth century the Indian population num-bered perhaps 2,000, of which fewer than 1,000 were Powhatan. Military conflict and the ensuing social disorganization thus played the major role in the decline of Virginia's Indian population.

Smallpox, which contributed to depopulation elsewhere, was not significant. Virginia experienced an isolated epidemic in 1667, but the absence of densely populated settlements and commercial centers limited the spread of epidemic diseases. The introduction of liquor among the Powhatans by the colonists may have hastened the disinte-gration of their society. One official posited a link between the use of alcohol by the Powhatans and elevated morbidity and mortality rates. "The Indians of these parts decrease very much," he noted, "partly owing to smallpox, but the great cause of all is their being so

devilishly given to drink." No doubt this was an overstatement designed to place responsibility for the population decline upon the indigenous inhabitants rather than the English.[23]

A quite different picture prevailed in Massachusetts. In 1620 a
group of English dissenters known as the Pilgrims landed in the Bay
State. Weakened on the long voyage by dietary deficiencies, they were
at risk in their new environment, and half of them perished during
the first winter. Yet they faced no threat from the native population.
The Indians had little love for Europeans, because earlier contacts,
beginning in 1605, had been distinctly unfriendly. But they were in no
position to harm the newly arrived Pilgrims. From 1616 to 1619 a
devastating epidemic, accompanied by famine, struck a mortal blow
to the Indians. Mortality, according to contemporary accounts,
ranged between 75 and 90 percent of the total coastal population of
perhaps 7,400. Even assuming that the mortality data were exaggerated, there is little doubt that the coastal tribes were beyond recovery.
Upon arrival, for example, the Pilgrims found the Wampanoag village of Pawtuxet abandoned and the corn fields overgrown with vegetation.

The epidemic—probably introduced by European voyagers around
1616—raged for at least three years. The symptoms included headaches, body sores, lesions, and scabs. The generalized nature of the
symptoms and the elevated mortality rates have been the subject of
innumerable discussions and debates since the early seventeenth century. Retrospective diagnoses have included yellow fever, measles, typhoid fever, chickenpox, typhus, plague, cerebrospinal meningitis,
and smallpox. The diagnosis that perhaps best matches the symptoms
is malignant confluent smallpox, which has a mortality rate of about
70 percent. Paleopathological evidence from skeletal remains provides some—but by no means definitive—confirmation for the smallpox hypothesis. Given an incubation period of twelve to fourteen
days and another two weeks for the active stage of the disease, it
would have been possible for infected but asymptomatic persons to
travel beyond their villages and thus act as carriers. Limited contact
with other regions may have also confined the epidemic to a specific
geographic region spanning the coastal area from Narragansett Bay
to the Kennebec.[24]

The pace of colonization accelerated after the Puritans settled in
Massachusetts in 1630. About 20,000 persons, consisting mostly of

entire families, including young children, arrived in New England by 1640. Since the Atlantic crossing took slightly less than two months, a ship leaving England with a case of smallpox could arrive in the colonies with active cases still aboard. A major outbreak began in 1633 and did not run its course until 1641.

In England smallpox was a disease of young children; virtually every adult had already been infected and therefore had acquired lifetime immunity. In the Americas, by contrast, the entire Indian population was susceptible. Following its initial appearance, it spread rapidly throughout the Northeast. By 1634 it appeared among the Narragansetts and Connecticuts, and then moved to New York and northward to the Great Lakes and St. Lawrence region in Canada. Increase Mather, the eminent Puritan minister, observed with some satisfaction that the dispute over boundaries had been ended when God sent "the Smallpox amongst the Indians of Saugust who were before that time exceedingly numerous. Whole Towns of them were swept away, in some not so much as one soul escaping the Destruction." The disease, according to another figure, "was so noisome & terrible to these naked Indians, that they in many Places, left their Dead unburied, as appeared by the multitude of the bones up & down the countries where had been the greatest Numbers of them."[25]

The epidemic of 1633 began a process that resulted in the virtual destruction of long-established Indian communities. At that time, for example, about 8,100 Mohawks—who were part of the Five Nation Iroquois Confederacy in New York State—resided in four communities. By the end of the epidemic only 2,000 survived. Nine northeastern groups (including the Mohawks) had a combined population estimated at 156,200 in 1633. By midcentury only 20,000 remained alive—a decline of about 87 percent. Nor was the epidemic confined to the British Northeast. The experiences of the Hurons in the Great Lakes–St. Lawrence River region in Canada followed a similar pattern after 1633. Smallpox epidemics were interspersed with outbreaks of other diseases among the Hurons. Food deficits from time to time exacerbated the situation. Their ranks were so thinned that they were vulnerable to attacks by hostile Iroquois. In the early 1600s there were between 20,000 and 35,000 Hurons settled in twenty-eight villages; by 1640 their number had shrunk to perhaps 10,000. The virtual destruction of their social structure led to their dispersal and absorption by other tribes.[26]

Although smallpox was responsible for a majority of deaths, other diseases—less evident or spectacular—added to the toll. The importance of respiratory infections and gastrointestinal disorders was probably magnified among people under severe stress from smallpox. High mortality rates, periodic famines, and the social dislocations that accompanied these crises also reduced fertility to such low levels that population recovery was impossible. The demographic experiences of the Indians residing on the island of Nantucket are in many ways symbolic of what occurred in all the colonies. Between 1659 and 1674 population fell from 3,000 to 1,500, and to 1,000 by 1698. The decline continued during the eighteenth century. In 1763 only 348 were alive, and by 1792 only 20 remained. A once-thriving community had all but disappeared.[27]

Depopulation in the seventeenth century was greatest along the East Coast, largely because of the presence of large numbers of Europeans and more frequent commercial contacts with Europe, the Caribbean, and Africa. In more remote areas in the far interior, mortality from such infectious diseases as smallpox was less significant because contacts between Indians and Europeans were more sporadic and infrequent. But as more and more Europeans migrated to the colonies during the eighteenth century, earlier patterns reappeared. The increase in the number of susceptible colonists ensured that periodic epidemics would recur in more densely populated areas. These epidemics would ultimately follow established lines of commerce and thus infect Indian communities. Even the South, where the disease had not played a major role before 1700, was affected. South Carolina experienced four epidemics beginning in 1711; the outbreak in 1738 killed nearly half of all Cherokees. In the late seventeenth century the South below Virginia had about 200,000 inhabitants; 95 percent were Indians. By the American Revolution the region had a population of about 500,000, but only 10 percent were Indians.[28]

Although European infectious diseases undoubtedly took the greatest toll, epizootics (wildlife epidemics) may have added to the burdens of disease. Sketchy evidence from fur trade records indicates the presence of such wildlife diseases as tularemia. A bacterial disease (sometimes referred to as rabbit or deer-fly fever), tularemia can be transmitted to humans by contact with infected animals. *P. tularensis* can also survive in water and thus infect such animals as beaver, which in turn could serve as a source of transmission to Indian hunters and trappers. Plague may also have been present (although there is scholarly disagreement on its existence at this early date).[29]

The toll exacted by disease was undoubtedly magnified by the military conflicts that followed the westward expansion of white settlers in the nineteenth century. The forcible removal and relocation of the native populations after passage of the Indian Removal Act in 1830 exacerbated the impact of disease. The relocation of the Cherokees in 1838 involved about 17,000 persons. Nearly half of the Cherokees perished during and immediately following their move to Indian Territory, a journey that came to be known as the "Trail of Tears." James Mooney, an ethnologist who interviewed some of the survivors, concluded that the Cherokee removal "may well exceed in weight of grief and pathos any other passage in American history." The behavior of federal soldiers was brutal and callous in the extreme. The long march overland began in October and did not conclude until the following March. "In talking with old men and women," Mooney wrote, "the lapse of over half a century had not sufficed to wipe out the memory of the miseries of that halt beside the frozen [Mississippi] river, with hundreds of sick and dying penned up in wagons or stretched upon the ground, with only a blanket overhead to keep out the January blast." Other tribes suffered the same fate.[30]

Even where removal was not a factor, depopulation was characteristic. The first contacts between Europeans and native people on the Northwest Coast proved deadly. Smallpox epidemics occurred roughly every generation. Fever and ague—probably malaria—became established in western Oregon after 1830 and took the heaviest toll. David Douglas, who spent four years journeying through the region, wrote on October 11, 1830: "A dreadfully fatal intermittent fever broke out in the lower parts of this [Columbia] river about eleven weeks ago, which has depopulated the country. Villages, which had afforded from one to two hundred effective warriors, are totally gone; not a soul remains. The houses are empty and flocks of famished dogs are howling about, while the dead bodies lie strewn in every direction on the sands of the river." Transported into a region that had suitable mosquito vectors, the malarial plasmodium was quickly disseminated among the natives. Perhaps 80 percent or more of the Indian population perished during the first century of contact, the majority from malaria and associated secondary diseases.[31]

The experiences of the Southern Plains Indians—such as the Cheyennes, Arapahoes, Kiowas, and Comanches—were similar. The Medicine Lodge Treaty of 1867 forced these nomadic tribes that relied on hunting to relocate on reservations and become farmers. The efforts to transform their culture and economy, however, proved a dismal failure. The federal government rarely lived up to its obligations to provide clothing, food, and other supplies. Nor were Indians able to adapt to a sedentary way of life. In expressing their feelings to the Peace Commission of 1867, the plainsmen noted that they "know nothing about agriculture. We love the chase. You may farm and we will hunt. You love the one, we love the other." The lack of a stable and balanced food supply and the presence of gastrointestinal disorders, malaria, typhoid fever, consumption, and other maladies resulted in high mortality rates.[32]

During the nineteenth century the Indian population continued to decline. There were at least thirteen identifiable epidemics of smallpox among the indigenous inhabitants who resided between the Appalachian mountains and the Pacific coast. Measles may have also become more important in rising mortality. Other diseases, including influenza, cholera, typhoid, scarlet fever, tuberculosis, and malaria, added to the risks to health and life. By 1890 the Indian population reached its nadir. Federal government statistics indicate that their numbers in the contiguous United States fell from 600,000 in 1800 to a mere 248,000 in 1890.[33]

By the end of the nineteenth century, epidemic diseases such as smallpox that had taken such a high toll had begun to decline in virulence. The surviving Indian population then began a remarkable recovery. From the low of 248,000 in 1890, population reached 1.42 million in 1980 (including Eskimos and Aleuts) and 2.242 million in 1995. In this respect native Americans benefited—along with other groups—from the decline in infectious disease mortality that played such a significant role in twentieth-century America.[34]

▾   ▾   ▾

That infectious diseases played a major—if not *the* major—role in decimating the indigenous population of the United States and the rest of the Americas is indisputable. Yet the explanations for the extraordinarily high mortality rates remain more problematic. Most populations, to be sure, are at higher risk when confronted with new diseases. The extreme vulnerability of the peoples of the Americas, however, is unique in recorded history. Even the Black Death of the thirteenth and fourteenth centuries was not accompanied by the mortality levels prevalent in the Americas following 1492. Europe and Eurasia also eventually overcame the destructive impact of the Black Death. What accounts for the inability of the inhabitants of the New World to accommodate themselves to new pathogens and thus to begin the process of demographic recovery?

The most powerful explanation involves the concept of "virgin soil" epidemics. Such epidemics, according to Alfred W. Crosby, "are those in which populations at risk have had no previous contact with the diseases that strike them and are therefore immunologically almost defenseless." Writing in 1976, Crosby rejected a genetic weakness hypothesis and pointed out that the scientific community inclined "toward the view that native Americans have no special susceptibility to Old World diseases that cannot be attributed to environmental influences, and probably never did have." He pointed instead to the fact that native Americans were subjected to successive epidemics that had devastating demographic consequences. The absence of acquired immunity, moreover, meant that virtually everyone was susceptible. During epidemics the entire community often became ill, thus complicating the essential tasks of providing everyday necessities. Equally important, native Americans had no experience with many imported diseases. Their systems of care for the sick were either inadequate or else collapsed during epidemics that affected virtually entire communities.[35]

The concept of virgin epidemics focused attention on the impact of disease on society, as well as on the ways in which people perceived of and reacted to morbidity and mortality crises. However valuable, the concept does not explain all the available data. Not all indigenous native communities were equally affected by epidemic disease; time and place sometimes shaped differential outcomes. The very inclusiveness and symmetry of the concept is so alluring that on occasion it leads to neglect of other elements that play a role in mortality. The concept of virgin epidemics must therefore be employed with some caution and a recognition of its limitations.

If the "virgin epidemic" theory is insufficient, what accounts for the steep mortality rates from smallpox (and measles) among the peoples of the Americas? Recent findings in genetics and epidemiology offer some clues to this fascinating question. Genetic research has not demonstrated that inhabitants of the Americas were genetically "inferior" or even that they manifested unusual susceptibility to new infectious diseases. Indeed, it is not possible to distinguish between Europeans and inhabitants of the Americas on the basis of genetic markers. Taken as a group, however, populations of the Americas were different. Having lived in isolation from the rest of the world for thousands of years, they were genetically much more homogeneous than populations that had intermarried outside their groups over long periods. Their more uniform blood types and their more homogeneous gene pool rendered them more vulnerable to diseases common in Europe, Asia, and Africa.[36]

Epidemiological research on measles has added still another important hint. In studying mortality rates from the disease, Peter Aaby and colleagues found that such host factors as malnutrition or age of infection were not significant elements in mortality. They did find, however, that mortality rates were much higher when the disease was contracted from a member of the household or a relative than when it was contracted from others in the community. In Guinea-Bissau, in Africa, for example, the mortality rate for isolated cases and index cases (the first case contracted outside the home) was 8 percent, as compared with 23 percent for secondary cases in the household. In a study in Senegal that took 1.0 as the mortality rate for cases contracted in the community, Aaby found that the rate would be 1.9 if contracted from a cousin, 2.3 from a half-sibling, and 3.8 from a full sibling. Other data demonstrated the absence of any relationship between severity of measles and the dose of virus to which the individual was exposed.

On these basis of these findings, Francis L. Black has suggested that high death rates in the Americas from European infectious diseases are related to the fact that the virus grown in one host became adapted to the immune response of that individual. When introduced in a genetically similar host, it gained in virulence and resulted in higher mortality rates. Thus the inhabitants of Greenland, though culturally Eskimo, did not experience high mortality from measles, because they had had sexual contacts with, and exposure to the disease from, the early Vikings. Genetic homogeneity, in other words, enhanced viral virulence as it passed through ingrown communities and households.[37] This phenomenon is by no means unusual. A household effect holds true for other diseases as well (e.g., polio-myelitis). Indeed, there is abundant evidence demonstrating that repeated passage of viruses can increase (or decrease) virulence.

Housing arrangements, culture, and tradition further magnified the virulence of European infectious diseases. Close living conditions and the absence of concepts of contagion ensured the rapid spread of disease with the concomitant increase in virulence. Having had no previous contact with these diseases, Indian systems of care also proved inadequate. When entire communities were infected, little attention could be devoted to caring for the sick and providing nourishment. Demoralization was common, especially in light of the fact that Europeans appeared immune to the diseases ravaging the indigenous population. In 1634 some natives living adjacent to the Plymouth colony fell ill. These Indians, noted William Bradford in his famous chronicle,

> fell sick of the small pox and died most miserably . . . For usually they that have this disease have them in abundance, and for want of bedding and linen and other helps they fall into a lamentable condition as they lie on their hard mats, the pox breaking and mattering and running one into another, their skin cleaving by reason thereof to the mats they lie on. When they turn them, a whole side will flay off at once as it were, and they will be all of a gore blood, most fearful to behold. And then being very sore, with what cold and other distempers, they die like rotten sheep. The condition of this people was so lamentable and they fell down so generally of this disease as they were in the end not able to help one another, no not to make a fire nor to fetch a little water to drink, nor any to bury the dead. But would strive as long as they could, and when they could procure no other means to make fire, they would burn the wooden trays and dishes they ate their meat in, and their very bows and arrows. And some would crawl out on all fours to get a little water, and sometimes die by the way and not be able to get in again.

Despite the Pilgrims' involvement in helping the sick and burying the dead, added Bradford, "by the marvelous goodness and providence of God, not one of the English was so much as sick or in the least measure tainted with this disease."[38]

The process of depopulation, however, cannot be attributed solely to the devastation that followed the introduction of new infectious diseases. The Pawnees, Choctaws, and Navajos, for example, suffered large losses during epidemics; yet the former two recovered and the latter actually increased in population. So long as their subsistence systems functioned and their culture remained intact, they were able to survive. Indeed, the Navajos never experienced the catastrophic epidemics that decimated other native groups throughout the Americas. The pastoral nature of their society enabled them to adapt to reservation life, and hence to avoid many of the health problems that other groups experienced.[39]

In general, the introduction of a market economy was followed by a rapid deterioration of the fabric of Indian society. In return for such manufactured goods as axes, knives, tools, and clothing, northern tribes began to engage in the fur trade. To encourage their participation in the emerging market economy, traders offered liquor and credit. Overhunting, the destruction of the traditional economy, alcoholism, and dependency upon Europeans and Americans followed. Dependency on whites was synonymous with the destruction of a communal culture, social dislocation, and the loss of subsistence systems.[40]

European contacts not only led to a decline in autonomy among Indians, but also disrupted their sophisticated cosmology, which spiritualized the material world. Europeans, by contrast, elevated human beings above nature. Native Americans were thus transformed; they became, Calvin Martin has argued, "despoilers" rather than "conservators" when they hunted animals for trade rather than subsistence. Martin's characterization is undoubtedly overdrawn. Yet as Europeans replaced traditional native beliefs with Christian cosmology and market values, they disrupted established lifestyles; alcoholism and the acquisition of material goods began to dominate the lives of many Indians.[41]

Vulnerability to disease seemed in many instances to follow the forging of dependent relationships. The history of tuberculosis is a prime example. Though present in the precontact period, the disease was not of major importance. By the second half of the nineteenth century, however, the prevalence of tuberculosis increased dramatically among Indians. In the name of progress, the federal government began to change their ancestral way of life and force them to live on reservations. Social disorganization and privation led to elevated morbidity and mortality rates. When 2,800 Sioux prisoners of war

were confined to army barracks in a prison camp in 1880, acute tuberculosis became rampant. High mortality rates followed; at the
peak the rate was ten times higher than that observed during the
worst of the nineteenth-century European epidemics. Even more destructive was the epidemic at the Qu'Appelle Valley Reservation, in
western Canada. Mortality leaped to 9,000 per 100,000—a rate un-
matched anywhere else.[42]

Whatever the precise reasons, the contacts between Europe and the
Americas had devastating consequences for the indigenous population. New infectious diseases, compounded by pressures that led to
social demoralization among peoples who were genetically homogeneous and therefore at greater risk, destroyed entire societies. The result was a precipitous decline in their numbers from the sixteenth
through nineteenth centuries. To Europeans the disappearance of the
native population provided opportunities to colonize the Americas
and to exploit its seemingly boundless natural resources. To the native peoples the coming of foreign settlers and entrepreneurs proved
catastrophic.

CHAPTER 3

Colonies of Sickness

When William Wood returned to England from Massachusetts in 1633, he published one of the earliest descriptions of that colony. In this account he described an environment in which the infectious diseases that had played such an important role in Europe were largely absent. Wood pointed to the "healthful bodies" of the indigenous inhabitants, who seemed to be free of such European maladies as "fevers, pleurisies, callentures, agues, obstructions, consumptions, subfumigations, convulsions, apoplexies, dropsies, gouts, stones, toothaches, pox, measles, or the like." Indeed, they lived long lives "numbering threescore, fourscore, [and] some a hundred years."[1]

Wood's portrayal of this utopia was quickly supplanted by a quite different reality. The settlers who migrated to the Americas from the British Isles and the Netherlands in the early seventeenth century found themselves in a totally new and different environment. The world they left behind had long-established institutions, structures, and cultivated landscapes; the land to which they came had been largely unaltered by humans. Indians, to be sure, lived in villages and cultivated the land; but their relatively sparse numbers ensured that much of the territory they inhabited bore little resemblance to the European landscape.

From the standpoint of health, the first settlers faced formidable and arduous challenges. They had to clear the land, grow a stable food supply, find dependable sources of water, build houses for shelter, and adjust to an unfamiliar climate. At the outset they experienced extraordinarily high morbidity and mortality. The harsh conditions of life in a new environment increased vulnerability to infectious diseases. In Europe infants and children had the highest death rates. In the earliest stages of settlement in America, adults also faced an omnipresent threat of death.

Accommodation to a new and unfamiliar physical and disease environment—what in the sixteenth and seventeenth centuries was called "seasoning"—was not a uniform process. All the colonies experienced extraordinarily high mortality rates at the beginning. Some adjusted quickly, and death rates fell within a few years. But in other colonies death rates tended to remain high. Existing mortality differences had little to do with the biological characteristics of those who migrated; they grew out of the interaction of new climatic, environmental, economic, and social forces. Before the colonies could begin a sustained period of growth, their inhabitants would have to adjust to new conditions. The process of accommodation during the seventeenth century offers insights into the complex relationships between disease and environment.

▼ ▼ ▼

Those individuals who migrated to America encountered a quite different climate. Western Europe's climate is oceanic in character; daily and seasonal fluctuations in temperature are relatively small, and rainfall is generally adequate in all seasons. Eastern North America has a continental climate, with far greater temperature extremes. Summers are warmer and winters colder; rainfall is less regular and more unpredictable. River and stream levels may vary greatly with the season and with cycles of high runoff or rainfall and drought, which frequently contaminate the water supply. The ecological and health consequences of these conditions were far-reaching.

Many of the early settlers assumed that the climate in their new surroundings would not differ from that of their homeland. This belief often led them to try to transplant crops grown in comparable European latitudes, sometimes with disastrous results. Massachusetts, for example, is situated at about the same latitude as Spain, but the climate of the two areas differs sharply. Moreover, between 1550 and 1700 the Northern Hemisphere experienced what sometimes is called the "Little Ice Age," which compounded the climatic challenges faced by settlers.[2] The harsher and unforgiving weather—extremes of cold and heat and humidity—added to the burdens of adjustment and played a role in shaping morbidity and mortality patterns. Years would pass before settlers abandoned their belief that weather patterns in North America were determined by latitude.

As a result of these facts, several of the earliest attempts (excluding the Norse presence in Newfoundland centuries earlier) to establish permanent communities in the Northeast and Middle Atlantic regions ended in failure. The famous settlement at Roanoke Island in Virginia in 1585 is a case in point. The learned Thomas Hariot spent a year at Roanoke and reported that only 4 (including "three . . . feeble, weake, and sickly persons before ever they came thither") out of 108 died. Yet when a second expedition arrived in Roanoke several years later, all traces of the settlement had disappeared. Recent analysis of bald cypress tree-ring data suggests that extraordinary drought conditions prevailed from 1587 through 1589; they constituted the driest three years in an 800-year period from 1185 to 1984. Such a severe drought could have led to severe food shortages. More important, it may have contaminated the water supply, leading to fatal enteric diseases. Extreme cold elsewhere led to the abandonment of other settlements. In 1607 the Virginia Company established a colony in Sagadahoc, Maine. The experiment lasted less than a year. Although poor management was partly responsible, an "extreame unseasonable and frostie" winter also played a major role. Sir Fernando Gorges subsequently recalled that "all our former hopes were frozen to death." More than a decade would pass before others attempted to establish a colony in this seemingly inhospitable region.[3]

▼   ▼   ▼

English colonization of North America, according to one scholar, "resembled an epic geographical comedy." Given the prevailing belief that latitude determined climate, those who promoted colonies created an imaginary America in their minds. That New England was named after the mother country was no accident. Similarly, the climate of Virginia and the Carolinas presumably resembled that of Spain and other Mediterranean lands.[4] Such environmental models led to counterproductive behaviors in a new and quite dissimilar setting that had a decidedly adverse affect on the health of early settlers.

Many newcomers in fact underwent what was known as a process of "seasoning," which meant a physical adjustment to the new environment. Settlers' bodies, as Joyce E. Chaplin has written, were comparable to "trees felled in the Old World, shipped like so much lumber to America, then dried, hardened, and proved durable in a new climate." A seasoned colonist had survived local hazards. The "change of ayre [in the Chesapeake]," noted John Hammond in 1656, "does much alter the state of our bodies."[5]

Nowhere were the difficulties of adjusting to a new environment more evident than in Virginia. In December 1606 three vessels and 144 individuals left England. Before reaching American shores the group stopped in the West Indies, where they rested, ate fresh fruits and meat, and replenished their supply of water. As a result, the lengthy voyage apparently had few negative effects; neither dietary deficiency diseases such as scurvy nor respiratory disorders took a toll as they had on other seafaring ventures. At the end of April the expedition reached the Chesapeake Bay, and on May 13 settled on a site for the colony at Jamestown, located some fifty miles from the mouth of the James River. When the vessels departed for England in late June, 104 healthy persons remained behind at the first permanent English settlement in North America.

The seemingly happy state of affairs proved short-lived. Within weeks nearly 20 percent of the colonists died. George Percy, one of the founders of the colony, provided a graphic description of events that fateful summer. "Our men," he lamented,

> were destroyed with cruell diseases as Swellings, Flixes, Burning fevers, and by Warres, and some departed suddenly, but for the most part they died of meere famine. There were never Englishmen left in a forreigne Countrey in such miserie as wee were in this new discovered Virginia . . . our men night and day groaning in every corner of the Fort most pittifull to heare, if there were any conscience in men, it would make their harts to bleed to heare the pittifull murmurings & outcries of our sick men without reliefe every night and day for the space of sixe weekes, some departing out of the World, many times three or foure in a night, in the mornings their bodies trailed out of their Cabines like Dogges to be buried: in this sort did I see the mortalitie of divers of our people.

John Smith observed that "God plagued us with such famin and sicknes, that the living were scarce able to bury the dead." By the end

of September nearly half of the group had perished. When the first
supply ship arrived in January 1608, only 38 of the 104 original settlers remained alive.[6]

From 1608 to 1624 Virginia remained a deathtrap for Europeans.
Morbidity and mortality, however, were by no means constant. By
October 1608 perhaps 244 individuals had come to Jamestown, and
144 had died. The number of deaths then fell, especially as population was dispersed away from the original settlement. During the
winter of 1609–10 mortality rose dramatically. From 1613 to 1616
the colony appeared to have overcome the demographic disasters of
its early years. But from 1618 to 1624 death rates again reached catastrophic levels. During these years about 5,145 persons lived in or
came to Virginia. Of this number only 28.4 percent survived, 49.3
percent died from disease, and 25 percent perished from other causes
or returned to England. In 1625 the population was only slightly over
1,000.[7]

What accounts for the Virginians' inability to adjust to a new environment during the first two decades following 1607? Contemporaries such as George Percy attributed the high mortality rate to lack
of food, a claim that has found a measure of acceptance among contemporary scholars.[8] Such explanations, however, are clearly inadequate in light of the abundance of fresh fish and other indigenous
sources of food. Even a diet that was less than optimal would hardly
have led to starvation, particularly among a group that was composed overwhelmingly of relatively young adults. Moreover, most of
the clinical descriptions of those who perished scarcely support the
claim that famine led to such devastation.

The extraordinary mortality rates were undoubtedly related to the
physical environment of the Jamestown settlement. The water supply
came from the James River and from shallow wells dug in the middle
of the fort in which the colonists resided. High precipitation, low
evaporation, and the runoff from upstream sources resulted in a relatively safe supply of drinking water for a good part of the year. In the
summer, however, river discharges fell precipitously, water levels receded, and Jamestown became a peninsula bordered by pools of stagnant and brackish water. The probability of contamination from salt,
sediment, and fecal matter increased proportionately. The concentration of the colony's population inside a small fort that drew its
water supply from the adjacent river or from shallow wells in their

midst provided optimal conditions for the proliferation of bacterial organisms.[9]

Dysentery and typhoid fever were the most likely causes of high mortality during the first summer. The former was often fatal and always debilitating, and respected neither class, gender, race, nor age—although the disease posed the greatest risk to infants, children, and the elderly. A generic term, dysentery has multiple causes and symptoms. Depending on the invading organism, dysentery can be marked by diarrhea, cramps, fever, sepsis, and bloody feces. Death from dysentery often follows electrolyte fluid loss and the ensuing dehydration; vascular collapse is also not uncommon. It can be caused by a large variety of bacterial, viral, and parasitologic pathogens. Bloody stools generally have bacterial and occasionally amoebic origins and almost never have a viral cause. Pathogens that cause dysentery are often spread by contact with infected humans as well as by healthy carriers. Environmental factors play a crucial role as well: the disposal of organic wastes can contaminate water supplies; improperly handled food can encourage microbial replication; and the absence of personal hygiene can create conditions conducive to infection. Dysentery tends to peak in warmer months and is more prevalent in southerly climates; high temperatures and humidity provide greater opportunities for rapid pathogen proliferation.

The symptoms of typhoid fever, caused by the *Salmonella typhi,* include fever, intestinal hemorrhaging, skin rash, enlargement of the spleen, and a low white blood cell count. It is spread by contaminated food and water, and hence can appear in epidemic form. An asymptomatic healthy carrier can also disseminate the disease. Typhoid fever occurs most commonly in the late summer and early fall, especially when water levels are low, and can have a mortality rate of 30 percent or higher. Given the environmental conditions that prevailed in Jamestown, the likelihood is that a combination of dysentery and typhoid fever was responsible for the death of so many inhabitants. Certainly the clinical symptoms described by Percy—"Flixes" and "Burning fevers"—are consistent with both disorders. A bacterial organism—perhaps the Shigella—was the most likely cause of the dysentery that decimated Jamestown; Shigellosis is marked by fever and diarrhea with blood and mucus, and has a mortality rate that can approach 30 percent.

The experiences of those who settled in Massachusetts provide a fascinating contrast to the colonization of Virginia. The Pilgrims, who relocated to America in 1620, were the first group to plant a permanent colony in Massachusetts. Their journey proved somewhat arduous. Originally they were to come in two ships. When one of the vessels proved unsatisfactory, its passengers, together with some of the provisions, were transferred to the *Mayflower*. The expedition did not leave England until September and arrived at Cape Cod Bay in early November. During the two-month voyage there were no major health problems. The shortage of provisions relative to the number of passengers, however, may have led to the beginnings of scurvy (a dietary disease caused by a lack of vitamin C)—a common problem during long sea voyages.[10]

The group explored the region for nearly a month before finding a suitable harbor. During that time many settlers fell ill from exposure to the colder climate. The newcomers initially focused on the construction of housing and ensuring an adequate food supply. Despite the mild winter, the death rate began to climb. By the end of December six persons had perished, probably from respiratory disorders. During the first quarter of 1621 nearly half of the group died, and virtually everyone was sick. William Bradford attributed the travails of the colonists to the lack of housing, scurvy and other diseases, and the debilitating effect of the transatlantic crossing. "In the time of most distress," he observed, "there was but six or seven sound persons who to their great commendations, be it spoken, spared no pains night nor day, but with abundance of toil and hazard of their own health, fetched them wood, made them fires, dressed them meat, made their beds, washed their loathsome clothes, clothed and unclothed them." The crew of the *Mayflower*, hitherto friendly, abandoned the settlers, "saying they would not hazard their lives for them, they should be infected by coming to help them in their cabins." The timing of the deaths and the general sickness indicates the presence of a respiratory disease, probably influenza. Weakened by the long journey and an inadequate diet, the settlers were vulnerable to an outbreak of epidemic influenza. Adult mortality reached 58 percent, whereas child mortality was only 10.7 percent. Once the epidemic passed, the colony did not experience further threats to health. Its location on high ground, on land that had already been cleared by Indians (who had disappeared as a result of a devastating epidemic from

1616 to 1619), access to a supply of uncontaminated water, and a varied food supply provided optimum health conditions.[11]

The major settlement of Massachusetts began in earnest in 1628. Two groups, numbering nearly 400 persons, settled around Salem in 1628 and 1629. A third wave of between 700 and 800 arrived during the latter half of 1630 and located in Charlestown. By 1640 more than 20,000 settlers had come to New England. Despite what appeared to be careful planning, both communities initially experienced high mortality: Salem lost 21 percent of its population and Charlestown about 30 percent. Nevertheless, there were significant differences between them even though geography and climate were similar.

At Salem lack of leadership and planning inhibited the development of an adequate food supply. John Smith was particularly critical of the settlers. He emphasized the absence of effective governance, failure to plant crops and construct adequate housing, and dependency on England for food supplies. The colonists "lived merrily of that they had, neither planting or building any thing to any purpose, but one faire house for the Governour, till all was spent and the winter approached." The result was "many diseases." Although specific descriptions of the symptoms of those who died are largely lacking, there is little doubt that nutritional diseases, particularly scurvy and perhaps beriberi (caused by a vitamin B_I deficiency), weakened the settlers. The comparatively harsh New England winters and crowded, poorly ventilated, and cold houses created conditions conducive to respiratory disorders among an already vulnerable population. Had epidemic diseases spread by contaminated water been present, more individuals would have fallen ill at the same time and the death rate would have been much higher.[12]

The larger settlement around Charlestown, Boston, and surrounding areas suffered proportionately more than Salem. The greatest number of deaths occurred in the summer months of 1630. Of all the Massachusetts settlements, Charlestown was the hardest hit; about one-third of its population of 600 perished. That its residents suffered from nutritional disorders is clear, but these would not of themselves have caused such devastation. Nor was dysentery widespread; the absence of descriptions of "bloody flux" in contemporary sources militates against the argument that such organisms as the Shigella were responsible.

A contaminated water supply at Charlestown may have been the cause of the numerous deaths. The Charlestown settlement bore some significant resemblances to that of Jamestown. It was located on the north side of the mouth of the Charles River. The only source of water was an adjacent spring, which sometimes failed to provide a sufficient supply for the residents. More important, it often overflowed at high tide and was generally brackish. Equally significant, human and animal wastes were left on the hill at Charlestown and were carried into the bay only during runoffs following rain. The ensuing high tide might very well have contaminated the town's only well, thus leading to a deadly outbreak of typhoid fever. Edward Johnson, a resident of New England during these years and author of a history of the colony, noted the "want of fresh water, for although the place did afford plenty, yet for present they could finde but one Spring, and that not to be come at, but when the tide was downe." Johnson and others emphasized the dangerous hygienic state of the Charlestown settlement and the ensuing movement of population to Boston proper. A smaller number died during the following winter, but their deaths were due to the familiar combination of nutritional diseases and inadequate housing, which heightened the incidence of respiratory disorders.[13]

The process of adjusting to a new environment was inevitably fraught with dangers. Yet some settlements managed to avoid the catastrophic mortality rates found in Virginia and Massachusetts. New Amsterdam, founded by the Dutch in 1625, for example, did not experience a mortality crisis in its early years. Careful planning by the Dutch West India Company ensured an adequate food supply. The location of the colony on Manhattan Island also proved fortunate. The soil was porous and sandy, pure water was plentiful, and rivers on both sides of the island provided convenient sewage and garbage disposal. Dysentery, typhoid fever, and other enteric disorders that took a heavy toll elsewhere were insignificant in the early days of this settlement.[14]

South Carolina is another case in point. Of the 130–150 original settlers who arrived in 1670, only 4 died in the first six months, and the annual mortality rate during the first two years was 5.6 percent. How did they manage to avoid diseases that elsewhere threatened colonies' very existence? In South Carolina the food supply, though tenuous, proved adequate, and nutritional diseases were largely absent. More important, the colony escaped those enteric disorders that ravaged other colonies. The settlement at Charleston was located on sandy soil with a rapid percolation rate. Many of its residents lived outside the fort, thus minimizing congestion. Finally, the nearby Ashley River had an adequate flow even during the summer months. These elements combined to reduce the risks of a contaminated water supply.[15]

The settlement of Georgia diverged from that of its neighbor. The first contingent from England arrived in 1733; two years later a group of German Salzbergers followed them. In the planning stages James Oglethorpe and his fellow trustees attempted to avoid the problems that had plagued earlier colonies. Each colonist was provided with land, farm implements, seed, and sufficient food for twelve months. The assumption was that at the end of a year most of the settlers would become self-sufficient farmers. The outcome, however, proved quite different. Many lacked farming experience as well as the skills to construct houses. Within two years most had adequate housing as the settlers mastered the requisite skills. The problem of providing the colony with a balanced diet, on the other hand, was not as easily resolved. There was insufficient time to clear land and plant crops, and for nearly two years food remained in short supply. More important, the diet was unbalanced. There was enough salt meat and flour, but a shortage of fruits and vegetables.

Both the English and German settlers suffered from nutritional diseases, including beriberi and scurvy. Nevertheless, the latter experienced far higher mortality rates. The diets of the two groups were similar, but the English arrived in better health. Their journey across the Atlantic was shorter, and they were provided with a satisfactory diet aboard ship. By the time the symptoms of beriberi and scurvy appeared, the first crops were being harvested, thus inhibiting a major outbreak. The Germans, by contrast, had a much longer and arduous voyage. Their diet was inadequate, and conditions aboard ship proved less than satisfactory. Given their more problematic health status upon arrival, it is not surprising that the characteristic symptoms of beriberi and scurvy appeared relatively early. Within a brief span 18 of the 47 settlers died from these diseases or secondary infections. In Georgia's formative stage, many settlers drew water from

shallow wells that were easily contaminated, and thus suffered outbreaks of dysentery and typhoid fever. Between 1733 and 1752 about
30 percent of the 5,600 settlers who arrived in Georgia perished.[16]

Although the concept of seasoning generally referred to new settlements, it applied as well in other contexts. In many ways the history
of the American people is a history of migrations of different groups
from distant lands. Each group faced the necessity of adjusting to an
environment, society, and culture that differed from their place of origin. The complex process of change frequently had dramatic if un-
equal consequences for health.

The experiences of two groups—German immigrants and African
slaves—in eighteenth-century Philadelphia are especially suggestive.
The travails of the former began during the difficult Atlantic crossing;
surprisingly, mortality at sea was only about 3.8 percent. Debarka-
tion morbidity was in the same range, and the rate tended to fall over
time. Those who settled in Philadelphia, however, remained at a severe disadvantage. From 1738 to 1756 the annual average death rate
for first-year German immigrants was 61.4 per 1,000, compared with
only 37 for established residents. The reasons for the difference are
not entirely clear. Native Philadelphians were at higher risk of dying
from smallpox; Germans were at lower risk, since they came from an
area in which the disease was endemic and hence were already immune because they had had the disease in childhood. Yellow fever
and malaria took a greater toll among immigrants than among natives.[17] The complex nature of migration and adjustment precludes
simple explanations.

African slaves in Philadelphia in the late seventeenth and early
eighteenth centuries faced quite different circumstances. From 1682
to the 1760s they accounted for perhaps a quarter of the city's workforce. Most came from the Caribbean or southern colonies and had
been exposed to semitropical infectious diseases. But they were unaccustomed to the harsher climate characteristic of the Northeast.
Many were also undernourished and afflicted with a variety of
chronic infectious diseases.

Although there were some similarities between the experiences of
European and African Philadelphians, the process of adjustment for
the latter proved both longer and more difficult. Black mortality was
about 50 percent higher than that of European immigrants. Seasonal
patterns played an important role in accounting for some differences.

White mortality tended to peak in the summer, when malaria and enteric diseases were the major causes of death among Europeans unaccustomed to a warm and humid environment. Black mortality peaked in the winter; respiratory disorders were the leading causes of death.

Climate by itself was not the only variable in shaping differential mortality patterns; diet played an important role as well. In cold winters with overcast days, the ability to utilize vitamin D is reduced, since it is synthesized by the body as a result of exposure to sunlight. A vitamin D deficiency also increases vulnerability to respiratory disorders. In the harsher northern climate dark-skinned people in particular suffered from this deficiency unless dietary sources compensated for the absence of exposure to the sun. The practice of feeding slaves an inferior diet, combined with the harsher winter climate, may have increased their vulnerability to respiratory disorders. Death rates for blacks were likewise higher during epidemics of measles, smallpox, whooping cough, and other diseases. For African Philadelphians the seasoning process was both harsh and long-lasting. Although the abolition of slavery in Pennsylvania in the late eighteenth century improved their lives, the persistence of institutionalized racism and segregation continued to cause deprivation and to have a negative impact upon their health.[18]

▼   ▼   ▼

After the initial stage of seasoning, new morbidity and mortality patterns appeared. These patterns reflected a complex blend of environmental, economic, social, and cultural variables. Climate, topography, and geographic location played a critical role in the distribution of human settlements. The same was true of those bacterial and viral organisms that gave rise to infectious diseases. Trade and commerce also played a significant role, for the movement of goods was accompanied by the movement of pathogens.

Of all of the areas settled in the seventeenth century, New England proved the healthiest. Once its residents had adjusted to their new environment by constructing adequate housing, assuring a sufficient and nutritious food supply, and developing safe sources of water, they were spared from the epidemic infectious diseases that took such a high toll at the outset.

By the end of the seventeenth century New England's population was about 90,000, with the greatest concentration of population in the southern part of the region. The overwhelming majority of residents were white. On the eve of the American Revolution, Rhode Island's black population was 8.5 percent of the total (many of whom were slaves working on large farms in the southern part of the state), whereas New Hampshire, Massachusetts, and Connecticut had less than 3 percent.[19] The rate of population growth in New England was higher than that of England and other European countries. Most New Englanders lived in small, compact, and cohesive villages. Boston was becoming a center of commerce, whereas the inland settlements were primarily agricultural in character.

The circumstances of life in seventeenth-century New England had a dramatic impact on health. Mortality rates, as compared with Europe, were extraordinarily low and life expectancy correspondingly higher. Such epidemic and endemic diseases as smallpox that exacted a heavy toll in England and on the Continent were largely absent in the colonies before 1700. A typical Atlantic crossing took two to three months. Given the relatively brief incubation rates of most infectious diseases, it was obvious that even if an epidemic broke out after a vessel had left its home port, it would have run its course before reaching New England. If epidemic diseases reached the port of Boston—as they did toward the end of the seventeenth century—slow communication with the interior and a dispersed population ensured its containment within the town's borders. Since infectious diseases remained the single most important cause of mortality at that time, the inability to disperse infectious organisms in America limited their impact.

Living conditions in small agricultural villages with low population densities also proved propitious to health. The typical diet was adequate, and the risk of contaminating water supplies by human and animal fecal matter and other organic wastes was relatively small. Cold winters and shorter summers made it more difficult for infectious diseases spread by insect vectors to become established. With some exceptions, drainage in much of the region inhibited the presence of such diseases as malaria, which exacted a heavy toll in the marshy and estuarine districts of southern and eastern England as well as in the southern colonies.[20] Malaria was present in New England, but it never became a major factor and had largely disappeared before the end of the eighteenth century.

Although aggregate data are nonexistent for the seventeenth century, local data provide some insights into prevailing health patterns. The demographic history of the Plymouth colony is instructive. After a disastrous first year, the colony grew steadily. Between 1630 and the early 1640s population tripled, to about 1,000. By 1660 it had passed the 3,000 mark, and at the time of its merger with Massachusetts toward the end of the century Plymouth colony had between 12,000 and 15,000 people. On average its population doubled about every fifteen years. Population growth was largely a function of low mortality among infants and children, which rarely exceeded 25 percent—an extraordinarily low figure for that era. A male surviving to age 21 could expect to live to age 69; the corresponding figure for a female was 62 (a disparity due in part to the risks of childbirth). For both men and women who lived to age 50 life expectancy was nearly 74.[21]

Nor was Plymouth unique. Dedham, founded in 1636 and located some nine miles from Boston, remained mainly agricultural until the nineteenth century. On the basis of admittedly incomplete records, Kenneth A. Lockridge estimated that its death rate before 1700 was between 24 and 27 per 1,000; the rates for some comparable English and French villages were as high as 30 or 40. In European communities demographic crises were sometimes severe. Periodic famine and epidemics could destroy a quarter to a half of their population. Although Dedham experienced years in which deaths exceeded births, the magnitude was far less.[22]

Ipswich, a small seaport north of Salem, and Andover, located some thirty miles north of Boston, demonstrated comparable patterns. Infant and child mortality rates in Ipswich were about half of those in Colyton, England. Of 1,000 men and women alive at age 21, about three-quarters survived to 60 and nearly half to 70. Indeed, a quarter lived into their 80s. In Colyton about 41 percent lived to age 60 and 18 percent to 70. Andover also had exceptionally low infant and child mortality and high birthrates in the seventeenth century. Average age of death of first-generation males was 72 and females 71. The lifespan of their children was also impressive; more than half of those born between 1640 and 1669 and surviving to age 20 lived to 70 or more.

Generally speaking, rural communities enjoyed advantages over their English counterparts, especially insofar as infant and child mortality was concerned, though for those who survived to age 20 the advantage diminished somewhat. Approximately 30 percent of New England males and 25 percent of females perished between birth and age 17. In England, by contrast, more than 25 percent died by age 10 and over 30 percent by 15. In France the situation was even more dismal; fully half died by the age of 20.[23]

The demographic experiences of New Englanders, however, were by no means uniform. Life expectancy in Rhode Island, New Hampshire, and Maine, as well as Plymouth, was higher than in the rest of Massachusetts and Connecticut, largely because their more rural character resulted in fewer contacts with larger commercial port towns, where infectious epidemic diseases took a higher toll. Similarly, mortality in such port towns as Boston, Salem, and New York was higher than in rural villages. At age 30, for example, Salem males could expect to live an additional 29 and females 20 years; the figures for Andover were 39 and 36, respectively. Communities that engaged in overseas trade were at higher risk from imported diseases than their counterparts in the interior. During the second half of the seventeenth century smallpox arrived in the colonies as a result of commercial contacts with other regions. By then the disease had assumed a more virulent character; the result was epidemics with significantly elevated mortality levels. The density of population and susceptibility of inhabitants—most of whom had had no prior exposure—facilitated its spread in epidemic form. Enteric disorders disseminated by contaminated water and personal contact also made their appearance. Although governing authorities in Boston and New York became more active in dealing with health-related issues, they tended to concentrate on paving and draining streets, imposing quarantine to prevent the importation of infectious diseases, and regulating certain "noxious" trades; they were less concerned with the purity of the water supply or the disposal of organic wastes.[24]

The health advantages of New England and the Middle Atlantic region were not replicated in the Chesapeake areas of Virginia and Maryland or in other southern colonies. Indeed, the more southerly regions experienced far higher mortality rates than their northern neighbors for virtually all of the seventeenth century and thereafter. Virginia is a case in point. In 1625 the colony had only about 1,300 residents despite the fact that as many as 6,000 had migrated. By 1699 population had increased to about 63,000. Yet, according to recent estimates, somewhere between 50,000 and 100,000 persons had migrated, a large majority of them young males. Even with the significant disparities between the numbers of men and women (which would have resulted in a relatively low birthrate) taken into account, the colony grew only because of immigration. Virginians experienced a mortality rate comparable to that of severe epidemic years in England. Nor were deaths concentrated among recent immigrants; older inhabitants perished in large numbers as well. Although mortality was not constant, and probably declined during the latter half of the seventeenth century, life in Virginia remained at best tenuous.[25]

In Virginia some areas presented greater risks to life than others. Charles Parish, established around 1645 at the eastern end of York County, is one such example. Even when the fact that males outnumbered females by wide margins is taken into account, the greatest impediment to growth was the area's low life expectancy. Infant and child mortality remained high between 1665 and the turn of the century. Overall child mortality for ages 1–14 was 145 per 1,000 for males and 198 for females, as compared with 95 for New England communities. Those who survived to age 20 could expect to live an additional 21 years; the comparable figures for Plymouth and Andover were 44 and 48 years. Even when compared with other Virginia counties, Charles Parish in tidewater Virginia proved exceptionally dangerous in the seventeenth century.[26]

In many respects Maryland resembled Virginia. A study of Charles County in the latter half of the seventeenth century found that the life expectancy for males at birth was slightly under 26. The native-born fared somewhat better than immigrants, but both lagged far behind New England residents. Indeed, life was probably shorter in the Chesapeake than in England; relatively few males lived to the age of 50. Even those who were economically advantaged and survived longer had much lower life expectancies than New Englanders. On average the latter lived a decade longer than individuals who served in the Maryland legislature, a group that represented the region's elite. High mortality was characteristic among all segments of the population in that colony.[27]

Those who settled in the Chesapeake region—even though in the prime of their lives—faced a seemingly inhospitable environment. Diet played at best a minor role. There were no reported shortages of food, and the ability to grow crops and gather a variety of plants, animals, and fish assured a reasonably balanced diet. Lack of knowledge about nutritional requirements may have caused some deficits, but these were of minor consequence once the initial stage of settlement passed.

What accounts for the dismal demographic experiences of seventeenth-century Chesapeake residents? The preponderance of available evidence, admittedly incomplete, suggests that malaria was of major importance in the history of this region. Malaria is a disease of ancient lineage; it is found among amphibia, reptiles, birds, and mammals. Climatic changes and the transition to sedentary patterns and agriculture promoted its dissemination among humans. It was probably present in the ancient Near East and the Greco-Roman world as well. High mortality rates and contemporary descriptions of the disease indicate that malaria had a firm foothold in the marshlands of southeast England by the age of colonization.[28] Malaria was and remains one of the world's most common serious infections.

Malaria is a complex disease that involves parasites of the genus *Plasmodium,* an insect vector, and human hosts. Malarial parasites of four species, each with a different biological pattern, may affect humans: *Plasmodium vivax, P. falciparum, P. malariae,* and *P. ovale.* Infection occurs when a female *Anopheles* mosquito, feeding on a person with malaria, ingests blood containing gametocytes. After undergoing sexual development (ending as sporozoites in the salivary glands), the insect injects a susceptible person, and the parasites multiply asexually in the liver. After maturing, merozoites are released into the blood and attack red cells. At that point the clinical disease begins as the immune system responds. The symptoms include fever spikes, chills, headaches, diarrhea, vomiting, and an enlarged spleen and liver. Ultimately the immune system prevails, but the parasite can remain in the liver and begin the cycle of infection anew. *P. vivax* and *P. falciparum* are the most common forms of the disease; *P. malariae* is uncommon, and *P. ovale* is rare and found only in Africa. Although it can recur, the *vivax* form is relatively benign and has a mortality rate of less than 5 percent; *falciparum* is generally nonrecurring but has a mortality rate of 20 to 25 percent.

Diseases rarely exist in isolated or ideal form, and malaria was no exception to the rule. Repeated attacks of the disease often result in a chronic state of ill health, thus rendering an individual vulnerable to other infections. Indeed, the debilitating effects of malaria may be as important as, if not more so than, its direct consequences. Malaria,

Mary J. Dobson has observed in her study of disease and mortality in early modern England, "appears to have set up a train of consequences which had a significant impact on the outcome of other variables in the marshes. The links between malaria and intercurrent infections, chronic illness, poor diet, reduced energy levels and destitution were all part of these important indirect effects." The disparity in seventeenth-century death rates between unhealthy wetland parishes in southeast England and salubrious upland farming localities was striking.[29]

When the number of humans with malaria is low, transmission is only occasional. But when the number of infected persons reaches a high threshold, larger numbers of mosquitoes become infected, thus setting the stage for malaria in epidemic form. Environmental factors also play a crucial role, for without the insect vector malaria will remain nonexistent. Consequently, semitropical weather provides an opportunity for insect proliferation. In regions with cold winters and short summers (such as New England) the life cycle of the mosquito is interrupted, thus inhibiting the transmission of the disease and ultimately leading to its eradication.

Whether or not malaria was present in the Americas prior to contact with Europeans has long been a subject of debate. The most recent scholarship suggests that it was absent in America. The "sickle cell" trait—which provides some protection against the *P. falciparum* form of malaria but which also leads to a chronic hemolytic anemia that can be fatal—is found only among populations (both black and white) living in regions where the disease is endemic. Abnormal hemoglobins, on the other hand, are absent among Indians who have not intermarried. Moreover, the extreme malignancy of malaria among them, as compared with its effect on Africans, suggests that malaria did not exist in the Americas before 1492.[30]

Whatever the case, it seems highly probable that the *vivax* form of malaria was imported from England, where the disease was already well established, by the early seventeenth century. The *falciparum* form, on the other hand, seems to have arrived from Africa after midcentury. The movement of malaria to the Chesapeake required people, the *Plasmodium*, and the insect vector. It is highly likely that infected persons were on the first ships that arrived in Jamestown in 1607. Some came from Kent, Essex, and parts of London where malaria existed in endemic form. Slowly but surely the mix of infected persons and insects created localized malarial environments in the Chesapeake. The process was slow, and symptomatic morbidity rose only gradually. In Virginia sharp geographic differences in morbidity were evident. Those in the older tidewater areas in Gloucester County were more likely to suffer from fevers and agues bearing a striking resemblance to malaria. In time, however, newly settled areas underwent environmental transformations and migrations that resulted in the same endemic levels experienced by older communities.[31]

The presence of malaria seems to have been a key factor in the differential life expectancies of the Chesapeake and New England. Malaria admittedly does not have a terribly high fatality rate. Nevertheless, it is debilitating and lowers the body's ability to respond to other infectious diseases. Indeed, there is a close relationship between malaria morbidity and overall mortality rates. After the introduction of malaria control operations in Guyana and Sri Lanka, for example, the fall in the death rate was two to four times the direct reduction of deaths from this disease. The differences between New England and Chesapeake mortality, therefore, may have reflected the relative unimportance of malaria in the former and its significance in the latter.[32]

In their classic study of malaria in the Chesapeake, Darrett and Anita Rutman pointed out that the town of Salem had significantly higher mortality rates than surrounding Massachusetts rural communities, particularly among women in their childbearing years. Indeed, Salem in Massachusetts and Middlesex in tidewater Virginia shared a common experience in this regard. Modern malariologists have found that pregnant women have attack rates four to twelve times greater than nonpregnant women. Both pregnant women and their fetuses are at risk from malaria. Salem was a community in which endemic malaria was present. When the disease disappeared from the region in the eighteenth century, its death rate fell while other nearby towns were experiencing an increase. Such findings tend to confirm the significance of malaria in the dismal demographic history of the seventeenth-century Chesapeake.[33]

The health problems experienced in the Chesapeake region were in many ways replicated in the Carolinas. To promote immigration, the colony's proprietors emphasized its delightful climate, fertile soil, and salubrious and healthful environment. The initial impressions of the first settlers and the absence of high mortality in the early days seemed to confirm such claims. The author of *A True Description of*

Carolina, published in 1674, wrote about the colony's environment in rhapsodic terms typical of promotional literature. "The Heavens shine upon this famous Country the sovereign Ray of Health; and has blest it with a serene Air, and a lofty Skie, that defends it from noxious Infection." Nor was there "any known Distemper . . . whereby to terrify and affright" inhabitants.[34]

The early years of the Carolina settlement were relatively uneventful. There were in fact no reports of fevers, agues, or excessive deaths. Although the presence of insects during hot weather was bothersome, there is no evidence of malaria among either the settlers or the indigenous Indian population. The disease may have been introduced into Florida by the Spanish in the sixteenth century, but their inability to colonize the Carolinas prevented its spread into that region.[35]

Within a decade the settlement had begun to experience outbreaks of malaria. By 1682 the colony had more than 2,200 inhabitants. The migration from southeast England probably included individuals infected with the *vivax* form, and hence the early epidemics that may have begun in the late 1670s did not result in high mortality. Nevertheless, fever and ague—the seventeenth-century terms for malaria— began to take a toll from June through October, especially in the areas of settlement adjacent to wetlands and marshes. By the 1680s the *falciparum* form probably was brought to the colony either by English sailors or by slaves from the West Indies born originally in West Africa. The mix of infected and susceptible persons laid the foundation for an especially virulent epidemic in 1684. After a voyage of about two and half months, a group of Scottish immigrants arrived in Charleston on October 2. "We found the place so extrordinerie sicklie," wrote two leaders, "that sickness quickly seased many of our number and took away great many." Moving to higher ground "free of swamps and marshes" on a high bluff led to the recovery of many, "and none have contracted sickness since we came tho many died of the sicknes they contracted at Charlestoun at our first arravell."[36]

The malaria epidemic that plagued the colony in 1684 ultimately diminished immigration, and the number of susceptible persons declined to the point where it became difficult to sustain a new outbreak. In addition, those who had been infected and survived developed partial immunity that modified in significant ways the clinical course of the disease (although this immunity has a modicum of strain specificity). The movement of population away from wetlands also served to mitigate the possibilities of new outbreaks. Consequently, the colony remained relatively free from major epidemics until the importation of other diseases—notably smallpox and yellow fever—toward the close of the seventeenth century. The introduction of rice cultivation in the early eighteenth century, however, created ideal conditions for the spread of malaria because of the proliferation of breeding grounds for the insect vector and the migration of both susceptible and infected persons into the colony. Whites and Indians were harder hit than black slaves because the sickle-cell trait provided some protection. Malaria, in conjunction with a variety of other infectious diseases, made the low country a graveyard, and its white population was unable to sustain itself through natural growth for most of the eighteenth century.[37]

Data from several South Carolina parishes reveal the impact on life of a disease that—if it did not kill its victims—left them in such a debilitated state that they were vulnerable to a host of other infectious diseases. Robert Maule, assigned to St. John's Parish by the Society for the Propagation of the Gospel in Foreign Parts, reported in 1709 that his health was good upon his arrival. But then, he wrote, "I was Seized with a very severe fit of Sickness; being held for near three Months together of a fever and Ague which at length concluded in a most Violent Belly Ache; so violent indeed that I verely believed it wu'd have ended my days; but I thank God I am now pretty well recover'd again." In another parish a minister reported that after a particularly virulent outbreak of malaria in 1716 "not many Children [have] been born this year and most that were are already deceased." During the eighteenth century 86 percent of all those whose births and deaths were recorded in the parish register died before the age of 20. The bulk of infant and early childhood deaths occurred in the late summer and early fall, the season when malaria mortality tends to peak (although enteric disorders played a major role as well). Of those born between 1680 and 1720, three-quarters of all males who survived to the age of 20 died before reaching 50. Female mortality was also high, particularly among women in their childbearing years.[38] Although a variety of infectious diseases took a heavy toll, malaria was undoubtedly a major element in the disastrous demographic history of South Carolina following its establishment in 1670.

By the early eighteenth century the process of seasoning for many of the colonies was largely complete. In a larger sense, however, the process of accommodation remained a perennial theme in American history. Successive generations would face challenges as they moved into new environments that varied in the extreme.

CHAPTER 4

The Promise of Enlightened Health

As settlers surmounted the difficulties encountered in moving to a new environment, they found that morbidity and mortality rates began to decline. Appearances, however, were deceiving; the health advantages enjoyed by colonial Americans proved transitory. Slowly but surely the increase in population and economic growth during the eighteenth century created conditions conducive to a wider dissemination of those infectious diseases that played such an important role in European mortality. Consequently, the seemingly good health characteristic of many colonies once the seasoning stage had passed slowly but surely gave way to a somewhat less favorable disease environment. To be sure, most colonies had lower morbidity and mortality rates than western Europe (including England). Despite population growth, the rural character of colonial America provided quite different environmental conditions, and the pattern of infectious diseases followed a somewhat dissimilar course. Yet the economic, environmental, and demographic changes that were transforming the lives of colonial Americans were also narrowing the magnitude of these differences. Indeed, the gains in health and life expectancy that occurred in many of the colonies in the late seventeenth and early eighteenth centuries slowly ground to a halt and would begin to be reversed after 1800.

▼ ▼ ▼

After the initial stage of settlement, population growth in the American colonies accelerated rapidly. Between 1700 and 1770 there was a ninefold increase from 250,000 to an estimated 2.15 million. Population distribution, despite disparate accommodations to particular environments, remained relatively even; 581,000 resided in New England, 520,000 in the Middle Atlantic region, 685,000 in the Chesapeake, and 345,000 in the Carolinas and Georgia.

Although population was equally distributed, the demographic characteristics of individual colonies varied in the extreme. New Hampshire, for example, was predominantly white; blacks constituted less than 1 percent of its population. By contrast, nearly one-third of Maryland and over 40 percent of Virginia residents were black. Blacks constituted about one-fifth of the total population. The overwhelming majority were slaves residing in the Chesapeake region and the Carolinas. Ethnicity proved to be less of a factor because the growth of the native population reduced the significance of immigrants.

Eighteenth-century America was distinctive by virtue of its peculiar marriage patterns and the youthful character of its population. In England and northern Europe women married in their middle or late twenties; perhaps 15 to 20 percent were unmarried by the age of 45. In the British mainland colonies, however, age at marriage was in the low twenties, and only about 5 percent were unmarried by age 45. The number of children per completed marriage, therefore, was correspondingly higher in the colonies, which grew more rapidly.[1] Children accounted for perhaps half of the total population. The number of aged persons was small by modern standards. The imbalance of males and females that had existed for much of the seventeenth century had diminished significantly; by 1750 there was a rough balance between the sexes.[2]

Population growth and economic development had a profound influence on morbidity and mortality rates. Acute infectious diseases remained the major threats to health and longevity in the eighteenth century. Their pattern, however, began to assume different shapes in response to environmental changes. The increase in the size and density of population, the expansion of internal and external trade and commerce, the development of new forms of agriculture, and transformation of the landscape, all combined to alter the complex relationships that existed between pathogens and their human hosts.

Throughout the eighteenth century there was an increase in mortality from a variety of infectious diseases, particularly among infants and children and those who resided in the larger towns and urban port areas. The first to experience the ravages of infectious epidemic diseases were urban port communities. Small if not infinitesimal by modern standards, they nevertheless brought significant numbers of people into close living conditions. The maritime character of Boston, New York, Philadelphia, and Charleston—the most important colonial ports—brought them into contact with each other and, more importantly, with Europe, the Caribbean, and Africa. The ports also tended to be the entry point for both sailors and individuals migrating to the colonies. Such population movements became the means of transporting a variety of pathogens capable of causing epidemic outbreaks.

In the early stages of settlement, migrants tended to be young adults who had already been exposed to a variety of infections, and thus were immune. A high proportion of immune persons in a community generally precluded epidemic diseases, because the capacity to transmit the pathogen from person to person was impaired. Over several generations, however, the increase in the number of susceptible persons created conditions conducive to the spread of infections. In particular, the physical environments of port villages—crowded living conditions, crude sewage disposal, and stagnant or contaminated water—produced settings in which outbreaks of infectious epidemics became possible.[3]

The history of smallpox is illustrative. In the early seventeenth century smallpox epidemics were sporadic. Massachusetts was struck by a relatively mild outbreak in 1648–49. For the next two decades the disease was absent. In 1666, however, smallpox was introduced into Boston either from England or Canada (where it had struck during the previous five years). Perhaps 40 to 50 persons died, while a much larger number were infected. A decade later smallpox made its appearance in Charlestown and quickly spread across the Charles River to Boston. Between 200 and 300 persons died. The adoption of measures to quarantine the community prevented its spread to adjacent towns.[4] "Boston burying-places never filled so fast," noted a youthful Cotton Mather. "It is easy to tell the time when we did not use to have the bells tolling for burials on a Sabbath morning by sunrise; to have 7 buried on a Sabbath day night, after Meeting. To have coffins crossing each other as they have been carried in the street . . . To attempt a Bill of Mortality, and number the very spires of grass in a Burying Place seem to have a parity of difficulty and in accomplishment."[5]

By the late seventeenth century smallpox was assuming a more virulent form in Europe. Either a lethal strain of *variola major* had been imported from Africa or the Orient, or else the virus mutated. Whatever the explanation, the relatively benign form of the disease that existed before 1630 was superseded by a more malignant one. London's large population, for example, permitted the disease to exist in endemic form. Between 1731 and 1765 the average number of deaths per year was 2,080, or 9 percent of total mortality.[6]

The pattern of smallpox in the colonies was different because no colonial town approached the size of metropolitan London. In the British mainland colonies an epidemic was succeeded by a period of years in which the disease was absent. During the interval between epidemics the number of susceptible persons gradually increased, and the stage was set for another outbreak. In the summer of 1702 the disease appeared in Boston and did not run its course until the following spring. The precise mortality figures are unclear, but out of a population of about 7,000 perhaps 300 deaths were recorded. Between 1721 and 1792 Boston experienced no less than seven epidemics, of which the first proved the most devastating. In a population of 10,670, there were 6,006 reported cases and 850 deaths. During the epidemic a fierce controversy developed concerning the risks and benefits of inoculation. Though not new, inoculation had been popularized in England a few years earlier. The technique was simple: smallpox was induced in a susceptible healthy person by making an incision and introducing into it material from the pustule of an infected person. The favorable outcome seemed to validate the effectiveness of the procedure. The death rate among those inoculated during the epidemic of 1721 was 2.4 percent, as compared with 14.6 percent among those who were naturally infected. The practice of inoculation became more common as the century progressed.[7]

Despite efforts at containment, it was difficult to prevent the spread of smallpox to neighboring towns and colonies with a high proportion of susceptible persons. The movement of people engaged in trade and commerce provided a convenient means of transporting the virus. Moreover, many fled from epidemic areas despite quarantine measures, and thus facilitated the dissemination of the virus. The war with the French in the 1760s merely exacerbated the problem.

Susceptible soldiers—many of whom came from areas untouched by smallpox—were infected and acted as vectors upon their return. "During the late war," noted Dr. Benjamin Gale in 1765, "the smallpox was brought into divers towns, in this and other colonies, by the return of our soldiers (employed in his majesty's service, in the pay of New England Colonies) for winter quarters, and by seamen employed in our navigation to the British Islands in the West Indies, where small pox was universally present."[8]

New England had little contact with the interior and therefore was spared from the outbreaks that were prevalent among the French and disseminated by Indians through trade and war. This was less true for New York, New Jersey, and Pennsylvania. In those colonies Philadelphia and New York served as ports of entry for the smallpox virus. Equally important, the entire region had close commercial and social ties that reached up to the Canadian border from the Hudson Valley. The large Indian population in this area served as a point of contact with Canada, and their roles as traders and warriors helped to spread smallpox. On average, Boston had an epidemic once every decade. New York, by contrast, experienced more frequent visitations, and the disease was present annually from 1756 through 1766. In Philadelphia smallpox was the single largest cause of mortality during the third quarter of the eighteenth century. Rarely was the disease confined to port areas of the Middle Atlantic region; trade and commerce assured its presence in inland areas as well.[9]

Although sporadic epidemics were common, smallpox was less significant in the Chesapeake and the South. A more dispersed population, an agricultural rather than a commercial economy, and the absence of port towns inhibited the introduction and spread of epidemics. South Carolina was an exception, since Charleston was an important seaport and commercial center with trade links to areas where smallpox was endemic. Like Boston, New York, and Philadelphia, it served as a port of entry for infectious diseases. The first outbreak of smallpox occurred in 1697 and took an estimated 200 to 300 lives. The town was hit by additional epidemics in 1711, 1718, 1732, 1738, and 1760. The long period between epidemics meant that most residents had never been exposed. In 1760 no less than 6,000 out of a total population of 8,000 were infected, and the estimates of mortality ranged from a low of 730 to a high of 940. Over 90 percent of all deaths in Charleston that year were due to smallpox.[10]

Smallpox was by no means the only imported disease. Yellow fever was another and in many respects was more terrifying. Aside from its higher mortality rate, it was a relatively "new" disease to Europeans and colonials, and consequently aroused greater fears than older but more familiar diseases because of its unpredictability. The characteristics of yellow fever reinforced anxiety and fear. Its symptoms were dramatic; its appearance and disappearance was random; and it respected neither class, status, nor gender. Yet it was not transmitted by infected individuals who moved from an epidemic area. Absalom Jones and Richard Allen, two African Americans who organized a major relief effort during the Philadelphia epidemic of 1793, provided a graphic description of afflicted individuals. Patients, they wrote,

> were taken with a chill, a headach, a sick stomach, with pains in their limbs and back, this was the way the sickness in general began, but all were not affected alike, some appeared but slightly affected with some of these symptoms . . . In some it raged more furiously than in others . . . Some lost their reason and raged with all the fury madness could produce, and died in strong convulsions. Others retained their reason to the last . . . Numbers died in a kind of dejection, they concluded they must go, (as the phrase for dying was) and therefore in a kind of fixed determined state of mind went off.[11]

Yellow fever is a viral disease transmitted by the bite of an *Aedes aegypti* mosquito infected about fourteen days earlier by feeding on a viremic person. The incubation period lasts between three and six days. The three characteristic clinical features are jaundice, albuminuria, and black vomit. Its sudden onset is accompanied by fever, headache, muscle pains, and prostration. Fatality rates can range from 10 to 50 percent, but this figure is a generally inflated one because of the inability to identify mild cases. The disease affected diverse subgroups differently. Children were usually more resistant and suffered only mild or subclinical forms. Blacks had less dramatic symptoms than whites as well as lower mortality rates. Those who managed to survive yellow fever acquired lifetime immunity. The disease was endemic in West Africa, and its presence in the colonies required the transportation of infected persons.[12]

Unlike smallpox, yellow fever was intimately related to climate and geography. One of the critical variables was temperature and moisture, for the *Aedes aegypti* breeds in stagnant water adjacent to homes and feeds only when the temperature is above 60°. The insect is not especially mobile, and its life cycle takes place in an area limited to a few hundred yards. In the British mainland colonies, therefore, the disease could never become endemic (as it was in West Africa), because the mosquito could not survive winter temperatures. Its eggs, to be sure, could hatch in the spring, but the virus had to be reintroduced for an epidemic to begin anew. Yellow fever, at least before the nineteenth century, was a disease confined to port cities with commercial ties to tropical areas, as well as to communities located on rivers that flowed into these ports. Moreover, by the time an epidemic was recognizable, large numbers of individuals were already infected.

Yellow fever was absent from the mainland colonies for most of the seventeenth century. The disease struck Barbados in 1647, where it resulted in an estimated 5,000 deaths, and appeared in Yucatán the following year. Ultimately it spread to other Caribbean islands as well as to Central and South America. The first epidemic in the colonies occurred in Boston in 1693 following the arrival of British vessels from Barbados. Six years later yellow fever appeared in Charleston and Philadelphia. In Charleston as many as 300 persons perished, and with one exception all were white. One correspondent found it difficult to describe "the terrible Tempest of Mortality" in the city. The "high and low, old and young" perished. The dead were piled into carts, business activity came to a virtual standstill, and little was done except to carry medicines and dig graves. In Philadelphia 220 died out of a population of about 4,400. New York was equally devastated by an outbreak in 1702.[13]

During the first two-thirds of the eighteenth century there were at least twenty-five major yellow fever epidemics, although the number of minor ones added substantially to the total. Charleston and New York experienced six each and Philadelphia four. But the disease could strike any port community, as its presence in such widely distant towns as New Haven, Norfolk, Pensacola, and Mobile indicated. Moreover, if the affected community was located on a river, the disease could be transported into the interior. Oddly enough, yellow fever seemed to disappear after 1765, perhaps because of the interruption in trade that occurred during the Revolutionary crisis. But the disease reappeared in devastating form in 1793 and persisted for much of the nineteenth century. Though arousing terror among the inhabitants of port towns, where life was brought to a virtual standstill for several months, yellow fever in the aggregate had little impact upon population growth or overall mortality. Its presence simply illustrated the complex relationships that existed among pathogens, insect vectors, humans, and contacts between different regions of the world.[14]

The history of yellow fever also suggests that public fears and apprehensions may bear little or no relationship to the actual impact or demographic significance of a specific disease. When mortality from "normal" diseases is regular and predictable, there is relatively little concern; death is accepted as a part of life. When "abnormal" epidemics appear at irregular intervals and result in mortality spikes, public fears often reach a fever pitch. Under these circumstances community life is disrupted, and often a search for explanations leads to the stigmatization of socially marginal groups as the cause of the disaster. Oddly enough, the high mortality rates associated with epidemics that appear irregularly generally have a much smaller impact on population size than does mortality from "normal" diseases.

▼ ▼ ▼

Periodic smallpox and yellow fever epidemics tended to overshadow other diseases that played a far more significant role in shaping population development and increasing risks to life during the eighteenth century. Indeed, the health advantages enjoyed by many seventeenth-century settlements once the period of seasoning passed began to disappear after 1700. Toward the close of the eighteenth century the disease environment of the colonies began to resemble in some respects the higher mortality regime of Europe.

The initial portrayal of the colonies as a health utopia, often used to encourage immigration, slowly gave way to acknowledgment of a harsher reality. The rise in morbidity and mortality rates occurred at the very time that internal and external conflicts were becoming more common. As the colonies matured, the preoccupation with survival and adjustment gave way to social divisions based on class, occupation, and geography. Mobility became more problematic; generational and group divisions became more visible; and tensions with British imperial authorities increased. The fear and disillusionment that followed these developments may have played an indirect part in fostering a willingness to break the bonds of empire and permit the colonies to pursue an independent destiny.

In the seventeenth century isolated agricultural communities in the colonies had relatively few contacts with each other. Travel routes were primitive and slow. Consequently, it was more difficult to spread many infectious diseases, given their brief incubation periods. The lower risk of contaminated water supplies in rural environments also reduced the prevalence of gastrointestinal disorders. In England and Europe, by contrast, travel and communication were more rapid, and the presence of densely populated urban areas provided opportunities for pathogens to maintain themselves among populations with relatively high birthrates. As a result infectious diseases often assumed an endemic character. Most urban environments had crude sanitation and water systems, and enteric diseases took a high toll.

In the eighteenth century infectious diseases traditionally associated with infancy and childhood became more common in the American colonies. Although these diseases can strike adults as well, the young were more susceptible simply because they had never been exposed to the organisms. Once newborns and infants (3 to 12 months) no longer enjoy the passive transfer of maternal immunity through breast feeding, they are vulnerable to a host of infections.

Diseases normally associated with infancy and childhood, however, occasionally exhibited quite different characteristics in colonial America. Many were not indigenous to the colonies. When they were imported, the entire population—young and old alike—were susceptible. The result was widespread epidemics with relatively elevated mortality rates even among adults.

The checkered history of measles in colonial America provides an example of the relationship between disease patterns and the larger environment. Before 1800 measles had not yet assumed an endemic character, nor was it a disease of the young. In the seventeenth century the disease appeared only sporadically. Boston had the first recorded outbreak in 1657, and the following year it was present in Connecticut. But nearly thirty years would pass before it reappeared. The brief incubation period and highly contagious nature of the disease reduced the odds of bringing the disease to the colonies; an outbreak at sea would generally run its course before a ship arrived in the colonies. After 1700, however, measles became more common. The growth of trade and construction of faster ships facilitated the importation of the virus into port communities, and in turn its transportation into interior regions. In 1713 the disease appeared in Boston and then spread southward into New York, New Jersey, and Pennsylvania. Mortality among those who are infected by a close relative tends to be higher than among those who are infected in the community at large, and the epidemic of 1713 was no exception. "The *Measles* are a distemper which in *Europe* ordinarily proves a light Malady." observed Cotton Mather in his pamphlet detailing the epidemic, "but in these parts of *America* it proves a very heavy Calamity; A Malady *Grievous* to most, *Mortal* to many, and leaving pernicious Relicks behind it in All." The epidemic devastated his own household; his wife came down with the disease, and four children and the maid died.[15] Although precise data are unavailable, contemporary accounts indicate that measles was prevalent among adults as well as children.

Throughout the eighteenth century sporadic epidemics of measles were common. The New England and Middle Atlantic colonies were the hardest hit; the Chesapeake and southern colonies were somewhat less affected. There was a steady decline in the intervals between epidemics. Between its initial appearance in 1657 and 1772, the interval in Boston declined from thirty to eleven years. Moreover, the growth in population and increase in commerce altered the local character of epidemics. In 1772 and 1773, Noah Webster reported, "the measles appeared in all parts of America, with unusual mortality." Though mild in New England, it was devastating in Charleston. According to Webster, as many as 800 to 900 children died in that city (out of a total population of 14,000). Although Webster's figures may have been grossly inflated, they do suggest the potential severity of the disease.[16]

Overall mortality from measles in the eighteenth century was extraordinarily high even though some epidemics were relatively benign. The epidemic of 1714 in New London, Connecticut, had a mortality rate of 45 per 1,000, and the rates for Philadelphia in 1747, 1759, and 1772 were 56, 63, and 62, respectively (equaling modern death rates for cardiovascular diseases and cancer).[17] Measles epidemics aroused fear because of their high mortality. Ebenezer Parkman, minister of Westborough, Massachusetts, from 1724 to 1782, underwent a "conversion experience" when at age 11 he recovered from a three-month ordeal from the disease. His diary, which he began keeping in 1719 while a student at Harvard, opened with a recollection of his illness.

I was visited with a Low fit of sickness beginning with a fever and attended with the Meazells, and after that with great weakness and

infirmities as also great pain. which Set me upon thinking upon
what would be the Estate, the Condition of My Soul after my Disso-
lution . . . Heartly wishing and praying that My many and great In-
iquities might be all so pardoned and washed away in the Blood of
the Lamb of God that taketh away the Sin of the World, Promising
allso that if God would in his great Mercy Spare my Life I would
Spend it more to the Glory and praise of his great Name.[18]

Nor was mortality from measles concentrated among the young;
adults were as vulnerable as children. Such excessive mortality may
have been the result of the susceptibility of entire families; contemporary data reveal that the transmission of measles within households
results in progressively higher mortality. But the variations among epidemics may have also reflected the presence or absence of other infectious diseases that increased the burden on health.

Elevated mortality rates may also have stemmed in part the failure
of measles to become established in endemic form. In England and on
the Continent, densely populated urban areas always included large
numbers of susceptible people. Consequently, many infectious diseases assumed an endemic character. Epidemics in relatively small
eighteenth-century colonial communities, by contrast, reduced the
number of susceptible persons to the point where no further outbreak
was possible.

The high mortality that accompanied outbreaks of measles was not
unique. The sudden appearance of diphtheria in epidemic form in the
mid-eighteenth century proved equally devastating. Diphtheria is a
human disease caused by the *Corynebacterium diphtheriae* and
spread by the secretions of infected persons. Often the disease is mild
and subclinical. But on other occasions one of its more virulent biotypes leads to lethal outbreaks in which the case fatality rate can
range from 30 to 50 percent. Ordinarily the organism infects the ton-
sil or nasopharynx. The toxigenic form of the bacterium may produce exotoxins lethal to the adjacent host cells. Carried by the blood,
these exotoxins can damage distant sites, including the myocardium,
nervous system, and kidneys. More often, death is caused by the presence of a pseudomembrane in the tonsillar area that obstructs breathing. Whether diphtheria was a new disease or an unrecognized older
one cannot be determined. In the eighteenth century, moreover, it was
not always possible to distinguish between diphtheria and scarlet fe-

ver, since both involved the throat (although the latter began with a streptococcus infection).

The first recorded outbreak of the "throat distemper"—the eighteenth-century term for diphtheria—occurred in 1659. In succeeding years diphtheria and scarlet fever were undoubtedly present, but the small number of cases limited their impact. In 1735, however, an epidemic of "throat distemper" swept through Kingston, New Hampshire. In the following five years it moved northward into Maine and southward into Massachusetts. Oddly enough, Boston was little affected; before reaching that town the epidemic turned to the west and southeast and eventually merged with an epidemic that had begun in New Jersey and moved northeast.[19]

At the time of this outbreak the majority of New Englanders lived in small and relatively isolated towns with populations as low as several hundred and as high as 5,000 (excluding Boston and adjacent areas). The epidemic that appeared initially in Kingston in the late spring of 1735 was extraordinarily virulent. The mortality rate among the first 40 cases was 100 percent. In the first few months the case fatality rate approached 50 percent, and by the end of the epidemic in 1736 more than a third of the town's children had perished. During the first year there were 984 fatalities in fifteen New Hampshire towns. Of this number 802 (81.5 percent) were under the age of 10, 139 (14.1 percent) were in the 10-to-20 age group, and 43 (4.3 percent) were over 20.[20]

News of the deadly outbreak spread quickly throughout the region. In one of the first printed descriptions, a writer in the *Boston Gazette* noted: "No Disease has never raved in *New England* (except the Small-Pox) which has struck such an universal Terror into People, as that which has lately visited *Kingston, Exeter Hampton* and other Parts of the Province of *New-Hampshire* . . . It has been among young People and Children, pretty universal and very mortal of Noise; and the next Day pays his Debt to Nature." In a contemporary broadside titled *A Lamentation,* an author called upon "Young and Old, to turn from Sin, and to seek GOD's Face and Favour."

> GOD smitten hath with sore Plagues
> Our Children young and small,
> Which makes me weep exceedingly
> And on CHRIST's Name to call.

> This mortal Plague doth much enrage,
>   Among our Little Bands,
> And sudden Death doth stop the Breath
>   Of these our little Lambs.
>
> What tears apace, run from our Face,
>   To hear our Children crying
> For help from pain, but all in vain,
>   We cannot help their dying.[21]

The origins of the epidemic will probably remain a mystery. Once present, however, it was disseminated within communities by personal contact. Ministers (who often practiced medicine as well) and physicians played a major role. In caring for and ministering to the sick, they unknowingly assisted in the spread of the disease. Some may even have been healthy carriers. Deaths in their own families, not surprisingly, tended to be more frequent. Another epidemiological characteristic of the disease was the multiple-death family; 40 percent of the families that lost children lost more than one. Conversely, less than 5 percent of families that did not lose a child during the epidemic ever experienced a year in which more than one child died.[22]

As the epidemic spread, the mortality rate underwent puzzling changes. New Hampshire had the highest rate; Massachusetts the lowest. The Connecticut epidemic either had independent origins or was part of the one that first appeared in New Jersey; it began along shore towns in the western region and then moved to the northeast corner of the colony. The most striking feature was the absence of any devastating epidemic in Boston, the town with the largest population.[23]

Such striking differences raise an array of questions. Why was diphtheria so lethal in New Hampshire and less so elsewhere? Why did Boston—a town with commercial links with interior regions—largely escape the epidemic? Why did mortality rates change as the epidemic progressed? Were high rates due to the presence of a more virulent strain? Did the pathogen undergo genetic reassortment that increased or decreased its virulence between 1735 and 1740? Did an earlier mild or inapparent epidemic diminish the number of susceptibles in some areas? If such was the case, why were mortality rates so different among those who were infected? Such questions, however, may never be answered with any degree of certitude.

After the epidemic of 1735—1740 subsided, diphtheria appeared periodically in many colonies. The pattern in New England was probably typical. Following an epidemic peak, there were occasional deaths in the next two or three years. In general, however, diphtheria reappeared at intervals of seven to ten years—a period sufficiently long for the nonimmune to become numerous enough to support an epidemic. Moreover, mild outbreaks would sometimes be followed by virulent ones. In Weymouth, Massachusetts, for example, about 150 persons (overwhelmingly children), or 12 percent of the population, perished from the "throat distemper" in 1751; from 1767 to 1770, 144 died in Oxford. In many instances communities had not experienced virulent outbreaks, and thus its inhabitants were unable to mount an adequate immune response. Oddly enough, the growth of population in the late eighteenth century in eastern Massachusetts and New Hampshire did not lead to an increased mortality rate from diphtheria. Indeed, there was a decline in the incidence of the disease after 1780. Yet by the early nineteenth century newer communities in western New England, Ohio, and Kentucky began to experience lethal epidemics, perhaps because their populations had not been immunized by earlier outbreaks.[24]

During epidemic years measles and diphtheria often proved fatal. But not all infectious diseases associated with infancy and childhood exhibited such dramatic outcomes. Scarlet fever, for example, was a comparatively mild disease in the eighteenth century. The disease is associated with Group A streptococcal strains that produce a toxin that leads to a diffuse pinkish-red flush of the skin that blanches on pressure. In the nineteenth century it became more dangerous, but before that time the case fatality rate ranged from 1 to less than 3 percent.

The first recorded epidemic occurred in Boston in 1702, and may have been imported from London; major outbreaks followed in 1735 and 1736. In *The Practical History of a New Epidemical Eruptive Miliary Fever* (1736), William Douglass provided a classic clinical description of scarlet fever. In that epidemic perhaps 4,000 (overwhelmingly children) out of a total population of 16,000 were infected. Douglass estimated that the case fatality rate was 2.8 percent; another observer put the figure at 1.7 percent. For nearly three decades there was no mention of the disease. After 1770, however, it became more common in virtually all the colonies, and by the end of the century began to result in much higher mortality.[25]

Pertussis (whooping cough) and chickenpox also made their presence felt in the eighteenth century. The causative agent of pertussis is the gram-negative coccobacillus *Bordetella pertussis*. Lasting about six weeks, the disease is characterized by a number of successive coughs followed by the whoop. It tends to appear in epidemic form, and a significant number of cases occur before the age of 2, since infants lack protective antibodies. By the middle of the eighteenth century the disease was present in all the colonies. Epidemics of pertussis lasted from one to three years, and the intervals between them ranged from three to six years. Although the disease was prevalent among the young, susceptible adults were also infected. Much the same was true of mumps and chickenpox, both of which are caused by viruses. These two diseases became more common in the mid-eighteenth century, and affected children and susceptible adults. Neither, however, was associated with elevated mortality.[26]

Colonial Americans were fearful of such diseases as smallpox, yellow fever, measles, and diphtheria, if only because of their visibility and dramatic nature of symptoms. Moreover, the infrequent appearance and the elevated mortality rates of epidemic diseases served to strengthen public apprehension and to create pervasive feelings of helplessness. Despite the high toll in lives, however, these diseases were by no means the most significant determinants of morbidity and mortality. Certain endemic diseases—notably dysentery and malaria—took a far higher toll even though their omnipresent nature tended to reduce public fear.

Dysentery was undoubtedly the most significant disease in eighteenth-century America. It played an important role when the colonies were being settled in the seventeenth century but became even more prevalent in the next. Outbreaks were especially common in such towns as Boston, New York, Philadelphia, and Charleston. These ports were the entry points for ships bringing thousands of immigrants to the colonies. Conditions aboard eighteenth-century vessels were particularly conducive to outbreaks of dysentery, and it was relatively easy for infected immigrants to serve as reservoirs for the causative pathogen upon their arrival. Although the perils of the North Atlantic crossing were often exaggerated, there is little doubt about the sporadic risks to health and life. "It is not surprising," wrote Gottlieb Mittelberger in 1756,

> that many passengers fall ill, because in addition to all the other troubles and miseries, warm food is served only three times a week,

and at that is very bad, very small in quantity, and so dirty as to be hardly palatable at all. And the water distributed in these ships is often very black, thick with dirt, and full of worms. Even when very thirsty, one is almost unable to drink it without loathing. It is certainly true that at sea one would often spend a great deal of money just for one good piece of bread, or one good drink of water—not even to speak of a good glass of wine—if one could only obtain them. I have, alas, had to experience that myself. For toward the end of the voyage we had to eat the ship's biscuit, which had already been spoiled for a long time, even though in no single piece was there more than the size of a thaler that was not full of red worms and spiders' nests. True, great hunger and thirst teach one to eat and drink everything—but many must forfeit their lives in the process. It is impossible to drink seawater, since it is salty and bitter as gall.[27]

Under such circumstances it is hardly surprising that enteric disorders took such a high toll among passengers during the voyage and after their arrival in the colonies. According to a contemporary account, the *St. Andrew,* which docked in Philadelphia on October 27, 1738,

> lost 160 persons; another that arrived the day before lost over 150; and one that came the day following was said to have had only 13 well persons on board. Meantime another has arrived, in which out of 300, only 50 fares are left. They have mostly died from dysentery, skin sickness and inflammatory fever; likewise some of the captains and many seamen . . . Many of the survivors die after landing, and thus diseases are brought into the country, so that many inhabitants and landlords become sick, are seized by the epidemic and quickly carried off.[28]

Outbreaks of dysentery occurred everywhere in the colonies, but especially in the more densely populated towns. Yearly epidemics were not uncommon, and rarely was there as much as a five-year interval between them. Lacking knowledge about the causes of dysentery, colonial Americans were unable to undertake preventive measures. Infected and healthy carriers transmitted pathogens; crude methods of disposing of organic wastes often contaminated drinking water; the absence of refrigeration permitted the growth of pathogens in food supplies; and prevailing hygienic standards enhanced the risk of exposure. Infants and young children were especially vulnerable.

The existing systems of care of sick persons, moreover, actually magnified the dangers posed by gastrointestinal disorders. Nor was there any understanding that dehydration could result in death. Local data reveal that during an epidemic, perhaps half of a community's population would become infected; of these, one of every six or seven would die. Noah Webster reported that in 1745 the town of Stamford, Connecticut, "was severely distressed by a malignant dysentery, which swept away seventy inhabitants out of a few hundreds." Local contamination in all probability was the source of the outbreak, since "the disease was confined to one street." Mortality during dysentery outbreaks ranged between 5 and 10 percent, to say nothing about the large numbers of individual deaths during nonepidemic years. Dysentery also contributed to overall mortality in indirect ways, for it weakened individuals and left them vulnerable to other diseases.[29]

Malaria had the same endemic characteristics as dysentery, although its impact was uneven. In the seventeenth century the disease was present in New England and the Middle Atlantic colonies. It was imported into such port communities as Boston, New York, and Philadelphia and quickly spread to interior regions. The clearing of land disrupted drainage patterns and created stagnant bodies of water. The presence of the *Anopheles* mosquito and the transportation of infected persons into an area set the stage for the appearance of malaria. The disease was present along virtually the entire East Coast. By the middle of the eighteenth century, however, malaria began to decline in New England, largely because the cold climate proved fatal for the insect population. In New York City, on the other hand, malaria persisted for much of the nineteenth century even though it never became a major problem.[30]

Nowhere was the impact of malaria greater than in the Carolina low country. The disease, to be sure, continued to pose a significant problem in the Chesapeake area. In South Carolina, however, the introduction of rice cultivation at the end of the seventeenth century magnified the impact of malaria. In 1699 1,500 barrels were shipped from Charleston. In slightly over three decades the figure soared to over 41,000, and by the close of the colonial era had reached nearly 120,000 barrels. Rice was not only the colony's most lucrative export but also the crop around which the economy, labor force, and culture revolved.[31]

The burgeoning rice industry had a devastating impact on morbidity and mortality. The cultivation of rice required flooding, since the crop flourished in wet and low-lying areas. Stalks of rice in still and shallow water provided the *Anopheles* mosquito with an ideal breeding site, and malaria quickly emerged as one of the leading causes of death. By the mid-seventeenth century indigo also accounted for about a third of the colony's total exports. The cultivation of this crop involved large amounts of water steeping in vats and stagnating behind dams, thus providing additional opportunities for mosquito breeding.

During the eighteenth century the system of agriculture in the low country gave South Carolina a deserved reputation as a graveyard. White mortality in the colony's lowlands can only be described as catastrophic. Mortality was highest from June to October, the months in which malaria tended to peak. For the black population the demographic situation was also grave, though less so than for whites. Neither group, as a matter of fact, could sustain a natural increase in their numbers. Without inmigration the colony would have faced virtual extinction. Environment, migration and trade patterns, and a particular form of agriculture combined to make South Carolina the unhealthiest colony in all of British North America.[32]

The establishment of malaria in endemic form also provided a rationale for the introduction and spread of slavery. In the eyes of whites, Africans seemed better equipped physiologically to labor in a sunny, hot, and humid climate, and such a belief was employed to justify slavery. "The utter ineptitude of Europeans for the labour requisite in such a climate and soil," the Reverend Alexander Hewat (an opponent of slavery) wrote in 1779,

> is obvious to every one possessed of the smallest degree of knowledge respecting the country; white servants would have exhausted their strength in clearing a spot of land for digging their own graves, and every rice plantation would have served no other purpose than a burying ground to its European cultivators. The low lands of Carolina, which are unquestionably the richest grounds in the country, must long have remained a wilderness, had not Africans, whose natural constitutions were suited to the clime and work, been employed in cultivating this useful article of food and commerce.[33]

Malaria flourished in warm and humid weather; colder temperatures diminished its prevalence. The seasonal decline in new cases, however, did not diminish the burden of disease. On the contrary, in the late autumn and winter respiratory disorders emerged as a major cause of mortality. Although it is virtually impossible to distinguish between viral and bacterial respiratory infections, it is clear that such disorders took a high toll, especially among the young and the elderly.

With the possible exception of dysentery, respiratory illnesses were among the leading causes of death in the eighteenth century. Prevailing patterns of care undoubtedly exacerbated the problems posed by respiratory disorders. Cold indoor temperatures—a characteristic of eighteenth-century homes—and failure to provide sufficient fluid intake increased the risks to life. Moreover, diseases often have a symbiotic relationship; the significance of respiratory disorders was magnified when they occurred in tandem with other diseases. In an essay published in 1742 John Tennent noted that "pleurisy"—a term used to describe respiratory disorders—was "the most fatal Disease that affects the Constitution of the Inhabitants of this Country."[34]

Most eighteenth-century respiratory disorders were endemic and seasonal in character. But the growth in population and expansion of trade began to render the colonies somewhat more vulnerable to influenza epidemics and pandemics. At the beginning of the eighteenth century distance protected the colonies from outbreaks occurring elsewhere in the world. Thus the European epidemic of 1708–09 did not reach the American colonies. In 1732–33 influenza was prevalent in the Northeast and Middle Atlantic colonies; it may have been a late flare-up of the 1729–30 pandemic that began in Russia and moved westward through Europe. Indigenous influenza outbreaks occurred periodically in many colonies. By the close of the eighteenth century the newly independent colonies had become part of a larger disease pool. In 1781–82 and 1788–89 influenza appeared in pandemic form, affecting millions of people in both Europe and America. Nevertheless, case fatality rates associated with influenza remained low. With the exception of the risks to elderly or chronically ill persons, influenza was not a lethal disease in the eighteenth century.[35]

Largely because of their spectacular appearances and cyclical character, epidemic diseases preoccupied colonial Americans. Other infectious diseases assumed a chronic rather than an acute form and hence tended to be less visible. Tuberculosis was one such example. Frag-

mentary evidence indicates that it was present in the early days of settlement. Contemporary accounts refer to deaths from "consumption," "scrofula," "pleurisies," and "phthisis." The symptoms—
coughs, fever, and bloody sputum—were consistent with the modern
understanding of tuberculosis, although eighteenth-century bills of
mortality were unable to distinguish between tuberculosis and other
pulmonary disorders. Journal P. Brissot de Warville, a perceptive foreign traveler, believed that the presence of consumption was often exaggerated. "Through ignorance this name is improperly given to
many other diseases that cause the same loss of weight that follows
pulmonary phthisis." Nevertheless, he conceded that of "all the diseases in the United States consumption undoubtedly wreaks the
greatest ravages." Even if we allow for the inability to distinguish between pulmonary disorders and tuberculosis, it seems likely that the
incidence of the latter rose during the eighteenth century.[36]

Many colonial accounts refer to "consumptions." Michael
Wigglesworth, the well-known Massachusetts clergyman, physician,
and poet, noted the death of a parishioner in 1668 "from a long and
tedious consumption." The colonies, he wrote in wrote a classic
poem, suffered from the same condition found in Europe.

> Our healthfull dayes are at an end,
>   And sicknesses come on . . .
> New-England, where for many yeers
>   You scarcely heard a cough,
> And where Physicians had no work,
>   Now finds them work enough.
>
> Now colds and coughs, Rhewms, and sore-throats
>   Do more & more abound:
> Now Agues sore & Feavers strong
>   In every place are found.
> How many houses have we seen
>   Last Autumn, and this spring,
> Wherein the healthful were too few
>   To help the languishing.[37]

Wigglesworth's observations were echoed by many others. In reviewing Philadelphia's irregular bills of mortality, Peter Kalm—a foreign visitor to the colonies—concluded that "consumptions, fevers,

convulsions, pleurisies, haemorrhages, and dropsies" were the leading causes of mortality in Philadelphia between 1730 and 1750. Another contemporary estimated that 19 percent of all deaths in that city in 1787 were due to this disease. Other communities exhibited similar patterns. In the ten-year period 1768–1777, 14 percent of all deaths in Salem were attributed to consumption, and in five small Massachusetts towns consumption accounted for between 18 and 20 percent of total mortality from 1784 to 1792. Data from southern colonies were not fundamentally dissimilar.[38]

By the late eighteenth century tuberculosis and other pulmonary disorders may have been among the leading causes of death in the new nation. What accounts for the rise in incidence and prevalence of a disease or diseases that have waxed and waned throughout human history? If a clear answer is not possible, certain factors undoubtedly played a role, especially population density. In his famous history of epidemic diseases, the ubiquitous lexicographer Noah Webster wrote that "pestilence has always been the *peculiar curse* of *populous cities.*" Of 200 general plagues, he added, "almost all have been limited to large towns." Webster's concept of crowding, however accurate, was too limited. Tuberculosis and pulmonary disorders were not confined to more populous communities; they were present in rural areas as well. The critical element was not total population, but household size. Eighteenth-century data reveal that, irrespective of town size, the typical dwelling (which was relatively small compared with contemporary structures) contained from 7 to 10 inhabitants. In 1741, for example, the average dwelling in Boston held approximately 10.3 persons, a figure that was fairly typical. Such crowding facilitated the household transmission of mycobacteria and other organisms. Other elements merely compounded the risks of contagion. Relatively inefficient heating led inhabitants to seal doors and windows during colder weather. Indeed, eighteenth-century colonial physicians advised against opening windows even in warmer weather. Moreover, caretakers often slept in the same bed with their patients. Behavioral patterns thus contributed to the spread of tuberculosis and pulmonary disorders during these decades. Finally, migration from England—where the incidence of these diseases had reached unprecedented heights—added to the risk of contagion in the colonies.[39]

In the eighteenth century the mortality rate was the measure of health, and acute and chronic infections the major causes of death.

Chronic degenerative or long-duration illnesses were undoubtedly present among older individuals, but they were minor causes of mortality because of the youthful nature of American society. Of approximately 3.9 million white males in 1800, for example, only 18 percent were age 45 or older, and the median age was about 16.[40] The relatively small proportion of older adults—to say nothing about the inability to diagnose many of these illnesses at that time—makes it virtually impossible to provide any realistic estimates of their prevalence.

▼ ▼ ▼

Acute infectious diseases posed the greatest danger to infants, children, and the aged. Yet unique circumstances had the potential to alter this demographic pattern. The experiences of the military during wartime are a case in point. Indeed, war provides a fascinating insight into the complex relationships between pathogens and humans, and demonstrates the crucial role of environment in shaping patterns of morbidity and mortality.

The Revolutionary War is a case in point. The circumstances of military life were quite different from those of civilian life. During the Revolution, large numbers of young males lived in crowded quarters that lacked even rudimentary sanitary facilities. The potential for contaminating water supplies from both human and animal wastes was high. Moreover, recruits came from predominantly rural areas, and many had never been exposed to common communicable diseases. Preoccupation with battlefield concerns often led military commanders and civilian authorities to pay inadequate attention to basic necessities, including food, clothing, and shelter. Neither camp nor personal hygiene was given high priority, even though authorities were aware of their significance. Under such circumstances the impact of pathogens was significantly magnified.

During the Revolutionary War perhaps 200,000 served in the military. According to the most careful estimates, 7,174 were killed in military engagements, 10,000 died in camps, and 8,500 perished as prisoners of war. The more than 25,000 deaths amounted to 0.9 percent of the population; only the Civil War had a higher proportion of fatalities. During World Wars I and II, by contrast, the figures were 0.12 and 0.28 percent, respectively.[41] Deaths in camps and among prisoners resulted from a variety of diseases, most of which were directly related to the circumstances of military life. Moreover, many battlefield deaths were the direct result of secondary infections associated with eighteenth-century surgical practices and the unsatisfactory conditions that prevailed in military hospitals.

At the beginning of the Revolutionary War smallpox emerged as a major problem, and large numbers of soldiers never previously exposed died. The ravages of the disease drastically impaired military effectiveness. In 1777, therefore, military authorities took the unprecedented step of ordering the inoculation of all recruits in order to reduce the threat of epidemics. This was the first time that any army had been immunized by command order. From 1776 through 1778, cold weather, clothing and food shortages, crude housing, and inadequate sanitation and hygienic practices combined to increase vulnerability to disease. Perhaps 90 percent of all deaths were due to disease; respiratory disorders and dysentery were the two leading causes of mortality. Typhus and typhoid fever were also present, though less significant. In the South and the Chesapeake malaria took its toll. Venereal diseases, scurvy, scabies (a parasitic skin infection more commonly known as "the itch"), and other infectious disorders and inadequate nutrition added to the health burden of the military and undoubtedly increased vulnerability. Given the nature of recruitment and the circumstances of military life during the Revolution, it is hardly surprising that mortality was overwhelmingly a function of the interaction of environmental conditions, pathogens, and human hosts. Military engagements accounted for only a small proportion of the total number of soldiers who died.[42]

▼ ▼ ▼

The general perception among European commentators was that Americans enjoyed a distinct advantage in terms of life expectancy. Brissot de Warville concluded that "the life of man is much longer in the United States than it is in the healthiest countries of Europe."[43] Yet aggregate mortality rates in the eighteenth century were rising, even in New England, which had lower rates than other colonies. Variations within this region, however, were striking. Port communities had death rates similar to those in England. Boston's mortality rate fluctuated between 30 and 40 per 1,000 between 1701 and 1774. During epidemic years the rate exceeded 60 on three occasions and reached 103 during the smallpox outbreak in 1721.[44] Commercial contacts with other parts of the world, higher population density, and crude sanitary conditions increased the risks to life in this community.

Boston, however, was not necessarily representative of the New England region. Data from other Massachusetts communities reveal a somewhat more mixed pattern. Mortality rates in Salem, which were high during the seventeenth century, fell during the eighteenth, particularly among infants and women of childbearing age. In Plymouth, Andover, and Ipswich, on the other hand, mortality rates among the very young increased as a result of increased contacts and the ensuing dissemination of infectious pathogens. Yet life expectancy among those who survived to adulthood remained relatively stable. More isolated western New England communities were less affected, and death rates in these areas for the most part remained lower.[45]

The overall increase in mortality in eighteenth-century New England, however, did not appreciably affect population growth. A 5 to 10 percent loss of population during infrequent epidemic years and an average annual loss in the range of 2 percent did not prove critical in limiting natural population increase even though the number of individuals migrating from New England to the west and south exceeded the number of immigrants. Oddly enough, New Englanders— perhaps because their memories were shaped by English experiences—believed that mortality remained high. Their religious beliefs, the appearance of periodic epidemics, and high levels of infant and child mortality led them to emphasize the precariousness of life despite the fact that their chances of survival were better than for those who remained in England.[46]

Our knowledge of demographic patterns in the Middle Atlantic region is far less complete than for Massachusetts. Nevertheless, a similar pattern seems to have prevailed. Aggregate mortality was marginally higher than in New England, but much lower than the southern colonies. Like Boston, Philadelphia (which has been studied in considerable depth) experienced high mortality rates as trade and commerce introduced recurrent waves of infectious epidemic diseases. Between 1680 and 1720 deaths exceeded births, and the share of individuals residing in Philadelphia relative to the total urban population in southeastern Pennsylvania fell dramatically. Between 1720 and 1760 the city became the center of a productive agricultural region as well as of foreign trade, particularly with the Caribbean. During these years its mortality exceeded that of Boston. Although both communities were centers of commerce and thus faced the threat of imported pathogens, Philadelphia had a much higher rate of immigration than Boston, a fact that compounded the risks posed by epidemic infectious diseases. Crude death rates in the City of Brotherly Love fluctuated greatly, between 30 and 60 per 1,000. Newly arrived immigrants were the most vulnerable; their mortality rates were nearly double that of native-born residents. For much of the eighteenth century Philadelphia remained a dangerous place in which to live; its death rates were even higher than those in many European cities. Although fertility was high, the growth of the city was possible only because of large-scale immigration of younger people.

After 1760 health conditions improved somewhat, especially among the white middle and upper classes. Among the poor—both white and black—mortality rose. An awareness of factors that increased health risks led Philadelphians to invest in public health measures, including street paving, garbage collection, safer water supplies, and smallpox inoculation. Rural areas in this region were healthier places to live. Nevertheless, increased population density and improved transportation after 1750 led to rising rural mortality rates.[47] Fragmentary data suggest a similar pattern for New York and New Jersey.

The demographic pattern in the South in the eighteenth century differed in fundamental respects from all the other British mainland colonies. Mortality rates in this region exceeded even those in Europe. Disease and death affected not only social relations but the very psychology of its inhabitants. The fragility of life gave rise to a sense of impermanence and a desire to amass wealth as quickly as possible. The devastation of the white labor supply and the inability of Europeans to adapt to a seemingly intractable disease environment promoted the enslavement of Africans.[48]

Mortality rates in the South were excessive even by eighteenth-century standards. In 1735–1739 the average crude death rate in Charleston reached nearly 130 per 1,000, largely because of the severity of the smallpox outbreak of 1738. But even in more "normal" years the death rate was slightly over 78. This figure was more than double the rates found further north. Indeed, the unhealthiest areas in England were well off by comparison with Charleston. In one Charleston parish only 19 percent of those born survived to the age of 20. In Andover, Massachusetts, by contrast, more than two-thirds of those born in the mid-eighteenth century survived to age 20. Moreover, Charleston residents who survived to age 20 had a 30 percent chance of living to 50, as compared with 66 percent in Andover. One percent of those born in Charleston reached the age of 80; the comparable figure for Andover was nearly 22 percent. The experience of the Chesapeake and North Carolina, though not as extreme, was far closer to that of South Carolina than to that of the Middle Atlantic and New England colonies. Without a constant flow of immigrants to replenish a population devastated by extraordinary death rates, not only would the southern colonies have failed to develop economically, but their very survival as a society would have become questionable. Nor did wealth or status confer a distinct advantage insofar as survival was concerned; mortality rates—admittedly unevenly distributed—remained high among all groups.[49]

Once colonial Americans had adjusted to their new environment, they enjoyed (with some exceptions) greater freedom from those infectious diseases that took such a heavy toll in the mother country and western Europe. All advantages, however, often give rise to unanticipated consequences. Rapid population and economic growth created conditions conducive to the spread of infectious diseases, and by the end of the eighteenth century the health advantages enjoyed by the newly independent nation were beginning to diminish. In the nineteenth century these advantages would diminish still further. The rise in the standard of living, paradoxically, would be accompanied by increases in morbidity and mortality.

CHAPTER 5

Threats to Urban Health

Half of New York City's population, Dr. Stephen Smith noted in 1865, lived in an environment that resulted in both physical and moral degeneration.

> Here infantile life unfolds its bud, but perishes before its first anniversary. Here youth is ugly with loathsome diseases and the deformities which follow physical degeneracy. Here the decrepitude of old age is found at thirty. The poor themselves have a very expressive term for the slow process of decay which they suffer, viz.: "Tenement-house Rot." The great majority are, indeed, undergoing a slow decomposition—a true eremacausis, as the chemists term it. And with this physical degeneration we find mental and moral deterioration.[1]

In his jeremiad Smith—who played an important role in public health—was implicitly acknowledging the rapid growth of urban areas and their deleterious effect on the health of residents. Although the United States was still a predominantly rural nation, cities were growing in number, size, and importance. In 1790 there were only six cities with more than 8,000 residents, and they held only 3.35 percent of the total population. By 1850 eighty-five such urban areas contained about 12.5 percent of the population. In 1790 no city exceeded 50,000, and only two had more than 25,000. By 1850 New York City had more than 500,000 residents, while five others had between 100,000 and 250,000, and twenty more ranged in size from 25,000 to 100,000.[2]

Urban growth reflected social, economic, and technological changes. The construction of canals and railroads hastened the creation of a national market economy that transcended local boundaries. Changes in the production of goods and services, the emergence of new occupations, and the creation of novel industries began to alter the lives of Americans in fundamental ways, although their full impact would not be felt until the latter part of the nineteenth century.

The growth of cities magnified the risks to health and life. Indeed, urban morbidity and mortality rates rose precipitously after 1800, and did not manifest significant improvement even in the post–Civil War decades. Although the same was true for many rural regions, the magnitude was not as great. Ironically, declining urban health occurred at precisely the time that real wages and the standard of living were rising. This seeming paradox runs counter to the intuitive belief that health and income are directly related. Yet for much of the nineteenth century the conditions of urban life promoted the dissemination of a variety of infectious diseases that took a heavy toll among residents.

▾   ▾   ▾

The increase in the size and number of cities and the simultaneous acceleration in economic activity, however beneficial in the long run, magnified the risks from infectious diseases. Urban growth during the first half of the nineteenth century tended to be somewhat haphazard. City governments, to be sure, began to assume responsibility for providing services previously handled by volunteer groups or individuals. By the 1840s, for example, there were indications that some cities were moving to assume responsibility for policing and firefighting functions, although the creation of bureaucratically organized and tax-supported departments would take several decades. The same was true for the building and paving of streets, which were considered vital for business. The protection of health, on the other hand, remained problematic, even though some urban communities adopted regulations to deal with public health concerns before the end of the eighteenth century. Nevertheless, the rapidity of change tended to overwhelm early health codes, which were generally designed to handle such obvious nuisances as "noxious trades" that created unpleasant odors, animal droppings that covered virtually every street, and the disposal of human and other organic wastes. Before the advent of the specific germ theory of disease, prevailing concepts of cleanliness tended to be chemical and mechanical rather than biological.

Provision of safe and widely accessible water supplies and removal of wastes presented municipal governments with their greatest challenges. At the beginning of the nineteenth century most residents drew their water from local sources. Some dug their own wells or took water from neighborhood streams and springs. Others purchased water from private suppliers. A number of municipalities had public pumps and assessed residents for their use.

Local water supplies, however, quickly proved inadequate. Surface water sources were easily contaminated. The lack of water to flush streets or control fires created other problems. Equally significant, human and other organic wastes as well as wastewater were generally drained into cesspools and privy vaults adjacent to homes. Such drainage systems soon became sources of biological contamination.

As urban population and density increased, the prevailing system of local water supply proved inadequate. By the early nineteenth century, therefore, larger cities, including Philadelphia, New York, and Boston, began to construct public systems that brought water from rivers and reservoirs outside their borders. As supplies increased, more affluent families began to install fixtures such as sinks and toilets in their homes. In the years following the opening of the Cochituate Aqueduct for Boston in 1848, the number of water-using fixtures rose from 31,750 in 1853 to 81,726 a decade later (of which 13,000 were water closets). The introduction of running water in cities resulted in a dramatic increase in per-capita water consumption, from about 2–3 gallons per day to 50–100.[3]

Population growth and rising per-capita water usage exacerbated the risks to health by overloading already inadequate means of water and waste disposal. The installation of water supply systems was not accompanied by the construction of sewer systems to remove the water in ways that would not threaten the health of residents. New York City, for example, refused to permit organic wastes to be disposed of in common sewers, which conveyed storm water out of the city. Instead it instructed its tanners and butchers to dispose of animal wastes directly "into the river or some other place where the same shall not be injurious or offensive to the inhabitants." The prevailing belief was that running water purified itself. Other industries using water in their operations added to health risks. Paper and woolen textile mills dumped industrial wastes into rivers from which water was drawn, and thus contributed to the contamination of household water. In a survey of water pollution in the Nashua River basin, the Massachusetts State Board of Health described a branch of the river in Fitchburg in dramatic terms:

> The water of the Nashua, in passing this city, is extensively polluted by the wash of nine paper mills, four woolen mills, two cotton mills, gas works, and other manufacturing establishments . . . The water presents a dirty appearance . . . It receives the whole sewage of the city . . . All the chemicals employed in paper mills and different manufacturing establishments—excrement, dyestuffs, etc., and street washings—find their way directly into the stream. The extent of the pollution is great.

Decades would pass before urban areas could provide residents with pure water.[4]

Prevailing systems of water and waste disposal were not alone in magnifying threats to health and well-being. In the nineteenth century urban transportation was based on the horse; the result was that city streets were covered with manure that produced "pestilential vapours" and attracted huge numbers of insects. Streets literally turned into cesspools when it rained. The paving of streets only exacerbated the problem, since the manure was ground into fine dust by wheels. Municipal codes, moreover, were silent on housing standards, and many buildings were constructed without regard to the health of inhabitants. No provisions were made for drainage or ventilation in most buildings. The accumulation of organic wastes on adjacent streets and their rising odors caused inhabitants to keep windows perpetually shut, preventing the circulation of fresh air indoors and facilitating the dissemination of infectious organisms.[5]

John H. Griscom, a physician whose investigations of the urban poor led him to espouse a variety of public health reforms, provided graphic descriptions of sanitary and housing conditions among working-class and poor residents in New York City. "The tenements," he wrote in 1845,

> in order to admit a greater number of families, are divided into small apartments, as numerous as decency would admit . . . These closets, for they deserve no other name, are then rented to the poor

. . . however filthy the tenement may become, he [the landlord] cares
not, so that he receives his rent . . .

In these places, the filth is allowed to accumulate to an extent almost incredible . . .

Another very important particular in the arrangements of these
tenements . . . [is that] *ventilation is entirely prevented.*

But the most offensive of all places for residence are the *cellars* . . .
1st, the dampness, and 2d, the more incomplete ventilation . . . they
are very often so situated, that the surface water finds its way into
them at every rain storm.

These terrible living conditions, Griscom noted, led to "much sickness and many premature deaths"; one-fourth of those born died before their fifth birthday, and one-half before their twentieth. Responsibility for the dismal housing conditions, he wrote a few years later,
lay with "those who build and own the tenements of the poor," and
he called for the enactment of laws that would protect the health of
New York's inhabitants.[6]

Although New York City grew rapidly in succeeding decades,
housing conditions failed to improve. Two decades after Griscom's
report, a committee of the Citizens' Association of New York described housing conditions in much the same terms. "It is true that
the tenant-houses of New York are rapidly becoming the nests of fever infection, and the poisoned abodes of physical decay. It is true
that in the tenant-house districts a worse than Spartan fate awaits all
children, and that cholera infantum, convulsions, scrofula, and
marasmus hover with ghoul-like fiendishness about the dismal and
crowded tenant-homes." The committee quoted with obvious ap-
proval a journalist who noted that the draft riots in the summer of
1863 originated in an area that could be described as *"hives of sickness and vice."*[7]

New York may have been the nation's largest city, but sanitary conditions there did not appreciably differ from those in other urban areas. Lemuel Shattuck's famous report to the legislature of Massachusetts in 1850 described similar conditions in Boston. Data from other
cities indicated much the same state of affairs. The location of Chicago, for example, created a variety of unanticipated problems. Sewage was disposed of in Lake Michigan, a body of water that lacked
currents. This practice often polluted water drawn from the lake for

domestic use, thus leading to epidemics of such water-borne diseases as typhoid and cholera. The land on which the city was built was flat, and inadequate drainage patterns created ideal breeding conditions for insects. From 1852 to 1859 the average annual death rate from malaria was 5.1 per 1,000, and the morbidity rate was probably far higher. Although data on infant and child mortality are not available, most contemporary observers agreed that their rates were excessively high.[8]

Large urban areas serving as centers of trade and commerce were magnets for rural residents as well as for European immigrants. The movement of large masses of people into urban environments magnified health-related problems. Rural migration had the unforeseen consequence of bringing into the city a steady supply of susceptible persons who had never before been exposed to many infectious diseases. Crowded housing, contaminated water supplies, and unhygienic conditions combined to facilitate the spread of infectious diseases.

▼   ▼   ▼

The expansion of foreign and domestic commerce that accompanied urban growth made possible the introduction of many different pathogens. The appearance of yellow fever in Philadelphia in 1793 was one such example. At the time the city had slightly over 51,000 residents, of whom 94 percent were white. The epidemic began in the summer and lasted until autumn. The virus was probably imported from Santo Domingo, which was then experiencing a slave rebellion. Perhaps 2,000 refugees came to Philadelphia from that strife-torn island, some of whom had yellow fever. A hot and humid summer provided ideal conditions for the proliferation of the mosquito population, and by August the city faced an epidemic of catastrophic proportions. "It was indeed melancholy," one resident subsequently recalled, "to walk the streets, which were completely deserted, except by carts having bells attached to the horses' heads, on hearing which the dead bodies were put outside on the pavements and placed in the carts by the negroes, who conveyed their charge to the first grave yard, when they returned for another load."[9]

A significant percentage of the population—perhaps half—fled during the outbreak. Of those that remained, between 9 and 12 percent perished. Adults had much higher death rates than children, African Americans much lower rates. Poor people were at greater risk of dying, but only because they lacked the resources to flee. The disease took its greatest toll in areas adjacent to the wharves; it diminished considerably in outlying areas and never extended beyond the city's boundaries. Although the epidemic had few lasting effects, it symbolized the vulnerability of densely populated urban communities.[10]

Yellow fever epidemics arose where certain conditions prevailed: the presence of the virus, the insect vector, a sufficiently large number of infected and vulnerable people, and a warm and moist climate. All these elements were present in American port communities with commercial links to regions of the world where yellow fever was endemic. The disease first appeared in the colonies in the 1690s and peaked in the middle of the eighteenth century. It disappeared until the 1790s. From 1793 to 1822 it was present in such cities as Boston, New York, Philadelphia, and Baltimore. The absence of a native *Aedes* mosquito population and a cooler climate, however, ultimately defeated the disease, and yellow fever did not reappear in the Middle Atlantic and New England states after 1822.

The environment in the South, on the other hand, presented fewer barriers to yellow fever. The region had an indigenous *Aedes* population, a semitropical climate, and large urban areas with appropriate breeding places for the insect vector. The appearance of a single case of the disease was capable of launching an epidemic. During the nineteenth century yellow fever recurred regularly in the South. Its visibility, irregular and unpredictable appearance, and occasionally destructive nature made it one of the most feared diseases even though its contribution to total mortality was relatively minor. Moreover, yellow fever epidemics had profound immediate consequences: commerce came to a halt, contacts with the interior were interrupted, and death rates rose precipitously.[11]

With the exception of Charleston, the South had no urban areas with large populations before 1800. Even New Orleans, destined to become a leading urban center, had fewer than 10,000 residents in 1800. After that date, however, the city grew rapidly and became a major commercial and trading center. It also attracted migrants from rural areas and Europe, as well as French refugees from the West Indies. By 1820 its population exceeded 27,000, and within two decades had quadrupled. Given population density, a warm and humid

climate, the accumulation of organic wastes, an abundance of breeding sites for mosquitoes, and perennial flooding, it was not surprising
that yellow fever flourished and appeared regularly. Just before the
Louisiana Purchase, a French visitor described the city in graphic
terms. "Nothing equals the filthiness of New Orleans," wrote Perrin
du Lac, "unless it be the unhealthfulness which has for some years
appeared to have resulted from it. The city, the filth of which cannot
be drained off, is not paved . . . Its markets which are unventilated are
reeking with rottenness . . . Its squares are covered with the filth of
animals which no one takes the trouble to remove. Consequently
there is seldom a year that the yellow fever or some other contagious
malady does not carry off many strangers."[12]

Between 1804 and 1819 New Orleans had five serious yellow fever
epidemics. But by midcentury the disease began to intensify; from
1848 to 1852 the average number of deaths each year from yellow fever was about 442. The epidemic of 1853, however, was unprecedented in scope and virulence. During the epidemic perhaps 30,000
to 75,000 of the more than 150,000 residents fled the area. Of the remainder, approximately 40,000 developed yellow fever. In a five-
month period, 9,000 of the 11,000 deaths were attributed to the disease, and the disposal of bodies became one of the most serious problems. "At the gates," the *Daily Crescent* reported, "the winds
brought intimation of the corruption working within. Not a puff was
laden with the rank atmosphere from rotting corpses. Inside they
were piled by fifties, exposed to the heat of the sun, swollen with corruption, bursting their coffin lids . . . What a feast of horrors!"[13]

More than two-thirds of the deaths were among white males between the ages of 20 and 39. While mortality among whites was 63
per 1,000, the comparable figure for blacks was only 1.4. Newcomers
had the highest death rates, undoubtedly because they came from areas in which yellow fever was absent, and hence were more susceptible than any other group. The epidemic spread to adjacent towns as
well as into interior regions. Major outbreaks followed in 1854,
1855, and 1858, although none proved as virulent.[14]

During the first six decades of the nineteenth century New Orleans
and yellow fever were inextricably linked. Nearly 58 percent of the
recorded deaths from the disease in the United States during these decades occurred in that city. Nevertheless, New Orleans was not the
only southern city to be ravaged. Other southern port communities,

particularly those on the Gulf coast, also faced periodic epidemics. Indeed, the extension of railroads and the development of faster steamboats after the Civil War, accompanied by the gradual spread of the *Aedes aegypti*, set the stage for the appearance of the disease in hitherto untouched areas. In 1878 yellow fever was carried up the Tennessee, Ohio, and Mississippi Rivers, eventually reaching St. Louis. About 10 percent of the population of Memphis (more than 5,000 people) died from the disease in that year.[15]

Climatic and environmental conditions inhibited the spread of the yellow fever virus and insect vector and limited the disease to specific geographic regions. Not all infectious diseases, however, were as sensitive to temperature and humidity, nor did their dissemination require an intermediate vector. The expansion of trade and commerce in the nineteenth century and development of ships that dramatically reducing sailing time between continents made possible the migration of pathogens that found environments conducive to their replication.

Cholera is one such disease that traveled from afar to American shores. The acute infection of the small intestine caused by the presence of the *Vibrio cholerae* results in an often fatal diarrhea. In severe cases the total number of stools in a twenty-four hour period can range as high as twenty to thirty. The organism, which replicates itself with astonishing rapidity in the small intestine, produces a toxin that inhibits the absorption of water and minerals and leads to extreme diarrhea. Untreated cholera can result in circulatory collapse and cyanosis, since the fluid is drawn from the blood, which consequently thickens. In addition to becoming dehydrated, infected persons are demineralized and dealkalinized. Mortality in adults can exceed 50 percent, and children and aged persons are at even greater risk of dying.[16]

Whether cholera is a relatively recent disease or an ancient one is a question that cannot be answered with any degree of certainty. The survival of the *Vibrio cholerae* in estuarine waters depends on the interplay of several variables, including temperature and alkalinity, salt content, the presence of organic matter, and the degree of bacterial contamination. No animal or human host is required. The organism appears to have been confined to the Ganges Delta in India, whose ecology provided an ideal environment. Though probably of ancient lineage, the disease may only have assumed a virulent character after the *Vibrio cholerae* underwent a genetic change that resulted in the production of a toxin that permitted rapid replication of the organism in the small intestine while inhibiting the growth of the normal enteric flora.[17] Cholera is transmitted by water contaminated by the feces of infected persons or by soiled bedding and clothing. It is not, however, passed directly from human to human.[18]

Cholera first appeared in pandemic form in Jessore, near Calcutta, in 1817. It spread rapidly eastward through China and Japan and as far west as the Syrian border, but did not reach Europe or the United States. More than a decade passed before a second pandemic appeared. By 1830 cholera was present in Moscow and then spread to central and western Europe. In the autumn of 1831 it appeared in England, and the following year arrived in Canada and in the United States. In 1849 and 1866 the United States also experienced cholera epidemics. Although each epidemic manifested distinctive characteristics, it is clear that emerging transportation systems—international, coastal, and internal—population mobility, and the rise of urban centers played crucial roles in the dissemination of the disease throughout the nation. The disease reappeared in 1873, but was neither as widespread nor as virulent as its three predecessors.[19]

The first epidemic appeared in Canada and spread from the St. Lawrence River to Lake Champlain. Once it reached New York City in the spring of 1832, it was dispersed to the west via the Erie Canal and the south via land and sea. Although urban areas provided ideal conditions for the rapid spread of the disease, small towns and villages on trade routes were not exempt. Cholera reached western regions by the Cumberland Road, which connected the East with western rivers. In most areas the pathogen was disseminated by the oral-fecal route. By the time the epidemic had run its course, between 50,000 and 150,000 people had died, though the number infected was far larger. The epidemics of 1849 and 1866 were less devastating; total mortality for the former was in the 100,000 range, and 50,000 for the latter.[20] Curiously enough, cholera was present from 1849 through 1854, but remained localized and did not contribute to overall mortality.

The distribution of fatalities within urban areas varied widely. The Five Points district in Manhattan, for example, had the highest case rate. It was among the most densely populated, impoverished, and unsanitary areas in New York City, thus rendering its residents extraordinarily vulnerable to a pathogen transmitted by contaminated water. The Five Points, according to the *Evening Post,* "are inhabited by a race of beings of all colours, ages, sexes, and nations, though generally of but one condition, and that . . . almost of the vilest brute. With such a crew, inhabiting the most populous and central portion of the city, when may we be considered secure from pestilence. Be the air pure from Heaven, their breath would contaminate it, and infect it with disease." Indeed, the death rate in this locale in nonepidemic years was three times the city's average. During the cholera epidemics Five Points residents had much higher mortality rates than those in other districts.[21]

New York was by no means unique. In Buffalo the epidemic of 1849 took a disproportionate toll among poor immigrants. The Irish suffered the most. Constituting less than a quarter of the city's population, they accounted for 42 percent of the cholera fatalities of known ethnic identity. The Germans—the city's largest immigrant group—accounted for 50 percent of the deaths. Deaths among native-born persons, on the other hand, were only 3 percent of the total. The disparity in mortality was a reflection of living conditions. The Irish and the Germans were concentrated in shanties and densely populated boardinghouses adjacent to the waterfront. Garbage and debris littered the streets, and dogs and pigs provided the major means of waste disposal. In hot and humid weather the odors emanating from privies and outhouses were overpowering, and these receptacles often overflowed during heavy rains. Water was drawn from adjacent shallow wells that were easily contaminated. In more affluent districts there were relatively few fatalities. These districts were generally located on higher ground some distance from the waterfront; population density was much lower; there was more open land; and its residents had fewer contacts with impoverished immigrant neighborhoods. Under such circumstances the risk of polluting wells from surface drainage was far less, and its inhabitants were generally able to avoid infection.[22]

After 1873 cholera no longer posed a threat to American society. Its disappearance was due neither to changes in virulence nor to personal behavior, but rather to a greater understanding of the means of transmission. In 1849 Dr. John Snow, a prominent London physician, published a brief pamphlet dealing with the spread of cholera. He suggested that the cholera poison was of a particulate character that reproduced itself in the alimentary tract. This poison was released in feces, which in turn contaminated the water supply and resulted in widespread epidemics. Five years later Snow provided empirical data that supported his earlier intuitive findings. He demonstrated that the incidence of cholera was far greater in an area of London served by a water company that drew its supply from the lower Thames, whereas the area served by another company that drew its water from the upper Thames had a far lower incidence. The former was contaminated by the discharge of sewage; the latter remained relatively pure. "All of the instances of communication of cholera through the medium of water," Snow concluded,

> have resulted from the contamination of a pump-well, or some other limited supply of water; and the outbreaks of cholera connected with the contamination, though sudden and intense, have been limited also; but when the water of a river becomes infected with the cholera evacuations emptied from on board ship, or passing down drains and sewers, the communication of the disease, though generally less sudden and violent, is much more widely extended; more especially when the river water is distributed by the steam engine and pipes connected with water-works.[23]

Snow's epidemiological analysis laid the groundwork for preventive measures. He recommended frequent washing when around an infected person; the cleaning of soiled bedding and clothing; the closing of pumps from contaminated water supplies; boiling of food; isolation of cases; and, in the long run, ensuring that water supplies remained free from contamination from sewers, cesspools, house drains, and the refuse of those who navigated rivers. Snow's work quickly came to the attention of prominent sanitarians, including Max von Pettenkofer in Germany. A movement to expand governmental authority in matters relating to public health slowly gained strength as a result. By 1866 New York had created a Metropolitan Board of Health, which employed a variety of measures, including quarantine, to limit the spread of cholera. The introduction of such public health measures during these years played a significant role in substantially eliminating the threat posed by cholera.[24]

Yellow fever and cholera aroused terror among urban residents, largely because of their episodic character and that fact that large numbers of people died within a very brief time span. Moreover, during these epidemics the routines and rhythms of daily life often came to an abrupt halt. One of the most striking characteristics of these outbreaks was the visibility of the dead. Many communities were unable to bury victims quickly enough, and the presence of cadavers, particularly in the warmer months, sometimes constituted a serious health problem.

Yellow fever and cholera epidemics, however spectacular, were not unique; other epidemic diseases also took a toll among urban residents. The introduction of vaccination in the early nineteenth century, for example, appeared to reduce the threat from smallpox epidemics that had played such an important role in the colonial period. Public apathy, a failure to recognize the need for revaccination, and the large tide of migration from Europe, which augmented the pool of susceptibles, who often resisted vaccination because of their suspicion of governmental authority, all tended to facilitate periodic smallpox epidemics. New York City, for example, experienced nine epidemics between 1804 and 1865. Fatalities from this disease increased sharply after the 1830s, and by midcentury accounted for nearly 25 out of each 1,000 deaths. During the first half of the century Philadelphia had eight epidemics, Boston six, and Baltimore three. Smallpox mortality was overwhelmingly a function of age. In 1850 children between birth and age 10 accounted for slightly over 56 percent of all deaths from smallpox in Baltimore; males and blacks were at higher risk of dying than females and whites. High population density and the presence of a sufficient supply of susceptible individuals helped to sustain the disease in urban environments.[25]

As terrifying as these epidemics were, few had a major impact on population growth and overall mortality rates. The total number of deaths from yellow fever and cholera, however pronounced in specific years, was relatively unimportant in the aggregate. Between 1800 and 1859 yellow fever resulted in perhaps 55,000 fatalities, or an average of slightly more than 900 a year. The three cholera epidemics between 1833 and 1866 accounted for 200,000 to 300,000 deaths, or an average of 5,900 to 8,800 per year. Similarly, smallpox, even though creating mortality spikes in epidemic years, contributed relatively little to overall mortality. Much the same was true of other minor outbreaks of epidemic diseases in specific years. In sum, epidemic diseases, however spectacular and feared, were not a major influence on aggregate morbidity or mortality.[26] Other forms of disease posed far greater dangers.

▼ ▼ ▼

The greatest threats to life in urban America during the first half of the nineteenth century were endemic infectious diseases that flourished in densely populated and unhygienic environments. Tuberculosis was among the more significant. An infectious disease caused by the *Mycobacterium tuberculosis,* it is particularly responsive to environmental cofactors, including crowded living and working conditions. With the exception of the bovine form, the bacillus is transmitted overwhelmingly by droplet infection. Upon entering the human body, the organism can lie dormant for long periods and then emerge in virulent form when host resistance is impaired. Although lungs are the most frequently infected organs, tuberculosis can infect any part of the body. Its course is irregular and unpredictable; episodic attacks can alternate with periodic remissions. Those in the active stage deteriorate slowly, and the process of dying can span months or years.

The wasting nature of the disease spawned a romantic literature in both the United States and Europe that associated it with genius and conferred upon its victims, often women, attributes of sensitivity and physical charm. To William Cullen Bryant the death of a beautiful young woman was a poetic theme that deserved to be celebrated.

> We wept that one so lovely should have a life so brief,
> Yet not unmeet it was that one, like that young friend of ours,
> So gentle and so beautiful, should perish with the flowers.[27]

The reality of tuberculosis, however, was a quite different matter. After four pregnancies that left her enervated, Harriet Webster Fowler—the daughter of the famous lexicographer Noah Webster—developed symptoms consistent with tuberculosis. In 1839 she had her first hemorrhage. "I began to cough," she wrote to her sister, "and the first mouthful I knew from the look and feeling was blood . . . I concluded to lay still and try what perfect quiet could do—swallowed two mouthfuls of blood and became convinced that if I could keep from further coughing I should be able to wait till morning without disturbing anyone. As soon as morning arrived, I looked at the contents of my cup. Alas my fears were realized." Fearing that she would suffer an early death, Harriet responded with stoicism. "I try to cultivate a cheerful spirit, to subdue every internal discontent and my prayer is *Thy will be done.*" For the next five years she continued to deteriorate, became invalided, and finally died in 1844.[28]

Tuberculosis was and is a disease of civilization. It has waxed and waned over the centuries. Possessing some features common to epidemic diseases, it manifested itself in slow-moving cycles. It peaked in England about 1650, declined until 1715, and surged to even higher peaks in the eighteenth and early nineteenth centuries. The greatest concentration of cases was found in densely populated cities such as London, where the disease at its height accounted for as much as 30 percent of total mortality. Indeed, in the nineteenth century tuberculosis became known as the "Great White Plague" and appeared to some to threaten the very survival of Western civilization.[29]

Data dealing with the incidence and prevalence of tuberculosis, however, are notoriously unreliable. In the nineteenth century the ability to differentiate between pulmonary diseases was highly problematic. Diagnoses were based on external signs and symptoms. Under these conditions there is little doubt that the categories then employed—pulmonary consumption and phthisis—included a variety of pulmonary and respiratory disorders. Nevertheless, it is clear that tuberculosis, whatever the precise data, accounted for large numbers of deaths.

In the United States the incidence of tuberculosis increased in the eighteenth century. High housing density, a susceptible population, and the migration of infected individuals from England facilitated the spread of the disease in both rural and urban areas. By the beginning of the nineteenth century tuberculosis reached its first peak, particularly in urban areas along the Atlantic seaboard. In New York City perhaps 23 percent of all deaths in 1804 were due to tuberculosis and other pulmonary disorders. Indeed, tuberculosis was one of the leading causes of death in the city in the nineteenth century.[30]

Data from other urban communities suggest a similar pattern. Nearly a quarter of all deaths in Boston between 1812 and 1821 were due to "consumption." Mortality from this disease peaked at the beginning of the nineteenth century, declined somewhat until the 1840s, and then increased until the 1860s. In his famous study of the sanitary condition of Massachusetts in 1850, Lemuel Shattuck noted that consumption accounted for one-seventh to one-fourth of all deaths. He also found that between 1820 and 1840 deaths from this disease declined, but increased thereafter. Comparable Baltimore data suggested a similar pattern; from 1812 to 1815 the death rate was 5.3

per 1,000; from 1836 to 1840 it had declined to 3.9; and from 1851 to 1855 surged to 4.7.[31]

Tuberculosis did not strike all segments of the population equally. African Americans in Baltimore in 1850 had higher death rates than whites (4.7 versus 3.2 per 1,000). The same was true in New York City. White mortality from the disease ranged from a high of 5.4 per 1,000 in 1836 to a low of 3.3 in 1859; the comparable figures for African Americans were 9.5 and 11.2, respectively. Although no data exist for the foreign-born before 1844 in New York, their death rates tended to fall midway between those for whites and African Americans. In Baltimore there were also few gender differences in mortality up to the age of 15; the risk of dying among this group was relatively low. After 15, however, the death rate rose precipitously; female mortality was nearly double that of males. The variability between urban areas and between regions, however, makes it difficult to provide firm generalizations about the United States as a whole. Shattuck, for example, found death rates in Massachusetts for females higher than for males aged 20 to 30 but then tended to become more equal. In New York and London, by contrast, males were at greater risk of dying of tuberculosis, and in Philadelphia rates were the same for both. Nor was tuberculosis a strictly urban disease; it was prevalent in rural areas as well.[32]

There is general agreement that the incidence and prevalence of tuberculosis and other pulmonary disorders are influenced by population density, nutrition, and occupation; a synergistic relationship between these variables may exist. Of the three, however, population density—and particularly housing—may well have played the most important role. Nineteenth-century tenements were constructed without regard to ventilation, and this fact had dire consequences for their residents. Moreover, as increasingly more impoverished immigrants arrived in the United States during the 1830s and 1840s, they tended to congregate in large numbers in confined dwellings. In Boston, for example, structures were remodeled to accommodate as many inhabitants as possible. In 1800 the average dwelling held 8.3 persons; by 1845 the figure was 10.6. A municipal committee concerned with health provided a dramatic description of housing conditions among the Irish in 1849.

> In such a state of things, there can be no cleanliness, privacy, or proper ventilation . . . and, with the ignorance, carelessness, and

generally loose and dirty habits which prevail among the occupants, the necessary evils are greatly increased both in amount and intensity. In Broad Street and all the surrounding neighborhood . . . the situation of the Irish . . . is particularly wretched . . . This whole district is a perfect hive of human beings, without comforts and mostly without common necessaries; in many cases, huddled together like brutes, without regard to sex, or age, or sense of decency; grown men and women sleeping together in the same apartment, and sometimes wife and husband, brothers and sisters, in the same bed. Under such circumstances, self-respect, forethought, all high and noble virtues soon die out, and sullen indifference and despair, or disorder, intemperance and utter degradation reign supreme.

The nativist sentiments of the committee members notwithstanding, it is quite evident from their description that crowding, lack of ventilation, and a generally unhealthful environment were characteristic of tenement housing and, as such, played a central role in the rising incidence of tuberculosis and other pulmonary disorders by mid-century.[33]

The part played by diet in tuberculosis morbidity and mortality is less clear. Protein deficiency can increase vulnerability to tuberculosis as well as to other infectious diseases. There is little evidence, however, to suggest that severe malnutrition was common during the first half of the nineteenth century, even among the urban poor. Indeed, the experience of Shaker communities indicates that crowding rather than diet was the key variable. Dedicated to prayer, celibacy, and pacifism, the Shakers by 1850 maintained twenty-one communities with 3,842 members. Despite residing in rural areas amid salubrious surroundings, they nevertheless had sharply elevated mortality rates from consumption between 1830 and 1870. The death rate from this disease in three Massachusetts Shaker communities was far higher than for the state as a whole. Shaker youths died at a much higher rate from consumption than did non-Shakers; Shaker women, like females in Boston, had higher death rates than men. The care provided for the sick was no different from the care provided by non-Shakers, nor were diets lacking in protein. Shakers, however, did tend to spend much of their time in communal activities in crowded quarters, thus creating optimum conditions for the spread of the pathogens responsible for tuberculosis and other pulmonary disorders.[34]

Mortality among prison populations in the 1830s and 1840s offers further evidence that crowding was probably a key variable. White prisoners during these decades had a mortality rate more than twice that of residents in seaboard urban areas. African Americans at the Eastern State Penitentiary in Pennsylvania were even more disadvantaged; they died at nearly four times the rate of white prisoners. Crowded prison quarters facilitated the spread of tuberculosis and other pulmonary diseases.[35]

Conditions of urban life during the first half of the nineteenth century were also conducive to the emergence of such infectious diseases as typhus. Known by a variety of names (e.g., jail fever, war fever, camp fever, or ship fever), typhus flourished amidst crowding and unhygienic conditions. Like viruses, the causative organism, *Rickettsia prowazekii,* requires living cells for growth. It is transmitted to humans by a body louse, which thrives when facilities to wash clothes and bathe are absent. Epidemic typhus is accompanied by high fever and a rash. Mortality rises with age and can reach 50 percent or more in adult populations.

In Europe typhus was especially prevalent in the military and in jails.[36] It was occasionally brought to the colonies in the eighteenth century by immigrants on crowded vessels, and was present in the military during the American Revolution. Epidemic typhus, however, did not become important until the mid-nineteenth century, when a combination of large-scale immigration and the rise of tenement housing provided ideal conditions for the disease to flourish. The relationship between crowding, housing conditions, poverty, and typhus was well known in the nineteenth century even though the etiology of the disease remained a mystery. Typhus was found largely in crowded urban tenements with large immigrant populations; it was generally not prevalent in less densely populated and more affluent districts, nor was it found in the Midwest or in rural areas. "In certain portions of the city," a New York City citizens' group reported in 1866,

> there exists an almost universal neglect of Sanitary regulations; the streets, courts, and alleys generally filthy, the gutters obstructed, the house-drainage defective, and the sewerage faulty; while in the tenant-houses of such localities are found numerous cases of typhus, small-pox, and all varieties of pulmonary and infantile maladies,

which can be perpetuated and rendered fatal by overcrowding, domestic uncleanliness, and lack of ventilation.

Typhus outbreaks often followed the migration of large numbers of persons from Ireland, which at that time was ravaged by famine and disease. The housing and environment of impoverished Irish immigrants in eastern seaboard cities provided optimum conditions for the pathogen and louse vector.[37]

Urban environments during the first half of the nineteenth century were also conducive to the spread of a variety of other infectious diseases. In addition to tuberculosis and pulmonary disorders (the largest single greatest causes of mortality among adults), pneumonia, diphtheria and croup, measles, whooping cough, and scarlet fever all added to the health burden of residents. Similarly, pregnant women were at risk from complications during delivery as well as from puerperal fever (a consuming septicemia). Diarrheal diseases took the greatest toll among infants and young children. From 1840 to 1845 the death rate from this category in New York City was 25.1 per 1,000 (as compared to 47.3 for consumption). With the exception of pneumonia, no other disease had a mortality rate that exceeded 5 per 1,000.[38]

Intestinal disorders, of course, can be caused by a variety of pathogens. In the nineteenth century they encompassed such diagnoses as cholera infantum, diarrhea, dysentery, and teething. The terminology of this era reflected an inability to distinguish between etiology and symptomatology. Lacking bacteriological tools, the authors of medical classification systems relied largely on descriptive categories. Such descriptions were by no means lacking in sophistication, but they did preclude the collection of data by etiological categories. The heterogeneous diagnoses of intestinal disorders during these decades, nevertheless, had several features in common: frequent and watery stools, general prostration, and rapid weight loss. Whatever the specific etiology, the typical mode of communication was by water or food that had been contaminated by inappropriate hygiene, spoilage, as well as bacterial transmission from feces by flies. The circumstances of urban life—crowding and inadequate sanitation—that led to high mortality from other infectious diseases played an equally significant role in enteric disorders. The storage and preparation of food in such environments posed serious problems. Given that the risks of severe dehydration were not clearly understood, it was inevitable that intestinal disorders would take a high toll.

Morbidity and mortality data for enteric disorders in the nineteenth century are fragmentary and confused. They suggest, however, that mortality varied sharply over time. Baltimore data, for example, reveal that cholera infantum, or "summer complaint" (generally understood as diarrhea in those under the age of 2), had very high death rates between 1818 and 1823, declined until 1827, peaked between 1828 and 1832, and fell to a low point in 1835. Rates remained low for nearly a decade but rose sharply from 1846 to 1856. During these years the rate per 1,000 ranged from a high of 43.9 to a low of 9.3. Diarrhea (a diagnosis generally used for adults and older children) showed similar peaks and valleys. Although satisfactory explanations for the changes in mortality over time are lacking, there is little doubt that intestinal disorders were a significant element in overall mortality.[39]

To demonstrate that infectious diseases were the major element in urban morbidity and mortality patterns is not to suggest that other disorders were absent. Chronic degenerative and long-duration diseases were present, including cancers, cardiovascular and renal diseases, and diseases of the central nervous system. Their incidence and prevalence, however, were low, if only because high mortality rates among the young meant that the older cohort constituted a relatively small percentage of the total population. Tumors (malignant and benign) did not play a significant role in Baltimore mortality before 1870, even when we allow for the unreliability of cancer mortality data. A similar pattern prevailed for diseases of the cardiovascular, renal, and central nervous systems. Only when infant and child mortality rates fell and more people survived to adulthood did chronic degenerative diseases emerge as significant factors in mortality.[40]

Urban mortality rates did not reflect only the paramount influence of infectious diseases; other contributory elements—suicide, homicide, accidents, and occupational diseases—also had an effect. Accidents, for example, played a relatively small role in mortality, but a larger role in the prevalence of chronic disabilities. The domestic technology of heating, lighting, and cooking in this period introduced new risks, and death or disability followed burns and scalding. The same was true for the development of urban transportation systems, which led to new categories of accidents. Though statistically the least important form of violent death, homicide was higher in mid-nineteenth-century than twentieth-century cities; the practice of carrying handguns contributed to the violent nature of urban life.[41]

No doubt a wide variety of chronic disorders and conditions were present that did not, at least directly, contribute to mortality but nevertheless affected the quality of life. Chronic infections, sexually transmitted diseases, physical deformities, to cite only a few categories, added to the health burden of urban populations. Finally, serious and chronic mental illnesses, though not unique to cities, created problems within households. Aside from behavioral disruptions that could threaten the integrity of the family, seriously and chronically mentally ill persons were often reduced to a state of dependency because of their inability to function or to work. A pioneering census of the insane in Massachusetts in 1854 by Edward Jarvis determined that there were at least 2,632 "lunatics" (as well as 1,087 "idiots") in a state with a total population of about 1,124,676. Of the severely mentally ill, 1,284 were at home or in public poorhouses, 1,141 were in mental hospitals, and 207 were other penal and welfare institutions. The pervasiveness of mental disorders in both urban and rural areas led to the creation of a large-scale system of public state and urban hospitals to provide care for this dependent population.[42]

▼ ▼ ▼

The burden of disease had profound consequences for urban populations during the first half of the nineteenth century. Infants and children were by far the most vulnerable group. Indeed, sanitarians dedicated to environmental reform claimed that infant and child mortality was rising during the first half of the nineteenth century. They also asserted that rates among the immigrant poor were three to four times higher than among the native population. Accurate data are unavailable to verify such claims. The improvement in death registration systems during the nineteenth century resulted in larger numbers of recorded deaths, thus rendering comparisons with earlier periods problematic. Yet there is little doubt that infancy and childhood in urban areas constituted the most dangerous years. Nor did class necessarily confer greater immunity from the dangers posed by acute contagious diseases. In Providence, Rhode Island, taxpayers enjoyed only a slight advantage over nontaxpayers; the death rate in

1865 from these diseases among the former was 33.5, and 39.5 among the latter.[43]

Data from pre–Civil War cities demonstrate the vulnerability of infants and young children. In Baltimore, for example, 1,974 deaths were recorded in 1830. Of these, 406 were under the age of 1 and 932 under 10. Three decades later the proportion remained similar. Of 4,866 deaths, 1,227 were infants and 2,616 under 10. In 1850 the death rate among infants was 167 per 1,000; a decade later it had risen to 188. Although the death rate fluctuated from year to year, the trend in pre–Civil War Baltimore was upward. Mortality, however, was not equally distributed among all groups. African-American infants and children were far more vulnerable than their white counterparts. The annual fluctuations in mortality among both groups were similar, but the rates for the former were consistently higher.[44]

Data from other urban areas, including Boston and New York City, exhibited somewhat similar characteristics; infancy remained the most dangerous stage of life. Young children had lower death rates, although by modern standards they were extraordinarily high. In New York City mortality for children between birth and 5 years between 1804 and 1865 ranged from 55 to 166.[45] The causes of death among infants and young children were also quite different. Infant mortality generally peaked in the summer and was generally caused by enteric diseases. Young children, by contrast, died throughout the year; the causes of death were far more varied.

Class also played a role in infant and child mortality patterns (although the absence of precise data renders broad generalizations problematic). In a study of Providence, Rhode Island, Charles V. Chapin—a major figure in public health at the turn of the twentieth century—linked the census and the income tax list for 1865. In a population of 54,595, there were 10,515 taxpayers and 44,080 nontaxpayers. Among the former (clearly the most affluent in the city) the infant death rate was 93.4 per 1,000; among the latter the rate was 189.8. The differential narrowed in the 1-to-4 age group; the figures were 40.3 and 66.6, respectively. For reasons that are not entirely clear, the mortality difference in the 5-to-9 age group virtually disappeared. Chapin noted that the city had no municipal water supply. Fecal contamination of water was therefore far greater among nontaxpayers, thus leading to a higher prevalence of diarrheal diseases, which had the greatest impact upon the very young. Overall the mortality rate among taxpayers was less than half that among taxpayers. Conceding that his was only a community study, Chapin suggested the need for "a study of the habits of life and of the environment which make for the longevity of the well-to-do."[46]

High infant mortality rates in urban areas might have been due to low birthweight (currently defined as newborns who weigh less than 5.5 pounds), which may account for as much as 90 percent of variance in the risk of perinatal mortality. Low birthweight is generally attributed to a variety of factors: genetic, gestational age, maternal health status, maternal behavioral patterns, class and status, and nutrition.[47] Yet there is little evidence to suggest that high infant mortality rates were related to low birthweight or inadequate maternal nutritional levels. At Philadelphia's Almshouse Hospital, for example, the nutritional status of infants—all of whom came from poor mothers—was surprisingly good. Average birthweights at the almshouse between 1848 and 1873 averaged 7 to 7.8 pounds; only 8.1 percent of the live births were less than 5.5 pounds. The mean birthweight at Boston's Lying-In Hospital in the late 1840s was just under 7.4 pounds; Boston data from three hospitals in the 1870s suggest a similar pattern. Indeed, the American diet, though unbalanced in some respects, was more than adequate and did not play a significant role in infant mortality.[48]

High death rates among infants were due neither to inadequate maternal nutrition nor to parental shortcomings or neglect. The fact of the matter is that there was little understanding that mortality from enteric disorders could be limited by preventive measures to minimize contamination of water, milk, and food and to ensure rehydration during acute episodes. This is not to insist that other elements associated with urban environments did not play a role. It is merely to assert that crowding, lack of sanitation, and poverty—all of which undoubtedly facilitated the transmission of infectious diseases—were less important than prevailing systems of infant care. Many infants perished because parents lacked the knowledge to deal effectively with intestinal disorders.

Infants and children raised in urban environments were also at greater risk of dying than their small-town and rural counterparts. Massachusetts towns with 10,000 or more had the lowest expectation of life in 1860. Expectation of life in infancy was 46.4 years for males and 47.3 for females for the state as a whole. The comparable rates for those living in towns of 10,000 or more was 37.2 and 41.0, respectively. These differences persisted throughout the age structure; urban residents always lagged behind those living in rural areas and small towns. The divergences were even more pronounced in larger urban areas.[49]

To be sure, urban mortality fluctuated from year to year. In general, however, mortality rates tended to rise, albeit unevenly, during the first two-thirds of the nineteenth century. Nor were the experiences of cities identical; some were safer than others. In New York City, for example, mortality rose from 28.1 per 1,000 in 1804—1809 to 40.7 in 1850–1854, and then receded slightly. New Orleans experienced the greatest fluctuations; rarely did its mortality drop as low as 40 per 1,000. Mortality levels in Boston, Baltimore, and Philadelphia, by contrast, did not for the most part reach the peaks attained in New York and New Orleans even though their rates were higher than those in small communities and rural areas. The differences between cities may very well have reflected varying circumstances. Climate was not the key variable, if only because Philadelphia and Baltimore are further south than New York City. Two elements may have shaped the mortality environments of New York and New Orleans. Both cities grew at a much more rapid rate than the other three, thus exacerbating those features of urban life that increased health risks. Moreover, New York and New Orleans were gateways to the interior; their ports received more transients and ships from other regions of the world, which made it difficult to prevent the entry of infectious diseases. The combination of these factors undoubtedly exacerbated their already harsh disease environment.[50]

In general, mortality rates rose in the antebellum decades and life expectation—even among adults—declined. One scholar has estimated that male expectation of life at age 20 fell from 46.4 in 1800–1809 to 40.8 in 1850–1859; the comparable figures for women were 47.9 and 39.5, respectively. Ironically, when mortality rates began to decline toward the end of the nineteenth century and more people survived, long-duration sicknesses—which are associated with aging—began to become more prevalent as the share of older people increased.[51]

Cities may have played a crucial role in creating the foundation of an urban industrial society that by the end of the nineteenth century

had made the United States a world power. Yet urban life, at least in
the formative stages, increased health risks. From the founding of
New York City in the early seventeenth century through the Civil
War, wrote Stephen Smith in somewhat hyperbolic terms, its residents were constantly confronted with an environment that threatened their very lives.

> The land was practically undrained; the drinking water was from
> shallow wells, befouled by street, stable, privy, and other filth; there
> were no adequate sewers to remove the accumulating waste; the
> streets were the receptacles of garbage; offensive trades were located
> among the dwellings; the natural water courses and springs were
> obstructed in the construction of streets and dwellings, thus causing
> soakage of large areas of land, and stagnant pools of polluted water.
>
> Later, in these centuries of neglect of sanitary precautions, came
> the immigrants from every nation of the world, representing for the
> most part the poorest and most ignorant class of their respective na-
> tionalities. This influx of people led to the construction of the tene-
> ment house by landowners, whose aim was to build so as to incur
> the least possible expense and accommodate the greatest possible
> number. In dark, unventilated, uninhabitable structures these
> wretched, persecuted people were herded together, in cellars and
> garrets, as well as in the body of the building, until New York had
> the largest population to a square acre of any civilized city.
>
> The people had not only chosen to conserve all the natural condi-
> tions unfavorable to health, but had steadily added unhygienic fac-
> tors to their methods of developing the city.
>
> The result was inevitable. New York gradually became the natu-
> ral home of every variety of contagious disease, and the favorite
> resort of foreign pestilences.[52]

Smith's vivid description of New York may have reflected a desire
to justify his own commitment to the principles of sanitary reform.
Nevertheless, his observations of mid-nineteenth-century New York
City were by no means inaccurate. To be sure, each urban area manifested its own unique pattern; morbidity and mortality rates often
varied. The differences, however, could not conceal the risks faced by
their inhabitants. Decades would pass before public and private actions would begin to reduce the dangers to health posed by urban life.

CHAPTER 6

Expanding America,
Declining Health

In his novel *Pierre,* published in 1852, Herman Melville expressed a
sharp dislike of the city. Pierre, the main character, had fortunately
"been born and bred in the country," untouched "by the dirty un-
washed face perpetually worn by the town." When Pierre arrived in
New York, he found himself accidentally in a police station. The
sights and sounds he encountered "filled him with inexpressible hor-
ror and fury . . . The thieves'-quarters, and all the brothels, Lock-and-
Sin hospitals for incurables, and infirmaries and infernos of hell
seemed to have made one combined sortie, and poured out upon
earth through the vile vomitory of some unmentionable cellar." Melville's portrayal of the evil, dirty, and disease-ridden city stood in
sharp contrast to his idealization of a healthful and bucolic countryside.[1]

The faith that rural life was superior to urban life was in part a
reflection of demographics. For much of the nineteenth century the
United States remained a predominantly rural nation. In 1800 no less
than 94 percent of the nation's 5.3 million people lived in rural areas.
The steady growth of urban areas during the first half of the century
slowly redressed this imbalance; yet on the eve of the Civil War fully
80 percent of America's 31.4 million inhabitants still resided in rural
regions.

Rural residents, moreover, enjoyed somewhat better health than
their urban counterparts. Low population density tended to inhibit
the dissemination of many infectious pathogens. Indeed, rural Americans generally had a better chance of surviving to adulthood without

experiencing many infectious diseases that were so devastating to infants and children living in congested urban areas. Life expectancy at birth was correspondingly higher for rural inhabitants than for their urban brethren. Yet the benefits of residing outside cities were only relative. Morbidity and mortality rates, which had declined for part of the eighteenth century, resumed an upward march in the early nineteenth century and affected all segments of the population irrespective of residence.

The urban-rural dichotomy, as a matter of fact, was less of a sharp break and more of a continuum with gradations that diminished over time. The westward movement of people over the Appalachian Mountains after the War of 1812, for example, created novel risks largely unknown to urban residents. The long journey was arduous; families had to travel over difficult terrain, endure harsh climatic conditions, and live with a marginal food supply until they reached their final destination. Moreover, the areas into which they moved lacked the amenities of more mature communities. The process of migration and settlement, the adjustment to new surroundings, and the environmental transformation that followed often resulted in higher morbidity and mortality than were found in older rural areas. Ecological changes also created conditions that fostered the appearance of new diseases previously absent.

It is ironic that the material progress characteristic of nineteenth-century America failed to translate into better health. Life expectancy and physical stature declined for both urban and rural residents and did not begin to recover until the latter part of the century. The concurrence of increasing prosperity and declining health poses a fascinating problem, for it runs counter to the intuitive and widely held belief that a rising standard of living leads to the improvement of health. It poses a puzzling paradox about the relation of material conditions to health.

▼ ▼ ▼

At the beginning of the nineteenth century there was a pervasive belief that Americans enjoyed a privileged position insofar as health was concerned. The causes that inhibited the growth of population in other countries, according to Adam Seybert, "have been more limited in the United States." Most people were engaged in agriculture, which in turn supported commerce. "Few of our citizens," he added, "are concerned in unhealthy occupations; our towns and cities are not yet so large as to endanger the health of their inhabitants; fatal epidemics have not been very prevalent; property is much divided amongst the people, and a very moderate share of industry will enable every individual to gain his support."[2]

The nation's rural character and wealth seemed to confer advantages that led to less morbidity and longer life expectancy than in Europe. The health of residents of rural areas and small towns in the New England and Middle Atlantic states outwardly confirmed Seybert's observations. Many infectious diseases were less common in more sparsely populated regions. Rural areas had fewer difficulties in dealing with the disposal of organic wastes and assuring a supply of pure water, thus minimizing but not eliminating the threat of waterborne diseases.

The experiences of the middle Connecticut Valley in western Massachusetts were typical. In that rural area mortality was lower than in the eastern part of the state and in southern Connecticut (both of which had much larger concentrations of people). Infants and young children in particular had a distinct advantage, since such infectious diseases as diphtheria, measles, and smallpox were relatively rare. Periodic outbreaks of gastrointestinal disorders, which took their greatest toll among young children, were the major cause of mortality after consumption. Mortality rates in this rural region tended to rise during the first half of the nineteenth century, but they were lower relative to other, more heavily populated, areas of New England.[3]

The national pattern was quite similar. In 1830 mortality rates among the white population were lowest in rural areas, somewhat higher in small towns, and highest in large cities. For the nation as a whole about 54 percent of those alive at age 5 survived to 60. In rural areas the figure was 57.5 percent, as compared with 43.6 in such small towns as Salem and New Haven and 16.4 in the large cities of Boston, New York, and Philadelphia. Though seemingly excessive when compared with contemporary standards, Americans—irrespective of where they lived—enjoyed a considerable advantage over Europeans. Half of all Americans surviving to the age of 5 had perished by 63. Life tables from several European countries (though not for identical years) provide a stark contrast. In Sweden (1755–1763) and the Netherlands (1840–1851) half of those surviving to age 5 had died by 55, and in Russia (1874–1883) the age was 54.[4]

Place of residence, however, was by no means the sole determinant of health status; numerous other factors shaped morbidity and mortality patterns. Mid-nineteenth-century New York State child mortality data illustrate this point. As in western Massachusetts, New York infant and child mortality to age 5 was approximately 20 percent higher in urban than rural areas. The urban-rural differential, however, cannot be explained solely in terms of population density and lack of a sanitary environment, although both were of major significance. In urban areas, for example, the mortality rates for children of foreign-born mothers were 24 percent higher than for those of native-born mothers. Such a difference suggests that a variety of factors were at work. A higher proportion of foreign-born admittedly lived in less healthy urban areas; but economic disadvantages and higher fertility rates were also contributory factors in elevating child mortality among this group.[5]

▼   ▼   ▼

Appearances, however, can be deceiving. By the early nineteenth century—and particularly after the War of 1812—what had begun as a trickle soon became a torrent as migrants began the process of westward expansion that reshaped the nation in profound ways. Between 1800 and 1860 sixteen states (excluding Maine, which was originally part of Massachusetts) were admitted into the Union. By 1860 their combined population was slightly over 13 million (or 41.3 percent of the total). This massive migration created unique risks and contributed to an increase in morbidity and mortality.

The travails of the famous Lewis and Clark expedition of 1803–1806 were by no means atypical. In early 1803 President Thomas Jefferson asked for and received authorization from Congress to send this group to explore the interior continent of North America and to find a transcontinental route to the Pacific Ocean. During their lengthy and arduous journey, the nearly four dozen members of the expedition experienced numerous illnesses. Gastrointestinal disorders were common, probably resulting from a combination of diet, fatigue, and exposure. Meat was the primary food, but living conditions precluded its proper preservation. Moreover, reliance on meat and the absence of fresh fruits and vegetables led to the appearance of scurvy. Drinking water sometimes came from polluted sources or else contained mineral contents that had a laxative action. Roots and other vegetation that were part of the group's diet also produced enteric disorders. "The party is much aflicted with Boils and Several have the Decissentary, which I contribute to the water which is muddy," Clark wrote in his journal. The next day several men had "the Disentary, and two-thirds of them with ulsers or Boils, Some with 8 or 10 of those Tumers."[6]

Exposure to the elements added to the hardships. Cold, dampness, and intense physical exertion led to arthritislike symptoms. "Some of the men," according to one member, "are complaining of rheumatic pains, which are to be expected from the wet and cold we suffered last winter; during which, from the 4th of November, 1805, to the 25th of March 1806, there were not more than twelve days in which it did not rain and of these but six were clear." Frequent respiratory illnesses, infections, fractures, gunshot wounds, bruises, cuts, lacerations, accidents, and insect bites were also prevalent.[7]

If the timing and length of the Lewis and Clark expedition were atypical, their experiences prefigured those of later migrants. Consider, for example, the medical problems faced by those who traversed the overland trails to Oregon and California. Two major routes and a number of alternate routes and cutoffs developed over time. The most famous—the Oregon–California and Santa Fe Trails —commenced at Independence, Missouri. The former led through South Pass, located on the Continental Divide in the central Rocky Mountains in Wyoming, and then divided into northern and southern routes. The latter followed the southern route and passed through El Paso, Tucson, and Yuma before ending in California. Both covered about 2,000 miles and on average took four and a half months to complete. Between 1841 and 1866 perhaps 350,000 people made their way through South Pass.

Travelers on both routes encountered similar health problems. Gastrointestinal illnesses were the most common and debilitating, and included dysenteries of unspecified origins as well as cholera (1849–50) and typhoid fever. "Becoming so weakened that I could no longer climb in and out of the wagon," a twenty-year-old pregnant woman suffering from dysentery wrote in her account of the journey, "I was compelled to keep my bed . . . the jolting motion of the wagon soon became a perfect torture to me, and at last became so unendurable, that I implored my husband to take me out, make my bed on the sand and let me die in peace." On occasion travelers, if they were not to dehydrate, were forced to drink from polluted sources of water. "Our drinking water," noted one Forty-niner, "*is living*—that is it is composed of one third green fine moss, one third pollywogs, and one third embryo mosquitoes." Another wrote that he had come to a puddle "where rain water had been standing til green on top and so muddy that if there had been a hog about, I should have set it down as one of their wallowing places. Yet this stuff which would have been rejected by my stomach at home, I drank with considerable relish by shutting my eyes and holding my breath." Many sources of water in the Southwest contained high-alkaline and sulphur compounds whose laxative effects magnified gastrointestinal problems. On the Oregon–California Trail in the Rocky Mountain region some of the diarrhea may have resulted from giardiasis, a protozoan infection caused by a pathogen residing in water.[8]

Migrants on the overland trails faced a variety of pathogens capable of causing other infectious diseases. On the northern route "mountain fever" was common. Its symptoms included severe headaches and muscle and joint pains. Peaking in the spring and early summer, this disease—now known as Colorado tick fever—was caused by an orbovirus transmitted by the bites of wood ticks. Malarial infections may also have been common. Many of the migrants came from malarial infected regions, and hence carried the malarial plasmodium. The presence of *Anopheles* mosquitoes in these regions completed the complex cycle of transmission. By 1830 malaria had spread to the lower Columbia River and Willamette Valley in Oregon. A hot and humid summer, the arrival of white settlers carrying the plasmodium, and the presence of the insect vector created conditions for an epidemic that within several years decimated the Indian population, which was especially susceptible to this imported organism. Military personnel in the Southwest were also hard hit. A battalion of 409 men sent from Illinois to New Mexico during the Mexican War reported 102 cases of malaria during the two-month journey. Undoubtedly many of the fevers that were common on both trails had other bacterial or viral origins. Whatever the source, "fevers" constituted a significant health hazard.[9]

Gastrointestinal and other infectious diseases, however important, were not the only threats to health. The long journey required that migrants carry their own food supply. At that time the typical overland trail diet was composed mainly of bread and bacon. Although many carried citric acid, pickles, and dried fruit and vegetables—all of which were sources of ascorbic acid—others did not. Those who failed to bring antiscorbutics or to eat some of the fresh vegetation found on both trails were prone to scurvy, a dietary disease that often proved fatal. "The amount of suffering on the latter part of the route," according to a San Francisco correspondent in 1849, "was almost incalculable . . . I saw men sitting or lying by the roadside, sick with fevers or crippled by scurvy, begging of the passerby to lend them some assistance, but no one could do it. The winter was so near, that it was sure death literally, and the teams were all giving out, so that the thought of hauling them in the wagons was absurd. Nothing could be done, consequently they were left to a slow lingering death in the wilderness."[10] Scurvy was particularly prevalent among California's Gold Rush immigrants in 1849; as many as 10,000 may have succumbed to the disease.[11]

The long journey over unfamiliar and often dangerous terrain posed other hazards. The vagaries of a continental climate that included summer droughts and winter storms added to the miseries faced by migrants. Most important, a variety of traumatic injuries led to lifelong disabilities or death. Large numbers were either injured or perished when crushed beneath wagon wheels. Accidental discharge of weapons, stampeding animals, drownings at the numerous river crossings, and fights between individuals whose tempers had already been strained by the vicissitudes of the journey added to the risks to life. Popular beliefs notwithstanding, deaths from Indian attacks were rare. Although accurate data are lacking, estimates put the overall mortality rate on the Oregon–California trail as high as 6 percent of the total; the actual number who perished may never be known.[12]

▼ ▼ ▼

Decades after the settlement of the Middle West, early pioneers in their reminiscences romanticized their experiences and forgot their hardships. Writing for the Old Settlers Society in 1881, one individual waxed rhapsodic about the pioneers' early experiences in Illinois. "Living in log houses, generally unplastered, with open fireplaces, they breathed pure air, and having regular sleep, and dressing healthfully, they were afflicted with but few physical ailments, save malarial ones."[13] But in fact most of the westbound settlers faced an environment that constantly endangered their health and lives. Indeed, there are striking parallels between the early experiences of the Jamestown and Plymouth settlers of the seventeenth century and their nineteenth-century midwestern counterparts. Those who moved to the Midwest and beyond confronted a variety of diseases that reflected the environment of that region. "Respecting the healthfulness of this country," according to James Kilbourne, a prominent Ohio journalist and legislator, "I have to repeat that it is in fact sickly in a considerable degree." He reported the presence of bilious fever in 1800 and 1801. "Almost all were sick, both in towns and country, so that it became difficult, in many instances, to get tenderers for the sick. In many instances whole families were down at a time and many died."[14]

Admitted to the Union in 1803, Ohio had a population of about 1.5 million in 1840, a time when Wisconsin had but 30,000 inhabitants. The initial pioneers were hunters, who rarely lived in one place for any length of time and who left little to suggest their presence. Eventually farmers, shopkeepers, lawyers, physicians, and other settlers moved into the region and established communities and towns. In so doing they transformed both the natural environment and the ecology of disease.

Before its settlement, the area drained by the Mississippi River— Ohio, Michigan, Wisconsin, Indiana, and parts of Illinois—was a region of forests and underbrush. When the leaves were out the sun rarely reached the ground, which remained waterlogged throughout much of the summer. In other areas, treeless prairies with high grass predominated. Whether in timber lands or prairie, streams and rivers often overflowed their banks in the spring, leaving large areas of stagnant pools in the already moist earth.

Such environments, particularly after settlers had moved in, created circumstances conducive to the prevalence of what was generally called the "ague." Among contemporaries there was general agreement that the ague was the most common of all diseases. Indeed, its omnipresent character led some to regard it not as a disease, but as an inevitable concomitant of frontier life. "He ain't sick, he's only got the ager," was the common expression.[15] Yet the symptoms were so dramatic that those who were afflicted recognized that they were indeed sick. The chills, recalled one old pioneer, came

faster and faster, and grew colder and colder as in successive undulations they coursed down your back, till you felt like "a harp of a thousand strings," played upon by the icy fingers of old Hiems, who increased the cold chills until his victim shook like as aspen leaf, and his teeth chattered in his jaws. There you laid shaking in the frigid ague region for an hour or so until you gradually stole back to a temperate zone. Then commenced the warm flashes over your system, which increased with heat as the former did with cold, until you reached the torrid region, where you lay in burning heat, racked with pain in your head and along your back, for an hour or so, when you began by degrees to feel less heat and pain, until your hands grew moist, and you were relieved by a copious perspiration all over your body, and you got to your natural feeling again.[16]

Such descriptions were characteristic of those who moved into this region. "You felt as though you had gone through some sort of collision, thrashing-machine or jarring-machine," noted one sufferer, "and came out not killed, but next thing to it . . . About this time you came to the conclusion that you would not accept the whole state of Indiana as a gift."[17]

What disease were midwesterners referring to when they spoke of the "ague"? In the nineteenth century there was a good deal of confusion about fevers, if only because the means of distinguishing between their causes were unavailable. To differentiate between malaria and typhoid fever (as well as a variety of other infectious diseases) was not a simple matter. Before the identification of the malaria plasmodium at the end of the nineteenth century, even autopsy findings could not always identify each with any accuracy; both involved pathological features in the spleen, liver, and bone marrow. The difficulties of distinguishing between malaria and typhoid persisted. When discussing camp fevers, Joseph J. Woodward (an assistant surgeon in the Union army during the Civil War who published an analysis of camp diseases) emphasized the presence of typhoid and malaria. He then went on to identify "a vast group of mixed cases, in which the malarial and typhoid elements are variously combined with each other and with the scorbutic taint." He proposed the diagnosis of typhomalarial fever, which then was adopted by the army in its sick reports.[18]

Despite the methodological problems involved in differentiating between some of the infectious diseases in the Midwest, there is general agreement that malaria was the most important disease in this region throughout much of the nineteenth century. Its periodicity (chills alternating with fever) and response to quinine provide persuasive evidence of its high incidence and prevalence. The data and shrewd observations presented by Daniel Drake in his classic work on diseases in the Mississippi Valley only reinforce this conclusion.[19]

Before the settlement of the Upper Mississippi Valley (comprising the present-day states of Illinois, Missouri, Iowa, Wisconsin, and Minnesota), malaria—which requires the presence of infected and susceptible persons—was nonexistent. Although the French had explored much of this region in the seventeenth century, they did not establish many settlements. As late as 1750 there were fewer than 3,000 French in Illinois. After the defeat of the French by the British in 1763, the movement of carriers and susceptible persons into the region accelerated. Consequently, there were sporadic outbreaks of malaria in the late eighteenth century.

The emergence of malaria as the most important disease, however, did not take place until the nineteenth century, when large numbers of emigrants began moving to the Midwest. By the turn of the nineteenth century Ohio and Michigan had already acquired a justified reputation as an area in which malaria reigned. Much the same was true of Indiana. The disease, however, did not appear at the same time in all areas. In Illinois, which was settled earlier than other states in the Upper Mississippi Valley, malaria assumed an endemic character and persisted for nearly a century following its initial appearance, in about 1770. In Missouri malaria peaked between 1820 and 1870; in Iowa and Wisconsin the high points were between 1830 and 1870; and the shortest peak occurred in Minnesota. Two factors played key roles in shaping this pattern. The first was the date at which large-scale migration into the area began. The second was location; in northern and upland areas malaria was less prevalent than in southern and lowland ones. When the disease assumed an endemic-epidemic character, mortality rose and reached a peak around 1860.[20]

As human beings interact with their environment, they can create conditions conducive to the emergence of new diseases or to the diminution of existing ones. The appearance of malaria is one such example. "Of all of our diseases," Drake observed, "it is the one which has the most intimate relations with soil and climate—that, in which peculiarities, resulting from topographical and atmospheric influences, are most likely to appear . . . It is, moreover, the *great* cause of mortality, or infirmity of constitution."[21]

The disappearance of malaria from the Upper Mississippi Valley in the latter part of the nineteenth century is even more fascinating; its decline occurred before an understanding of its etiology or mode of transmission had emerged or programs to prevent or suppress its presence. What elements, therefore, shaped the odd appearance and disappearance of a disease that was unknown in pre-Columbian America? Of key importance was the movement of people into the region. Migration brought both carriers of the plasmodium from areas in which malaria was endemic and susceptible persons from malaria-free regions. The presence of large numbers of human beings, however necessary, was not sufficient to create the conditions required for the introduction of the disease.

Besides carriers and susceptible persons, the presence of the *Anopheles* mosquito was necessary. The Midwest was always an ideal breeding ground for mosquitoes of all kinds, largely because the overflow from streams and rivers from melting snows, as well as poor drainage even on the prairies, created marshes and pools of stagnant water conducive to their reproduction. The initial pattern of settlement served only to increase still further the already large mosquito population. The absence of roads made the waterways, streams, and rivers of the Mississippi Valley the basic mode of transportation, especially after the introduction of the steamboat in the early nineteenth century. Hence early emigrants resided near waterways. Many recognized that they were living in intrinsically unhealthy places, and urged remedial measures. "The question of continued health or disease, of long life or premature death," wrote Noah Webster in 1799, "hangs very often upon the choice of a salubrious situation for a house." It was inexcusable to build "within a mile of the sources of disease and death." There were several ways of improving the salubrity of wetland areas—"by draining the lands and cultivating them . . . or by turning them into streams of running water." "Means too might be taken to enlighten the settlers upon the method of choosing the best sites for their dwellings," observed Benjamin W. McCready in 1837, "and the means best adapted to prevent the effects of malaria upon their constitutions."[22]

The advice of Webster, McCready, and others, however, was all but ignored. Since the construction of roads in a wilderness area was not feasible for much of the first half of the nineteenth century, virtually all the early settlements were along waterways. Such areas were natural breeding grounds for insects because flooding in the spring left many pools of stagnant water. Moreover, the clearing of lands and construction of dams for mill ponds compounded drainage problems by adding to stagnant water areas. The reduction of forests also removed the dense shade that inhibited insect breeding. These activities inadvertently provided ideal conditions for the proliferation of the *Anopheles* vector, which was indispensable to the spread of malaria.

Housing conditions also played a role in the transmission of malaria. Many of the early settlers constructed log cabins, which generally had no or one window (glass was a luxury on the frontier). In areas lacking timber, people built mud huts and sod houses for shelter. Given the fact that the malaria-transmitting species of the *Anopheles* prefer a damp, dark, and warm environment, it is obvious that early housing provided conditions that enabled the insect to live in close proximity to humans. All of these conditions—population movements, settlement in poorly drained areas, and housing—combined to make malaria the most important disease in the Middle West.

Just as early environmental change fostered conditions conducive to the spread of malaria, so later changes created circumstances that contributed to its disappearance. After 1850 railroad construction in the Upper Mississippi Valley began in earnest. The advantages of railroads were obvious. Unlike waterways (which were not navigable during certain seasons) they provided year-round transportation; they also expanded dramatically the area of settlement. The construction of railroads admittedly led to an occasional increase in malaria, for the ditches constructed alongside the tracks provided additional breeding grounds for insects. In the long run, however, railroads shifted population away from waterways and lowlands, where drainage had remained a perennial problem.

A variety of other developments contributed as well to the disappearance of malaria after 1870. Although the disease virtually disappeared before the introduction of state drainage projects, there is considerable evidence suggesting that individual and local drainage projects diminished the amount of stagnant water and thus reduced the mosquito population. Moreover, after the initial phase of settlement, housing improved. Newer homes were dry, better sealed, and included more windows, which provided a source of light. Screens, which became more common during the latter half of the nineteenth century, were also an important innovation, even though they were installed for comfort rather than health. All these changes tended to reduce the presence of the *Anopheles* in homes.

The introduction of cattle breeding into the region also played a role. In Iowa, Wisconsin, and Minnesota, farmers began to shift from raising crops over to dairy cattle because of soil exhaustion, competition from wheat growing states in the South and West, the need to use surplus feed for cattle, and high dairy prices. Between 1850 and 1870 the number of cattle in the five states of the Upper Mississippi Valley rose from 2 to nearly 5 million, and by 1890 had nearly reached 14 million. As many *Anopheles* species prefer to feed off cattle rather than human beings, the large number of cattle reduced the odds of malaria transmission by the insect vector.

The appearance and subsequent decline of malaria in the Upper Mississippi Valley is suggestive of the intimate relationship between environmental change and disease processes even though the nature of their interaction may never be fully understood. The region's temperate climate admittedly played a major role by shortening the infective season and ultimately interrupting the life cycle of the *Anopheles* species. Conscious human interventions were relatively insignificant, if only because the etiology of the disease was little understood. The use of quinine increased dramatically after 1850 but did not play a significant part in the disappearance of malaria. The drug neither prevented infection nor sterilized the carrier; it minimized the clinical attack and permitted people to function.[23]

Those who moved westward into open spaces and clear air enjoyed an advantage over urban dwellers. Yet the frontier environment was hardly a health utopia. The cabins in which settlers lived were small, and crowding was common. Nor did they have an aversion to dirt. Soap was a luxury, and relatively few washed or bathed with any regularity. Vermin, mosquitoes, and other insects lived alongside human occupants. A traveler in Illinois in the early 1840s provided a graphic but not atypical description of conditions. In the house, he observed,

> the room is almost darkened by myriads of house-flies . . . Molasses, sugar, preserved fruit, bread, everything on the table, is loaded with them, and the very operation of fanning them off drives numbers of them into the molasses and other things of an adhesive nature. It is not safe to open your mouth. It is evident too, on examining the

molasses, that the small red ant has been purloining it, and has left a number of his unfortunate companions enveloped in its mass; whilst ever and anon a cockroach makes a dash at the table, and, in nine cases out of ten, succeeds in scampering across over meat dishes and everything that comes in the way, and that too in spite of the bitter blows aimed at him with knife and spoon, he is "so t'rnation spry."[24]

Settlers rarely paid close attention to the sources from which they drew their water. Because wells required considerable labor to dig, they hauled their water from local streams, rivers, or stagnant ponds, many of which were contaminated from natural sources. The practice of using adjacent bodies of water to dispose of animal manure and other organic wastes only added to the risks of contamination. Finally, the abundance of insects made it possible to spread organisms from feces to food.[25]

Such conditions created an environment in which a variety of infectious diseases could flourish. Dysentery was common, and as many as 10 percent of those afflicted died. Typhoid was undoubtedly present during the first half of the nineteenth century, but the difficulty in distinguishing it from malaria makes it virtually impossible to estimate its prevalence. Whatever the case, it is evident that by midcentury prevailing sanitary conditions had made typhoid one of the region's most significant epidemic diseases, a position it retained until the end of the century. Similarly, there is evidence that erysipelas, a disease caused by Group A hemolytic streptococci, was present from the 1830s to the 1870s. Often associated with unsanitary hygienic practices, erysipelas appeared in epidemic form and often was accompanied by puerperal fever, a generally fatal postpartum infection in women generally transmitted by attending physicians.[26]

Many of the infectious diseases prevalent in the Midwest were the same as those found in the older settled regions on the Atlantic seaboard. The cholera epidemics that plagued the East on three separate occasions spread to the Midwest as well, where they took a devastating toll in small towns and newly established and growing urban areas. Infectious diseases associated with the young—measles, mumps, whooping cough, and others—added to the health burden. Respiratory and rheumatic disorders were common and affected children and adults alike.[27]

Infant and child mortality rates in the Midwest were high, although available data are unreliable. The federal census of 1850 included mortality data for the first time in its history, but the number of reported deaths was far lower than the actual total.[28] If it is correct to assume that underreporting was equal for all states, then newly settled states had lower rates than older midwestern states, but both enjoyed an advantage over the Atlantic seaboard. Illinois and Ohio, for example, had higher infant mortality rates than Iowa, Wisconsin, and Minnesota, but about a third lower than Massachusetts. Mortality among children aged 1 to 5 was also at elevated levels. In the Midwest, as in the East, urban mortality was higher than rural mortality. In Illinois in 1850 children between the ages of 1 and 5 accounted for 19 percent of all deaths. In Chicago, by contrast, the comparable figure was 36.7 percent, and by 1860 reached nearly 56 percent. The causes of death included dysentery, respiratory diseases, scarlet fever, and other diseases commonly associated with childhood.[29]

More recent studies, however, using other kinds of data, suggest a different pattern. In a national sample of 1,600 households taken from the 1860 census and traced back to the 1850 census manuscript schedules, Richard H. Steckel found that there were few regional differences in infant mortality, but that losses among children aged 1 to 4 were higher on the frontier. The number of children was also a significant variable; mortality was highest in larger families. A combination of poor nutrition, contaminated water supplies, new disease environments, congested housing, and the hardships of pioneer life, according to Steckel, may have been responsible. Another study of Utah Mormons and employing genealogical data found that during the initial stage of settlement, early marriage, early childbearing, brief birth intervals, and high age at last birth resulted in high levels of both fertility and infant mortality. When fertility declined because of delayed marriage and increased birth spacing, infant mortality fell as well.[30] Although the shortcomings of nineteenth-century aggregate mortality records prevent any definitive conclusions, it seems clear that infant and child mortality on the frontier was generally high.

There were also some differences in regional morbidity patterns. A case in point was an often fatal disease that in the nineteenth century played an important role in the Midwest and was present in the South as well. In North Carolina and Georgia it was known as the "trembles." In Ohio, Indiana, and Illinois it sometimes received other names, including "swamp sickness," "puking fever," "bloody mur-rain," and "distemper." But it was best known as "milksickness." It affected both cattle and humans and tended to be endemic rather than epidemic. The symptoms resembled those of arsenic poisoning: irregular respiration, subnormal temperature, constipation, and a bloated abdomen. Individuals experienced extreme thirst, muscular weakness, and nausea, all of which led to a comatose condition alternating with intense pain and ended in death. There were many theories about its etiology: some insisted that it had botanical origins; others described it as "severe Bilious remittent fever with a complication of gastro enteritis." In 1838 John Rowe, an Ohio farmer, declared that white snakeroot gave cattle the trembles and humans the milksickness, but his explanation was dismissed by Daniel Drake for lack of evidence. The riddle to the disease was finally solved in 1927 when the active ingredient in the white snakeroot was isolated and given the name tremetol (a poison found in such plants as the rayless goldenrod that grew in other regions). The poison was ingested by animals who had eaten the white snakeroot; humans who consumed their milk or ate their flesh became ill in turn.

Although few data are available on the incidence and prevalence of milksickness, early nineteenth-century medical sources provide rich descriptions indicating that entire communities were affected. Indeed, many believed that the presence of milksickness made the Middle West an uninhabitable region. In 1851, for example, the *Report on Practical Medicine* to the members of the Illinois Medical Society noted that the disease had "turned back many an immigrant from settling in our State." Soon afterward, however, the disease had begun to disappear. After 1858 milksickness was rarely mentioned at the meetings of the society. Its disappearance, like that of malaria, was due largely to environmental change. By cultivating land, farmers reduced forests where the snakeroot grew wild, and the confinement of cattle to enclosed fields further diminished the possibility of ingesting a plant containing a dangerous substance.[31]

The circumstances of frontier life added to the risk factors. The outdoor activities characteristic of farming led to frequent accidents. Even minor bruises and cuts could result in "blood poisoning" or "lockjaw" (tetanus). Living as they did in proximity to domestic and wild animals as well as to ticks and other insects, it is not surprising that settlers suffered from zoonotic diseases, although the absence of data does not permit any estimate of their prevalence. We do know that large numbers of venomous snakes posed a hazard; during local extermination efforts, inhabitants might kill hundreds of rattlesnakes ranging from three to ten feet in length.

More subtle in shaping health patterns was the sex imbalance that persisted in many frontier areas Young unmarried males, a group more prone to violent and antisocial behavior and much less likely to eat nutritious food or pay attention to personal hygiene, worked in mines and construction, frequently succumbed to disease and accidents, and perhaps fell prey to psychological despair. Infectious diseases such as syphilis and tuberculosis, violent behavior, accidents, excessive use of alcohol, and inadequate diets that resulted in scurvy combined to have a devastating impact upon their health and longevity. This sex imbalance was especially prevalent in the dry plains and mountains west of the 100th meridian.[32]

Areas with a more balanced sex ratio had quite different health patterns. Seventeenth-century Massachusetts, for example, had a rough balance between men and women; Virginia and the Chesapeake region a pronounced imbalance. New England enjoyed a distinct health advantage over its southerly neighbors. This pattern would persist throughout the nineteenth century as Americans moved westward. In fertile regions with adequate rainfall, settlement tended to be by families; in more rugged terrain less suited to small-scale agriculture young males predominated. As late as 1870 California and Oregon had twice as many males as females, Arizona four times as many, Nevada five times, Wyoming six, and Idaho and Montana eight times as many. In areas with a balanced sex ratio, male behavior tended to be more restrained. The needs of the family took precedence over those of the individual; prospective loss of life was less acceptable to married than to single men. "The men had a great deal of anxiety and all the care of their families," Martha Ann Morrison wrote in 1844. In an account of the journey to California in 1849, Catherine Margaret Haun observed that the presence of women and children on the Oregon Trail "exerted a good influence, as the men did not take such risks with Indians and thereby avoided conflict; were more alert about the care of the teams and seldom had accidents; more attention was paid to cleanliness and sanitation and, lastly but not of less importance, the meals were more regular and better cooked thus preventing much sickness and there was less waste of food."[33]

▼ ▼ ▼

Given the variable terrain, environments, and climates found within the continental United States, there were inevitably regional differences in health patterns. The South is illustrative. During the colonial period the Chesapeake, Carolinas, and Georgia experienced much higher morbidity and mortality rates than the New England and Middle Atlantic colonies. After 1800 the acquisitions of the Louisiana territories and Florida opened up new areas for settlement. During the nineteenth century the South came to include four somewhat distinct regions: the Atlantic coastal plain, the Gulf Coast, the Appalachian Mountains, and the interior.[34] Each had somewhat different epidemiological patterns, which reflected the influence of climate and geography. Most significant, the presence of large numbers of African Americans—most of whom were slaves—gave the region a distinctive character. Recent estimates indicate that the total black population of the United States increased from about 1.6 to 4.9 million between 1810 and 1860. On the eve of the Civil War perhaps 80 percent lived in the South.[35]

The absence of reliable data makes it difficult to provide accurate estimates of morbidity and mortality. It is clear, however, that many of the diseases present in the South were no different from other regions. Gastrointestinal disorders and respiratory infections were common. Given climatic differences, it is probable that the former were more important in the South and the latter more prevalent in the North and mountain regions. Periodic yellow fever and smallpox epidemics, however spectacular, were less significant than those endemic diseases that grew out of contaminated water supplies and lack of attention to sanitation. As in many other areas of the nation, infant and child mortality were particularly high. The federal census of mortality of 1850, for example, found that 21.4 percent of all deaths in Mississippi were among those less than 1 year old, and an additional 25.4 percent were in the 1-to-5-year category.[36]

Despite similarities with other regions, the South presented a different epidemiological environment related to its warm and moist climate and the importation of certain African diseases, namely, falciparum malaria, hookworm, and yellow fever. During the nineteenth century the latter ravaged southern port cities and from time to time spread to interior regions. Although it aroused fear among urban inhabitants, the actual impact of yellow fever on overall mortality was relatively small. Falciparum malaria, on the other hand, had a major impact on life and health. The disease was brought to the colonies in the late seventeenth century by slaves from Africa. Unlike vivax malaria (which was endemic in England and remained the dominant form in more northerly regions in the United States), the falciparum variety had a much higher mortality rate. A warm and rainy semitropical climate, the presence of an indigenous *Anopheles* mosquito population, and agricultural practices that created ideal insect breeding grounds made falciparum malaria one of the most important diseases in the South. Indeed, its presence played a role in the spread of slavery, for many Africans (like other populations living in malarial regions) had developed the sickle cell trait, which served as a partial protection against falciparum malaria even though it resulted in a shortened life span. Africans, moreover, were largely immune to the vivax form. Their relative immunity to malaria tended to reinforce the institution of slavery, since they appeared especially suited to agricultural labor in an environment that posed greater threats to the health and lives of whites.[37]

A variety of other infectious diseases, including guinea worm, filariasis, tapeworm, hookworm, and trypanosomiasis, were also carried to the Americas. Some took root in the Caribbean, where the importation of slaves into a region with a tropical climate reproduced a modified West African disease environment. With its warm but not tropical environment, the South in general did not support many of the infections that became endemic in the Caribbean. One exception was the filarial roundworm, the causative organism of elephantiasis. Transmitted by a variety of mosquitoes, the adult worm lives in the lymphatic vessels and lymph nodes, eventually causing obstructions and producing scrotal, labial, or leg and foot swelling. Oddly, the disease was limited to Charleston, South Carolina, and did not disappear until the early twentieth century; the city was the only place that harbored a sufficiently large number of infected persons to sustain the life cycle of the roundworm.[38]

Unlike filariasis, hookworm (though not identified until the beginning of the twentieth century) quickly became endemic through large parts of the rural South. Eggs of hookworm (*Necator americanus*) are discharged in the stool of infected persons and release a free-living larva that shortly becomes infective. Penetrating the skin and eventually reaching the intestine, hookworms attach by their mouths to the mucosa of the upper small intestine and suck blood. The disease is prevalent where people walk barefoot over soil contaminated with the feces of infected persons; it is clearly associated with improper sanitation and poverty. Symptoms include iron-deficiency anemia, lethargy, and growth retardation; the presence of the disease can increase vulnerability to other diseases. Antebellum medical accounts suggest that hookworm was widespread throughout the South, particularly in the Atlantic and Gulf coastal areas.[39]

By the middle of the nineteenth century data drawn from printed family histories (overwhelmingly white and perhaps biased toward the more successful) indicate that the sharp differences in regional colonial mortality rates had narrowed or disappeared. In the seventeenth and eighteenth centuries mortality rates in the Chesapeake and areas farther south were much higher than in New England. Cohorts born in the South in the mid-nineteenth century, however, had life expectancies similar to those born in the North.[40]

The morbidity and mortality experiences of slaves, however, was quite different from that of whites. The legal slave trade before 1808 and the illegal trade thereafter had always been perilous. The death rate during the middle passage from Africa to the New World was high. Though declining from the seventeenth to the nineteenth century, it ranged from 10 to 30 percent or more, depending on the place of origin, date and duration of the voyage, and presence of endemic disease.[41] The death rate during the first year after arrival was also excessive; in the lowcountry of South Carolina at the end of the eighteenth century perhaps a third perished.[42]

Once in the United States, African Americans faced a difficult process of adjustment. Most came from West Africa, where their diet generally lacked protein; meat, milk, and other dairy products were rarely consumed. Carbohydrates were the basic staple, and even vegetables were low in protein because the soil was acidic and deficient in nitrogen. Consequently, nutritional disorders were common, and the presence of a variety of tropical diseases left the indigenous population in a precarious position. Slaves imported directly from West

Africa to the United States were severely malnourished and shorter in stature than Creole-born slaves who came from the Caribbean.[43]

Genetically Africans had adapted to their environment; they evolved hemoglobin defenses against malaria and were less susceptible to hookworm infestations. What was an asset in one environment, however, became a liability in another. Africans had a higher frequency of lactose intolerance, a condition that occurs when individuals lack high levels of lactase enzyme and hence cannot break down milk sugars. In West Africa (as in many parts of the world) this deficiency was harmless, since milk was not part of the diet. In a cow-milk-drinking society such as the United States, Africans who consumed dairy products developed severe diarrhea and gastrointestinal discomfort. Africans were also especially prone to miliary tuberculosis, perhaps the most fatal form of the disease (largely because the tubercles are not confined to one organ but are spread throughout the body). Their susceptibility to tuberculosis may reflect the fact that they had not been exposed to the disease in Africa, and hence failed to develop a strong immune response. Thus genetic and environmental differences, at least in the short run, created health problems for Africans transported to America.[44]

Even after adjusting to a new environment, African slaves faced formidable health problems. Both Africans and whites suffered from similar diseases, but the conditions under which slaves lived magnified the significance of many diseases. Overcrowding, lack of ventilation, damp earthen floors and poor sanitary conditions in slave quarters—conditions generally found in congested urban areas—facilitated the transmission of respiratory and gastrointestinal diseases in both winter and summer. Even typhus, which was relatively uncommon in rural areas, struck antebellum Virginia several times. Yaws, syphilis, and gonorrhea were also present. In urban slave communities, overcrowding and poor housing conditions replicated disease patterns found on many plantations.[45]

Plantation working conditions often contributed to sickness. In the lowcountry rice plantations of South Carolina and Georgia slaves worked in knee-deep flooded fields and were exposed to a host of water-borne infections as well as sunstroke and heat prostration. Aware of the perils of their environment in the summer months, when sickness was particularly prevalent, many landowners migrated to healthier areas. "I would as soon stand fifty feet from the best Kentucky rifleman and be shot at by the hour," one South Carolina rice planter stated, "as to spend a night on my plantation in summer." Slaves were also exposed to diseases from the animals with which they worked. At industrial sites they faced other hazards. Tobacco factory environments posed the threat of lung diseases from tobacco dust and fumes; those who worked at coal mining faced similar conditions. And, of course, there was plantation discipline, which often relied on whipping. "I can' never forgit, how my massa beat my brothers cause dey didn' wuk. He beat 'em so bad dey was sick a long time, an' soon as dey got a smatterin' better he sold 'em."[46]

Slavery was a complex institution, and slaveowners behaved in ambivalent ways. Nowhere is this ambivalence better revealed than in the diet provided slaves. It is difficult to reconstruct typical diets. In recent years, however, scholars have begun to study diet by relying on a combination of traditional sources such as plantation and medical records and surviving anthropometric data. Research in physiology, anthropology, and nutrition has demonstrated that height-by-age data make it possible, within limits, to ascertain nutritional status.

In general, the food supply in the South was adequate for all people. The staples of pork and corn were supplemented by turnips, sweet potatoes, okra, and peas.[47] Nevertheless, surviving evidence suggests that African-American slaves manifested nutritional problems related to both their genetic endowment and the diet provided by owners. The work responsibilities of the mother and the presence of maternal and fetal infections exacerbated the problems of pregnancy. Moreover, after weaning, slave children were provided with a high-carbohydrate and low-protein diet. Lactase intolerance deprived many youngsters of such essential minerals as calcium, magnesium, and iron as well as certain vitamins. Slave infants weighed less than 5.5 pounds as compared with modern standards of 7.5. Their mortality during the first year of life was approximately 350 per 1,000; between the ages of 1 and 4 it was 201. The figures for the white antebellum population, by contrast, were 179 and 93, respectively. More than half of all slave infants and children, in other words, perished before their fifth birthday. Moreover, slave children were extraordinarily short, falling around or below the first centile of modern standards. Aside from nutrition, there is little doubt that infants and young children of slave mothers received less care than whites.[48]

After age 11 there was a rapid improvement, and young adults ranged between the 25th (males) and 30th centile (females) in height. The growth in the height of slaves during adolescence may have reflected a change in diet; slaveowners tended to provide young adult workers with more balanced and nutritious diets, and they reached heights exceeding 67 inches. Indeed, height-by-age profiles reveal that male slaves were taller than Europeans but shorter than American whites. Slaves were better fed on average than Europeans but less so than native-born whites. Data on ex-slaves who served in the Union Army and southern whites who served in the Confederate Army reveal that the latter were on average two inches taller. By ages 20–24 mortality rates for slaves and whites were virtually the same.[49]

That slaves had excessively elevated infant and child mortality rates is incontrovertible. To be sure, those who survived to adulthood had life expectancies that did not differ in fundamental respects from the general antebellum population. Nevertheless, there is some contemporary evidence that nutritional deprivation during early childhood can have lasting effects upon physical and mental development. Malnourished children tend to lag in motor skills; their emotional growth is retarded; they are apathetic, less aggressive, more dependent; and their cognitive skills are less well developed. The institution of slavery, therefore, had a profound impact because of its legacy of malnutrition and neglect.[50]

▼   ▼   ▼

In the nineteenth century the United States Army faced many of the same risks to health and life as those in civilian life. The infectious diseases that accompanied the westward movement were present among soldiers assigned to frontier posts as well as among migrants. Equally significant, the wars of this century, as in the American Revolution, created an ideal environment for the dissemination of infectious diseases that took an appalling toll in life and dwarfed actual battlefield casualties. Aside from waging the War of 1812, the Mexican War, and the Civil War, one of the basic responsibilities of the army was to establish and staff a series of defensive posts on the East and Gulf Coasts and on the ever-moving westward frontier. Some were designed to protect against Indians and British fur traders from Canada; others to prevent Indian raids into Mexico; others to protect migrants and settlers; and some to explore western territories. The isolated nature of many of these posts made resupply arduous, a fact that sometimes led to dietary illnesses such as scurvy. In warmer regions malaria posed a threat; in colder regions frostbite occasionally occurred. Dysentery and respiratory disorders were present everywhere. Cholera and yellow fever epidemics reached posts along well-traveled routes. Isolation, even in posts that included families, led to high rates of alcoholism. Military expeditions sent to explore new territories or to establish new posts were often decimated by dietary and infectious diseases.[51]

In general, morbidity and mortality rates were higher among soldiers stationed in lowland and southern regions than among those in higher and more northerly regions. The experiences of those who served on Texas frontiers (which included about 20 percent of the army in the 1850s) are revealing. Between 1849 and 1859 20,393 men saw duty in Texas (7,301 on the southern and 13,083 on the western frontiers). There were 66,486 cases of disease reported (26,245 in the former and 40,241 in the latter), and 703 deaths. Both morbidity and mortality rates were higher in Texas than elsewhere. The safest stations were in New England and the eastern interior from the fortieth parallel to the Great Lakes. In Texas, summer heat and fatigue took their toll. The principal diseases were fevers (especially malaria) and gastrointestinal disorders, which accounted for about two-thirds of all fatalities. The circumstances of army life on the frontier magnified the impact of disease. Though rarely fatal, outbreaks of scurvy contributed to debility and apathy. Crude housing only exacerbated other problems. Two years after the establishment of Fort Ewell in 1852, the surgeon reported that the place

> remains to this day a mere camp, in which the troops have been for somewhat more than two years, without flooring for the tents, without proper food, and often without sufficient clothing, exposed to the intense heat and malaria of summer and to the searching "northers" in winter, with no shelter but the canvas, which was sometimes carried away or blown into shreds by the hurricanes, which are not infrequent in this region, and from the force of which not a tree could be found to protect them. Sick and well have been alike subjected to this exposure.

Such conditions also produced bone and joint disorders; no less than 2,500 cases of rheumatism were reported in Texas.[52]

The exigencies of war exacerbated conditions that in the nineteenth century made military frontier life so arduous. Disease took a far higher toll in lives than did actual battlefield conflict in the three wars that America fought between 1812 and 1865. In the War of 1812 dysentery, respiratory disorders, malaria, and other infectious diseases took, in the words of General George Izard, a "prodigious" toll. General Edmund P. Gaines suggested that the "irregularity in the Supply and badness of the rations" had played the major role in retarding military operations. Although detailed statistical data on morbidity and mortality are lacking, scholars have estimated that perhaps two and a half times as many soldiers perished from disease or accident as were killed or wounded in battle. A sample from military records reveals that 3.2 percent of soldiers were killed or wounded in action, whereas 8.2 percent died from disease or occasional accidents.[53]

A similar situation prevailed in the Mexican War, from 1846 to 1848. In that conflict slightly more than 100,000 men served in the army. About 1,600 were killed in battle or died from wounds. Perhaps 11,000 men perished from what was known as diseases of the camp (overwhelmingly dysentery), and far more were incapacitated at one point or another. Mortality from disease among regular army troops was half that of volunteers. Regulars had adjusted to the discipline of military life; they were cognizant of the importance of personal hygiene and an appropriate diet, and were in a better position to meet the challenges of war. The same was not true of volunteers. Such men, observed an army surgeon,

> were for the first time in their lives subjected to all the dangers to health incident to camp life–half of them bivouacking at night, exposed to an almost tropical sun during the day–drinking brackish water, and compelled to subsist on the rations inartistically & carelessly cooked, and without vegetables, and, above all, suffering under the depressing influence of nostalgia. Under these circumstances, sufficient in themselves to decimate the whole Army of Volunteers, the measles broke out among them, and typhoid fever with its characteristic rosecolour eruption, and chronic diarrhoea opened each for itself a broad avenue to death.

Indeed, the proportion of deaths from disease exceeded that of any other conflict in which the United States was involved.[54]

Nowhere, however, was the impact of environmental conditions on disease better illustrated than in the Civil War, a conflict that anticipated the wars of the twentieth century because of the numbers of soldiers involved. From 1861 to 1865 more than 4 million men served in the military, and over 600,000 perished. Nearly two-thirds of the deaths were from disease. This conflict was an example of natural (as contrasted with deliberate) biological warfare and demonstrated the ability of pathogens to devastate human populations in the absence of effective preventive measures or therapeutic interventions.[55]

Oddly enough, the military weaponry of the Civil War was not especially lethal as compared with that of the twentieth century. The field artillery deployed in 1861–1865 was relatively ineffective; bullets from muskets accounted for the overwhelming majority of wounds and deaths. Far more dangerous was the lurking invisible biomilitary armamentarium. In the premicrobiological era the causes of infectious diseases were imperfectly understood. Moreover, concepts of field sanitation and hygiene were not based on microbiological principles, but often reflected aesthetic considerations. The result was a demographic catastrophe of major proportions.[56]

Army life during the Civil War magnified the risks of infection in a variety of ways. The majority of recruits came from sparsely populated rural areas, and perhaps half or more were susceptible to the acute infections of childhood that urban dwellers had already experienced. The conditions of military life provided an ideal environment for the dissemination of pathogens. The concentration of tens of thousands of men disrupted drainage patterns, and the accumulation of human, animal, and other organic wastes ensured that pathogens and insects had exemplary breeding grounds. Crowding and poor ventilation were common. Sanitary conditions were abysmal; fecal and other organic wastes often contaminated drinking water. Chronic and healthy carriers of various infectious diseases facilitated the spread of infections. During the conflict an overwhelming proportion of the army was made up of new recruits. The rapid buildup of the military in the early years of the war only compounded health-related problems. The rank and file as well as officers lacked the discipline and experience of regular troops, and hence were far more vulnerable to the ravages of infectious disease.

Lack of refrigeration, poor food handling, and inappropriate culinary practices further compounded the risks to life. Acute diarrhea/

dysentery and chronic diarrhea afflicted both the Union and Confederate armies. In addition to abysmal sanitary practices, the diet sometimes lacked nutritional necessities. Consequently men were often weakened and became vulnerable to a variety of other than gastrointestinal diseases. The presence of scurvy in the military confirms the likelihood that a nutritional deficiency syndrome plagued the armies throughout the war.[57]

It is difficult to overestimate the impact of disease on Union troops. According to the classic compilation prepared by Joseph K. Barnes, there were more than 6 million medical casualties between 1861 and 1866, which included slightly fewer than 300,000 deaths. About 44,000 died on the field of battle, and an additional 49,000 died of wounds and injuries. By contrast, 186,000 died from disease. Acute and chronic diarrhea and dysentery alone accounted for over 1.7 million cases and 44,568 deaths. More than 1.3 million cases (10,000 deaths) of malaria were recorded. Nearly 35,000 of the 150,000 men who came down with typhoid fever perished. Respiratory disorders took more than 20,000 lives. A variety of other infectious diseases were present, including measles, mumps, syphilis, smallpox, and tuberculosis. Of the noninfectious diseases, acute and chronic rheumatism were most significant. Revised data suggest much higher numbers of deaths, including 67,058 killed in battle and 43,012 dying of wounds, as compared with 224,586 from disease. Indeed, mortality from disease was 65 per 1,000.[58]

Morbidity and mortality rates from disease, however, were not constant. New recruits were often at greatest risk, largely because they had not yet adjusted to military life and learned from the experiences of regular or "seasoned" personnel. White personnel also seem to have had a distinct advantage over African Americans. For the war as a whole the death rate among the former was 53.48 per 1,000, as compared with 143.4 among the latter. The disparity between the two groups was largely a function of time of recruitment. Morbidity rates, for example, peaked early in the war among new recruits, and tended to fall over time. The induction of African Americans into the Union Army, by contrast, did not begin in large numbers until late 1863. Indeed, that summer one-half were sick. These recruits, according to Joseph J. Woodward,

were largely found among the escaped slaves who accumulated in large numbers within the lines of our armies, and who had suffered much from exposure and privation before they enlisted. Moreover, from want of discipline and other causes, the hygienic conditions which at first prevailed in their camps were of the most unfavorable character. With subsequent improvement in the discipline and hygienic management of the colored troops the mortality from diarrhoea and dysentery progressively diminished. This view is confirmed by the circumstance that the total mortality from disease among the colored troops was also proportionately greatest during the year ending June 30, 1864, and subsequently diminished in like manner.

By the end of the war morbidity and mortality rates of white and African-American personnel were similar.[59]

Confederate data, though far less complete because of the destruction of records in a Richmond conflagration, suggest that disease was also the major factor in mortality. Although we shall never be able to ascertain numbers with any precision, the Civil War provides a dramatic illustration of the intimate and inseparable relationship among environment, humans, and bacterial organisms and viruses.

▼   ▼   ▼

The increase in population, rapid economic growth, and territorial expansion were accompanied by faith in the inevitability of further progress. "In the history of the world the doctrine of Reform had never such scope as at the present hour," confided Ralph Waldo Emerson in his journal in 1840. Not "a kingdom, town, statute, rite, calling, man, woman, or child, but is threatened by the new spirit."[60] Social activists labored to eliminate existing evils and to create institutional structures that would ensure an even brighter future.

The optimism prevalent among antebellum Americans, however, was not reflected in better health or longevity. To be sure, the differences in regional life expectations, which had varied sharply during the colonial period, diminished; by 1860 life expectancy among whites in the North and South was similar. Yet health indicators during the first two-thirds of the nineteenth century offered little evidence that the future would be better than the past. Data from both census and genealogical sources indicate that life expectancy for both males and females began a decline about the turn of the century and persisted for much of the antebellum period. The advantages enjoyed by rural populations, as compared with urban residents, persisted, but the decline was evident among both. Immigrants, particularly those who settled in urban settings, had lower life expectancies than the native-born. Aggregate data reveal the magnitude of the decline. In the period 1800–1809 a white male and female aged 20 could expect to live an additional 46.4 and 47.9 years, respectively; in 1850–1859 life expectancies had fallen to 40.8 and 39.5. For the nineteenth century as a whole there was relatively little improvement in mortality, thus reversing the trend toward greater longevity that occurred for much of the eighteenth century.[61]

Declining life expectancy was accompanied by a decrease in height. By the American Revolution, oddly enough, Americans had achieved heights not fundamentally different from their twentieth-century successors. Revolutionary military recruits had a mean terminal height of 68.1 inches, a figure nearly equal to the height of those who served in World War II. Mean heights increased until the 1820s, and then declined. Males born in 1840 were half an inch shorter than those born in 1830, and those born in 1860 were shorter by slightly more than one inch. These figures admittedly conceal significant differences in height across occupations, regions, urban-rural residence, migrants, and birth cohorts. Data on body mass index (BMI; weight in kilograms divided by height in meters squared, a measure that is often used to predict productivity, morbidity, and mortality) for the early nineteenth century are sparse, and hence cannot be employed to predict mortality. Nevertheless, recent scholars have suggested that the decline in height reflects a comparable decline in health. Moreover, studies of Civil War veterans show that those born between 1840 and 1849 had progressively higher prevalence rates for a series of chronic conditions than those born between 1830 and 1839; the same was true of the latter group as compared with those born between 1820 and 1829. A study of Amherst College male students (an economically homogeneous but probably an atypical group) covering the period from 1834 to 1949, on the other hand, failed to establish a height-mortality risk (although the BMI was a better predictor of mortality). At present the absence of a longitudinal record of anthropometric and mortality data of economically heterogeneous groups renders linkages problematic.[62]

In recent years scholars employing anthropometric and life expectancy data have suggested a variety of answers to puzzling questions concerning the relation of economic expansion and progress to increased mortality rates. They have pointed to the increasing rate of urbanization, the rise in immigration, the decline in per-capita meat production because of the failure of the agricultural sector to keep pace with higher demands for food, the increase in food prices, the rise of a factory system that adversely affected workers, growing disparity in the distribution of wealth, and the heightened significance of infectious diseases that followed rapid migration and greater population density. Careful analysis, however, renders many of these global explanations problematic at best. By the time of the Civil War, industrialization, the factory system, and urbanization—to cite the most obvious—were still in their early stages. Given that the major decline in health indicators occurred in the antebellum decades, it is difficult to assign responsibility to them.[63]

Any interpretation of the decline in health indicators during the first two-thirds of the nineteenth century must be at best partial, given the complexities involved. Economic adversity, for example, probably did not play a direct role. The agricultural and commercial society of the eighteenth century was gradually being replaced by a more market-oriented economy even though the process was gradual. In 1810 72 percent of the workforce was engaged in agriculture; half a century later the share had fallen to 56 percent. The rise of a new economy was not necessarily directly related to urbanization; many of the early industrial changes occurred in rural and semirural areas. Not only was the economy growing, but real wages were increasing. To be sure, there were disparities between the wages of skilled and unskilled laborers as well as regional differences. Nevertheless, overall gains in wages between the 1830s and 1850s were in the range of 30–60 percent, a fact suggesting that the standard of living was rising rather than declining.[64]

If economic development had benefits, it also had costs that negatively affected health by intensifying the prevailing disease environment. The creation of a national transportation network increased both internal migration rates and interregional trade, and thus contributed to the movement of infectious pathogens from urban to rural and semirural regions, where more susceptible populations resided. Movement into new areas promoted environmental changes that enhanced the significance of such debilitating and sometimes fatal dis-

eases as malaria and various forms of dysentery. The diffused workplaces of the eighteenth century were slowly replaced by artisan
workshops and factories, which concentrated employees in surroundings more conducive to the spread of infectious diseases. Moreover,
the humid and dusty conditions that prevailed in many mills helped
to disseminate tuberculosis and other pulmonary disorders. Similarly,
the emergence of public schools facilitated the spread of infectious
diseases among children. Studies of children during these years also
demonstrate that morbidity and mortality rates varied inversely with
the birthrate; child deaths increased with the number of siblings. Immigration of lower socioeconomic groups from Ireland from the
1830s to the 1850s exacerbated the prevailing disease environment,
particularly in urban areas. Children of foreign-born parents in urban
areas, for example, were considerably smaller than children of native-
born parents; the same held true for birthweights. The Civil War
added to the burden of disease, although its effects were limited
largely to those born several decades earlier.[65]

For much of the nineteenth century infectious diseases continued to
play the major role in shaping morbidity and mortality patterns. Such
diseases not only resulted in high mortality rates, but also may have
had a significant impact on individual development. Certain infectious diseases in the mother could have easily damaged the fetus. In
infancy, moreover, exposure to certain pathogens retards growth and
reduces lung capacity, which in turn may result in respiratory disorders and heart disease in later life. The high prevalence of chronic diarrhea during these decades also served to deplete the body of vital
nutrients and reduce their absorption. The ensuing loss of appetite
only compounded nutritional problems. A decline in meat consumption in the antebellum period may have led to maternal malnutrition
and anemia and thus to fetal malnutrition. Above all, the increasing
prevalence of infectious diseases could have reduced the nutrients
available for growth by diverting them to the struggle against these
diseases. Infectious disorders, in other words, not only took a direct
toll in lives, but may have helped to create nutritional problems that
under other circumstances might not have existed.[66]

In the nineteenth century Americans manifested pride in the material advances that characterized their nation's development. It is
ironic that material progress had, at least in the short and intermedi-

ate term, a negative effect on health. The decline in morbidity and mortality that was evident for much of the eighteenth century was reversed during the nineteenth century. Fundamental changes would be required to alter the infectious disease environment and to create new patterns of morbidity and mortality.

CHAPTER 7

Threats of Industry

"In reviewing the various employments by which man obtains his bread by the sweat of his brow," Dr. Benjamin W. McCready noted in 1837 in a pioneering work on occupational diseases,

> we are struck by the fact that various as is their nature, there is nothing in the great majority of them which is not compatible with health and longevity. With the exception of a few occupations in which the operative is exposed to the inhalation which mechanically irritates the lungs, and a few others in which he suffers from the poisonous nature of the materials which he works in, his complaints arise from causes which might be obviated. It is inattention, ignorance or bad habits on his part, or a rate of wages so low as to leave him time insufficient for repose or recreation, or finally the faulty construction of his dwelling or workshop, that produce the majority of his ailments.[1]

Yet even as McCready was publishing his sanguine analysis, economic and technological changes were beginning to magnify some occupational risks to health. After 1800 the relatively simple rural economy of colonial America was replaced by a new agrarian and commercial economy, which in turn gave way after midcentury to an emerging industrialized society. The changes that were in the process of creating a new economy had a profound impact upon people's lives. To be sure, Americans enjoyed a steadily rising standard of living, even though periods of relative prosperity alternated with increasingly severe economic depressions. But the very forces that held out the promise of a better life also transformed the workplace in ways that sometimes had adverse consequences for many workers. The rise of new industries and technologies in the latter part of the nineteenth century magnified older, and created novel, occupational risks. These took a variety of forms. The most important were dusty environments, unsafe machinery, the use of toxic substances, and crowded workplaces that enhanced the ability to spread infectious diseases. Although the vastness and diversity of occupational diseases precludes comprehensive coverage, some representative examples will suffice to demonstrate the complex and close relationship between industrial change and occupational disease.

▼   ▼   ▼

Occupational and industrial diseases have a long history. All human activities, after all, have consequences, if only because there is an inseparable relationship among behavior, environment, and health. Some occupations only marginally affected health patterns; some had deleterious consequences; and in others the effects were beneficial.

Awareness of job-related health hazards was by no means unknown. Scattered references to the dangers of certain occupations began appearing with regularity as early as the fifteenth century. By 1700 Bernadino Ramazzini, an Italian professor of medicine, published *De Morbis Artificum Ciatriba,* one of the earliest works on the subject. Within five years the book was translated into English under the title *A Treatise of the Diseases of Tradesmen, Shewing the Various Influence of Particular Trades upon the State of Health; with the Best Methods to Avoid or Correct it, and Useful Hints Proper to Be Minded in Regulating the Cure of All Diseases Incident to Tradesmen.*[2]

In the early nineteenth century concern about some job-related diseases began to mount. This concern was particularly evident in England, a nation that had pioneered in creating new methods of production, altering work relationships, and transforming the workplace. A decade before Edwin Chadwick's famous *Report on the Sanitary Condition of the Labouring Classes* (1842), Charles Turner Thackrah, an English physician, published *The Effects of Arts, Trades and Professions, and of Civic States and Habits of Living, on Health and Longevity.* Thackrah called attention to medical problems associated with certain trades in Leeds, a burgeoning manufacturing community. He pointed out that in 1821 there was 1 death out of 67.5 persons in Ripon (a town that lacked manufactures) and 1 out of 74 in Pickering Lythe (an agricultural district). In Leeds, by contrast, the comparable figure was 1 out of 55, which amounted to an excess of 321 deaths. Thackrah estimated that "at least 450 persons die annually in the borough of Leeds, from the injurious effects of manufactories, the crowded state of the population, and the consequent bad habits of life!" Nor was it possible to overlook "the impaired health, the lingering ailments, the premature decay, mental and corporeal, of nine-tenths of the survivors."[3]

In the United States, by contrast, the contribution of diseases associated with the workplace was minimal from the seventeenth to midnineteenth century. In the South, to be sure, slaves employed in rice and hemp cultivation were at risk because of the conditions under which such crops were grown. Similarly, seamen faced a variety of hazards. Irregular and harsh climates, the absence of appropriate wearing apparel, long hours of work, inadequate diets, cramped and unsanitary living quarters, cruel treatment by superiors, and exposure to contagious diseases in foreign ports made seafaring a particularly dangerous occupation. The absence of social ties in port and high levels of alcoholism contributed further to high morbidity and mortality rates.[4] Though less fraught with dangers, other occupations—including some related to agriculture or associated with various trades—had their own unique risks.

Nor was the colonial period entirely free from the use of such toxic substances as lead. Exposure to high levels of lead has adverse effects on both the central and peripheral nervous systems, and there is evidence that renal functioning can be damaged. Lead poisoning among children leads to behavioral changes and impaired learning ability. "Dry gripes"—one of the original designations of lead poisoning—was associated with the production of rum. The use of lead in distilleries led to high levels of the mineral in the finished product. Those who drank large quantities of rum often suffered as a result. Pewter kitchenware (composed of tin and lead) employed in the preparation and serving of food also contributed to lead poisoning. Benjamin Franklin knew of lead poisoning among typesetters as well as those involved in other occupations in which lead was used. Qualitative evidence indicates that lead poisoning existed among colonial Americans. Although there was a substantial literature from earlier times describing the dangers of the metal, interest in controlling its use had waxed and waned over the centuries.[5]

In many ways the growing concern with occupationally related diseases in the early nineteenth century was part of a larger preoccupation with general health problems related to environmental and living conditions, particularly in urban areas. One indication of this concern was the decision in 1835 by the Medical Society of the State of New York to offer an annual prize for the best essay dealing with the "influences of trades, professions and occupations in the United States in the production of disease." Two years later twenty-four-year-old Dr. Benjamin W. McCready was declared the winner. McCready had received his M.D. from Columbia's College of Physicians and Surgeons in New York City and served briefly as a house physician at the New York Hospital.

Published in 1837 in the *Transactions of the Medical Society of the State of New York,* McCready's work was the first detailed analysis of occupational health written by an American. At that time industrial changes had yet to transform the workplace. Indeed, McCready suggested that the poor health of workers in certain occupations was due as much to external circumstances as to working conditions. Ill-ventilated housing, intemperance, lack of exercise, and inadequate diets were contributory factors that could not be ignored. A significant exception involved those employed as painters. "They are in general sallow and unhealthy in their appearance, and subject to nervous and gastric diseases," he wrote. Those who painted what was called "dead white" (a mixture of white lead and turpentine) were particularly vulnerable, and they suffered nausea, vomiting, dizziness, and headaches. Excessive use of alcohol by painters only compounded the poisonous influence of lead.[6]

McCready's treatise was based on a reading of medical authors, personal observation, common sense, and conventional wisdom. Like others of his generation, he believed that agricultural pursuits were the "healthiest, and the most natural of all employments." Pure air, moderate exercise, and an abundant and nutritious diet ensured that agricultural occupations would maximize health. Consumption, for example, was less prevalent in the country than in the city. "Pure air and active exercise . . . prevent the development of the disease; and experience is not wanting to prove . . . [that] the same agents afford the best means of retarding its progress."[7]

McCready conceded that certain occupations posed serious health risks. Those who labored on railroads and canals, he noted, were exposed to "malarious diseases." Similarly, the conditions under which seamen worked led to health-related problems. There was little evidence to suggest, however, that factory work per se was harmful. Unlike their English counterparts, American factories were not concentrated in cities, nor did they rely on steam power. They tended rather to be dispersed throughout the countryside and used water power from streams and rivers. Mortality rates in manufacturing villages, McCready suggested, were no higher than in rural districts.[8]

Each occupation, McCready observed, had unique circumstances that affected health. Tailors, for example, spent their days in confined quarters, and the position of their bodies was "exceedingly unfavorable." Digestive troubles and phthisis were common, and relatively few survived beyond the age of 60. In comparable occupations—shoemaking, dressmaking—similar conditions prevailed. Those in the printing trade, by contrast, were more favorably situated, although "varicose veins and ulcers of the lower extremities" were common because of the need to stand constantly. Butchers were "generally healthy" and often long-lived, "but the fulness of their diet exposes them to apoplexy, and renders them more liable to inflammatory disease." Carpenters usually lived to old age; their greatest risks came from work accidents. Professional men—physicians, clergymen, professors, literary figures—survived the longest. Because their "intellect" was "cultivated to the neglect and injury of the body," diseases of the brain were more frequent than among the laboring class, and "apoplexy and paralysis in many instances take the place of fevers and inflammatory affections."[9]

In this relatively sanguine analysis, McCready admitted that there were a few occupations in which workers were exposed to dangerous fumes or poisonous substances. But there was nothing in the great majority of occupations that was "not compatible with health and longevity." Most causes of ill health could be avoided. Bad habits, low wages, and inappropriate dwellings and workshops were responsible for a majority of ailments. Intemperance was also "an evil of wider influence."[10]

"Many of the evils incident to the occupations of civilized society," McCready concluded, could "be remedied, and others essentially alleviated." Yet a note of caution was in order. Anxiety and striving after wealth might have contributed to prosperity, but these very same attributes often had a negative effect upon health. "Every deterioration of the general health of the parent is transmitted to their offspring," and the consequences of a progressive deterioration could have devastating consequences. McCready had "little doubt that the pale and unhealthy appearance of our population" was due "to the very causes which have contributed to the rapid rise and unexampled prosperity of our country," notably the striving after wealth and the rage for speculation. Indeed, the preoccupation with business precluded leisurely meals and led to a general dyspepsia and permanent functional derangement of the stomach. In offering such an analysis, McCready was implicitly criticizing the materialism of his countrymen and calling upon them to behave in ways that were consistent with the moral and physiological laws that governed all human beings.[11]

McCready's pioneering work was less a commentary on occupational disease than a treatise on behavior and environment. He emphasized a public health approach that conflated working and living conditions. The diversity of the economy and the variety of settings in which people worked made it virtually impossible for him to develop a classification system that separated home and workplace and specified diseases that were strictly a function of occupation.[12] To be sure, the economy during the first half of the nineteenth century was beginning to experience modest structural and technological change, which in turn tended to sharpen divisions between workers and employers and to create new categories of labor. Nevertheless, industrial development at that time was at best uneven, and a large majority of laborers exercised considerable control over their workplaces.

At the beginning of the nineteenth century, for example, tradesmen constituted nearly half of Philadelphia's workforce, and no single occupation was dominant. Between 1800 and 1850 the city's population increased from 81,000 to more than 400,000. Although immigration was by no means insignificant, population growth was fueled primarily by migration from rural areas and by natural increase. At midcentury Philadelphia ranked second only to New York City as a center for commodity production. Yet industrialization was by no means synonymous with large-scale factories. In Philadelphia production took place in diverse work environments. Factories drawing power from steam or water employed less than a third of the workforce, and they were limited to textiles, machine tools, and iron. The remainder worked in manufactories (places that employed more than twenty-five persons, but were without power sources), small sweatshops, artisan or neighborhood shops, or else made their living by "outwork." Nearly 90 percent of the labor force worked in firms that employed fewer than twenty-five persons. Philadelphia, like many other urban and rural communities, was, in the words of Bruce Laurie, "a fascinating blend of the old, the new, and the transitional."[13] From these circumstances it is clear that many of the occupational diseases subsequently associated with industrial and technological change were not present before 1850.

To suggest that the factory system of production was not typical in the early nineteenth century is not to say that it was nonexistent. In Massachusetts, for example, the cotton textile industry, which emerged after the War of 1812, was organized in factories utilizing automatic machinery and water power. These factories employed a large number of young women between 17 and 24 years of age. The average length of service was four years, after which these women left the mills to marry. Contemporary descriptions of conditions in these mills varied sharply. Michel Chevalier, a Frenchmen who visited the United States in 1834, described conditions at the Lowell mill—perhaps the most famous of its kind in the United States—in favorable terms. "On seeing them pass through the streets in the morning and evening and at their meal-hours, neatly dressed; on finding their scarfs, and shawls, and green silk hoods which they wear as a shelter from the sun and dust (for Lowell is not yet paved), hanging up in the factories amidst the flowers and shrubs, which they cultivate, I said to myself, this, then, is not like Manchester; and when I was informed of the rate of their wages, I understood that it was not at all like Manchester." The companies, he noted, exercised "the most careful supervision over these girls," who were expected to be honest and industrious, observe the Sabbath, and avoid intoxicating beverages. Company housing was generally supervised by widows, who were responsible for the conduct of their boarders. Although Chevalier had little to say about the health of these laborers, the implication of his favorable portrait was that occupational diseases were generally absent. Eight years later Charles Dickens described Lowell in similar terms, but added a caveat. "It is their station to work," he observed. "And they *do* work. They labour in these mills, upon an average, twelve hours a day, which is unquestionably work, and pretty tight work too."[14]

Some descriptions of factory working conditions were less positive. Seth Luther, a famous labor reformer, was prone to point to the evils of the factory system and its deleterious effect on the health of workers. In 1834 the New England Association of Farmers, Mechanics, and Other Workingmen criticized the conditions under which factory operatives labored, and its members demanded regulatory legislation. Cheap manufactured articles "are no recompense for their injury to the health and the morals of the rising generation," their address read. "To look at the pale and dirty, and spiritless beings, as they pour out of the factory to their hurried meals at the sound of a bell; and, although inhumanly stinted as to time, to see the lazy motion of their jaded limbs, and the motionless expression of their woebegone countenances, must give a pang to the feeling heart which can never be forgotten." Dr. Charles Douglass, president of the association, was equally harsh in his portrayal of the conditions under which Lowell workers labored and of the adverse effects on their health.[15]

Many descriptions of mill conditions, Dr. Josiah Quincy noted in a study prepared for the newly established American Medical Association in 1849, came from "politicians and partialists," who "have made statements and counter-statements, and too often, such only as would best make capital in favouring the views of each." Despite the availability of morbidity and mortality data for mill operatives as well as Lowell residents, Quincy found it difficult to come to any definitive conclusions about the relationship between factory work and health. The mill-worker population was quite unstable. Although a small number had worked in the mill for more than a decade, the average was only nine months. Some went from one mill to another; some went to other manufacturing establishments; some married; and others returned to their original homes. Under these circumstances Quincy admitted that it was not possible to determine "how many leave on account of ill health, nor how many of these become ill while connected with the mills, nor how many of these can trace the cause of declining health to influences concomitant with their employment."[16]

Quincy conceded that mill labor was "light, but constant" and that workers had sufficient rest as well as an adequate diet. Nevertheless, he rejected the claim that the mills kept a constant temperature and provided well-ventilated facilities. In his eyes the variable temperatures and inadequate ventilation were "the most prolific source of deteriorated health in the adjuncts of factory labor." The air in both the factory and dormitories was stagnant. In the former the admixture of gases and suspension of dust particles contributed to pulmonary and respiratory disorders. Indeed, English physicians had already identified a category they designated "spinners' phthisis"—a "distressing pulmonary irritation from the dust and filaments" found in textile mills.[17]

In 1877 a British physician concerned with the breathing problems of textile mill workers created the new diagnostic category of byssinosis (subsequently given the name brown lung). This disease was related to the presence of cotton, flax, and hemp dust. In the acute form the symptoms included a cough and dyspepsia. In the chronic stage the pulmonary disease often led to total disability and death. Textile mill environments were also conducive to respiratory disorders and tuberculosis. Whether byssinosis was a serious problem in early New England textile mills remains an unresolved issue. Although few employees may have worked long enough to develop chronic lung problems, Quincy's preoccupation with ventilation and dust suggests that the mill environment was not unrelated to morbidity even though he also insisted that workers were "as healthy, perhaps, as the aggregate of all other classes."[18]

▾ ▾ ▾

Generally speaking, New England textile factories were atypical work environments in the early nineteenth century. Most production took place in smaller settings, and new occupational diseases were relatively rare. The most important factor limiting industrialization was the relative shortage of power. Before 1850 manufacturing enterprises depended on wood or water for power. Dependence on water to generate power circumscribed both the size and location of factories. To generate steam power by burning wood as an alternative source of power presented other formidable problems. Wood was used primarily in home heating and construction. Timber may have been bountiful, but it was not inexhaustible. As late as the mid-nineteenth century the average American family annually burned approximately eighteen cords of wood. Along the eastern seaboard forests slowly receded. The rising costs of transporting wood, its uses as a fuel for the developing railroad system and as a primary building material, and diminishing supplies meant that it could not become the foundation of an industrial economy.[19]

If America was to become an industrial nation, other sources of power had to be found. Sporadic fuel shortages in the early nineteenth century led to the exploitation of anthracite coal in Pennsylvania. The availability of rivers and subsequently canals to move coal and its use to generate steam power, which in turn drove factories, steamboats, and locomotives, hastened the emergence of the coal industry.

During the latter half of the nineteenth century coal became the foundation of the burgeoning industrial economy. In 1800 Pennsylvania produced 250 tons of anthracite and 87,000 tons of bituminous coal. A half-century later the respective figures were 4.3 and 2.1 million tons. In 1900 the state's anthracite mines produced over 57 million tons and employed about 144,000 individuals each day. That same year the nation's bituminous mines employed over 304,000 workers and produced 212 million tons. By the turn of the century coal was the preeminent source of energy, and served as the basis for the rapid growth of a variety of important industries, including those producing iron and steel.[20]

That the mining of coal—as well as such metals as tin, lead, and iron—was a dangerous occupation was well known. Agricola's classic *De Re Metallica,* published in 1556, had chronicled some of the dangers to life and health posed by mining, and his work was followed by many other treatises. Whatever their persuasion, all emphasized two primary risks—pulmonary disorders and accidents. Such threats to health and life, however, did not deter the exploitation of these natural resources, and during the seventeenth and eighteenth centuries the mining of coal and other metals increased dramatically in England and western Europe.[21] The foundation of industrialization, mining was perhaps the most striking example of an occupation that was associated with what may best be termed "dust" diseases. It also increased the frequency of industrial accidents and made them a more significant element in morbidity and mortality.

From the seventeenth to early nineteenth centuries coal was mined by cutting a pit into a hill in which there was an exposed vein or digging it out of the side of a ravine. By 1850, however, such simple quarries had been exhausted, and mining moved deep underground.

Four alternative methods of gaining access to coal were available, but all involved different ways of connecting underground tunnels to a surface access. A shaft was sunk to a vein of coal, and tunnels extending in all directions were constructed. The extraction of the coal was relatively simple; miners blasted coal in tunnels and loaded it onto cars, which were then conveyed to the surface.[22] Much of the work was done by hand; mechanization did not become common until the early twentieth century. The large capital investment required for the mining of coal contributed to the diminution of workers' control of their jobs.

Coal mining was (and remains) an especially dangerous occupation. The depth of shafts required adequate means of ventilation to assure a steady supply of oxygen as well as a means of disposing of the smoke and carbon dioxide from powder charges and miners' lamps, the effluvia from humans and mules, and the methane gas released from the coal. The latter was particularly dangerous, since it could produce explosions. The presence of coal dust only magnified the dangers of methane gas. Moreover, the constant accumulation of water from surface and underground sources required methods to prevent flooding. Roof and tunnel collapses added to these hazards.

The greatest risk to health and life in mines came from the omnipresent dusty environment. In the early nineteenth century there was but a vague recognition that coal mining as an occupation was detrimental to health, a reflection of the fact that surface mining was intrinsically less risky. Medical authors rarely made reference to the morbidity that was characteristic in this occupation. Indeed, when Thackrah published the first edition of his book in 1831, he noted that few occupations had been studied to determine their relationships to health and longevity. In reviewing his book, the prestigious *Edinburgh Medical and Surgical Journal* decried the inattention to occupational diseases. "English medical literature has been till now destitute of a single general treatise on the diseases of trades and professions."[23]

During the latter half of the nineteenth century medical investigators began to develop an awareness of the health risks posed by mining. Miners' disease went under several clinical labels—miners' asthma, miners' consumption, and anthracosis. There was general agreement that those who labored in mines suffered from a disabling chronic condition that often ended in death. Its symptoms—shortness of breath, chest pain, cough—were common to a variety of respiratory and pulmonary disorders. Anatomically, however, miners' disease was marked by the presence of necrotic cavities in the lung. Melanoptysius—black sputum from a ruptured lesion—was the clinical sign of what at present is known as coal miners' pneumoconiosis, or CWP. Yet etiological confusion, which was related in part to the absence of mechanisms to collect statistical data, continued to prevail. Some investigators attributed ill health among miners not to coal dust, but to a stagnant environment harboring decaying substances that gave rise to miasmas. More important, medical investigators were preoccupied with the internal damage to lungs at the individual level; epidemiological studies that would determine the distribution of miners' disease in the workforce were largely absent. Nor were state or federal authorities concerned with the collection of statistical data dealing with the health of particular occupational groups; they lacked the administrative capacity to study the prevalence of dust diseases. Indeed, in the early twentieth century almost all physicians denied that the dusty environment in coal mines was harmful. Some suggested that expectoration of black sputum was merely a way in which the lungs rid themselves of carbon deposits. Equally notable was the allegation that coal dust protected miners against tuberculosis. British research led to the conceptualization of CWP as a distinct clinical entity. Beginning in 1943, Britain accepted thousands of compensation claims by miners.[24]

Despite the lack of a diagnostic category for miners' disease and of data on the prevalence of dust hazards, there is persuasive evidence that coal mining was the nation's most dangerous occupation. "Any one," wrote journalist Henry Sheafer in 1879, "who has . . . watched the thick clouds of dust which sometimes envelop the huge coal-breakers of the anthracite region so completely as almost to hide them from sight can form an idea of the injurious effect upon health of constantly working in such an atmosphere." England, which had an elaborate data-gathering office in place by 1836, had amassed a substantial body of evidence about the health risks of mining. These data demonstrated that miners had far higher morbidity and mortality rates than those in other occupations. Moreover, the differences increased with the worker's age.[25] American physicians and other professionals were quite familiar with English data dealing with the risks of mining.

In 1918 Frederick L. Hoffman, an influential statistician at the Prudential Life Insurance Company, undertook a survey of the biomedical literature dealing with respiratory diseases in the dusty trades for the U.S. Bureau of Labor Statistics. Hardly a defender of workers or unions, Hoffman nevertheless concluded that "all inorganic dust in industrial occupations demands the most effective safeguarding of the employees against unnecessary hazards to health and life." In 1914 American mines employed a total of 921,000 individuals. Of this number, 793,000 worked in coal mines, and 639,000 were employed underground. Hoffman was critical of the methodology of those who insisted that the impregnation of coal dust was not injurious to their health. "Investigations made in this country," he noted, "are quite conclusive that more or less health-injurious consequences must in course of time result from an extensive coal-dust infiltration." Although Hoffman provided no prevalence estimates for CWP, he did allude to census and other data demonstrating that mining was an extremely dangerous occupation, a conclusion that applied to virtually all occupations in which dust was a factor.[26]

Without doubt the greatest threat to worker health in the late nineteenth and early twentieth centuries came from atmospheric pollution in mines, factories, and workshops. The growing application of machine technologies to production dramatically increased the amount of dust and fumes. These contaminants included metallic and mineral dust, vegetable fiber dust, animal dust, organic dust, and mixed dusts. Data from the census of 1910 indicated that approximately 4 million out of about 44 million workers were employed in settings in which exposure to harmful dusts was common; the actual figure was probably much higher. Although miners were at the greatest risk, workers in the metal trades, textiles factories, clothing workshops—to cite only some of the more obvious examples—worked in surroundings that maximized exposure. In his study of dust diseases, Hoffman identified 117 occupations in which exposure to dust was common.[27]

In the metallurgical industries, for example, ore (whatever its composition) had to be broken or crushed in preparation for smelting. Throughout the process workers were exposed to dust. Although the term silicosis was not widely used before World War I, it had long been known that hard-rock miners, cutters, potters, glassworkers, sandblasters, and foundry workers suffered from serious and life-threatening respiratory disorders. Indeed, the improvement of ore-re-duction methods in the latter part of the nineteenth century led to finer dust and a corresponding increase in the mortality rate of work-ers. "Whether we call the cases fibroid phthisis, chronic interstitial pneumonia, stonecutters' phthisis, miners' consumption, or chali-cosis, depending on the character and amount of foreign matter, or classify them under the generic name of pneumoconiosis, makes but little difference," Dr. William W. Betts wrote in 1900; all were part of a seamless pathological process. Indeed, some time generally had to elapse before symptoms appeared. In one instance an employee worked for eighteen months without manifesting any clinical symp-toms. At that point, according to Betts, "shortness of breath, loss of appetite, fatigue on slight exertion, and emaciation" became no-ticeable.

> The cough and expectoration were slight for months. He has now been in the city for about a year. The pathologic process continues and his symptoms do not improve, though from present indications he will live some months. His clinical history and physical examina-tion reveal a condition typical in fibroid phthisis, and in marked contrast to the poor fellows who after three months' exposure died within a year. Thus we have all grades . . . depending on the general constitution and natural resisting power of the men, also largely on the amount of foreign matter inhaled.[28]

Dust diseases were found as well in textile mills. Although milling involved a series of operations and a variety of machines, the process of turning baled cotton into yarn or cloth was not complex. Initially the baled cotton was cleaned and raked. The resulting slivers were converted into yarn, which was then woven into cloth. One of the pe-culiar characteristics of cotton is that it requires high humidity for snapping to be avoided. Consequently, moisture was constantly added to the mill environment. Southern mills were particularly damp and hot because the moisture and heat from the machinery was superimposed upon an already hot humid climate. The outstanding characteristics of mills were the never-ending presence of dust and an extraordinarily high level of noise. The humid, dusty, and noisy set-ting was also conducive to high accident rates involving the loss of fingers or limbs. Equally notable was the lack of concern for hygiene and sanitation. Most mills had sufficient water closets, but they were rarely maintained. In one southern mill the floor of the men's toilet was covered with "quids of tobacco and murky pools of tobacco juice together with pieces of paper . . . [and were] wet and slimy, and the odor decidedly offensive." Spitting, a characteristic behavioral trait, and the use of a common cup for drinking facilitated the dissemination of infectious diseases. Most early twentieth-century observers agreed that cotton mill workers suffered health problems even though the precise causes of elevated morbidity and mortality rates remained problematic.[29]

▼   ▼   ▼

An industrial economy rested on access to raw materials, many of which were extracted from beneath the earth's surface. The rise of mining industries was accompanied by a dramatic increase in accidents that maimed and sometimes killed workers. Coal mining perhaps best illustrates this generalization. Official statistics on mine accidents were not collected until 1869. But according to data gathered in 1858 by a correspondent for the *Miners' Journal,* a Pennsylvania mine worker had less than an even chance of surviving for twelve years, and could expect to be killed or permanently crippled in six. With about 600 workers in 1850, the St. Clair shafts could expect on average 108 accidents and 36 fatalities each year. Indeed, the fatality rate in Pennsylvania anthracite mines was two to three times that in England.[30] Those who labored in the mines had few illusions about their work. The reminiscences of one miner were revealing:

> Considering the numerous accidents in mining and the dangers involved, and comparing the risks of a miner with those of a soldier, Mr. Maguire used to assert that a miner is a soldier every day he works, while the man in the army is only taking risks when he goes to the front, which is only occasionally. Looking back over a long period of mining, the dangers he recalled having passed through were very, very many, and he realized that the miner may expect, in the natural course of events, to ultimately meet his death in the performance of his duties.

Mine accidents also had a ripple effect upon families. In one mining community in 1870, 72 of the 112 men killed had wives; their deaths left 72 widows and 252 children. For these families survival became uncertain, because the community provided no relief except confinement in the poorhouse.[31]

The worst American mine disaster up to that time occurred at the

Steuben Shaft at Avondale, Pennsylvania, in 1869, which had only recently opened. On a Monday morning 108 men began sending coal up from the bottom of a 300-foot shaft. A fire broke out, and the shaft quickly filled with burning timber and coal as well as twisted metal. Two rescuers descended but were themselves quickly asphyxiated. Three days later 110 bodies were recovered. A few had been harmed by the fire and blast, but most had been asphyxiated or killed by smoke inhalation. Avondale was but the first of many similar disasters. From 1878 to 1910, 242 major disasters took the lives of 5,835 workers.[32] The mood surrounding these disasters was graphically caught in the reminiscences of a West Virginia miner:

> Not a week passed but what tragedy touched some home. When a housewife . . . chanced to glance through the window and see a group of miners bearing an improvised stretcher between them, she spread the alarm. In a twinkling women were on the porches, wiping hands on aprons, calling to one another . . . Anxious, distraint women and children, uncertain of the fate of their loved ones, demanded to know the identity of the victim. When the dreaded news was revealed, the women gathered around their hysterical sister and offered comfort. Presently they returned to their household duties, thankful that a merciful God had seen fit to once again spare husband, or son, or brother.[33]

Major disasters, however, accounted for only a small proportion of mine fatalities. From 1884 to 1912 nearly 43,000 miners died from accidents. Of this number, roof and coal falls accounted for 20,287 deaths, explosions for 8,240, and haulage for 5,169. Mine fatalities were much higher in the United States than in Europe. Belgium, Great Britain, and Germany had fatality rates equal to those of the United States before 1900, but American rates rose in 1896–1908, whereas rates in the other nations declined because of the passage of regulatory laws pertaining to safety. By 1908 the fatality rate in the United States was 3.64 deaths per 1,000 workers, as compared with .88 for Belgium, 1.24 for Great Britain, and 1.71 for Germany.[34] The fatality rate grossly underestimated the risks of this occupation, for it did not include major injuries that maimed and incapacitated miners for life.

Some of the hazards presented by coal mining were to some extent replicated in other emerging industries. Railroad work is one such example. By the end of the nineteenth century railroads occupied a crucial place in the American economy. Before 1850 inland waterways (including canals) were the primary means of moving raw materials and finished goods. In 1845, for example, the Erie Canal in New York State carried about half of the 2 million tons of freight moved by waterways. Canals and rivers, however, had inherent drawbacks; they did not serve many areas, and many were closed during the winter months. Railroads had none of these handicaps, and track mileage expanded rapidly. In 1830 the United States had only 23 miles of track; sixty years later there were over 200,000 miles of track. Railroads not only moved people, raw materials, and finished goods, but also stimulated the development of basic industries, because they consumed large quantities of coal, iron, and steel. By the turn of the century railroads employed more than a million workers.[35]

Railroad work in the nineteenth century was inherently dangerous. The primitive character of railroad technology and the conditions of work combined to create a variety of risks to health and life. Most railroads operated on a single track. The absence of sophisticated scheduling and signaling systems magnified the frequency of collisions. Poorly constructed roadbeds, bridges, and overpasses only exacerbated occupational risks. Boiler explosions, fires from engine sparks, the lack of automatic braking and coupling systems, and exposed trains that in winter could lead to frostbite only added to the problems of work. Nor were those who labored in machine and repair shops, switching or coupling cars, or loading bulky freight insulated from the risks of the workplace. A veteran brakeman of twenty-five years described the hazards of his job to a congressional committee in 1890:

> Say, for instance, it is a bad night—what we call a blind night on the road—sleeting, raining, snowing, etc. We hear the call for "down brakes." Of course we cannot always be on top of the train. During cold weather we go into the caboose occasionally to warm ourselves. We are called out by a signal of "down brakes." We get out on top of the train. We find that the tops of the cars are completely covered with sleet. In attempting to get at those brakes a great many brakeman lose their lives, slip off the cars and again, even if they do reach the brakes, it is more often the case than it is not that they find that the brakes are frozen up, and they cannot twist them. That again occasions danger . . . As no brakes are set, all will depend on the engine to stop the train, and if the train was going with any speed it would take some time to stop it.[36]

Before the creation of the Interstate Commerce Commission (ICC) in 1887, aggregate statistics on accidents and deaths among railroad workers were nonexistent. Some states with railroad commissions occasionally collected data. In New York in 1855, for example, 1 worker out of 546 died, while 1 in 439 was injured. Four states in the 1870s reported a range from 1 in 272 to 1 in 695 killed and 1 in 97 to 1 in 571 injured. In 1889 the ICC began to collect data. During the year ending June 30, 1890, 749,000 men were employed at one time or another by the railroads. Among this group there were 2,425 fatalities and 22,396 injuries; 1 out of every 309 workers was killed and 1 in 33 injured. In addition, there were 3,884 deaths and 6,631 injuries among passengers and "other persons." Thus railroad work and travel appeared to become more dangerous toward the end of the nineteenth century, perhaps because of the increase in passengers and traffic.[37]

That the risks of accidents in many industries were increasing in the late nineteenth century is clear. But the absence of prevalence data tended to blur public concern. As late as 1926 Ethelbert Stewart, commissioner of labor statistics in the U.S. Department of Labor, admitted that machinery for the "collection of adequate and reliable reports on industrial accidents in the United States unfortunately does not exist." In 1921 his agency attempted to secure returns from the states of all fatal and reportable nonfatal accidents for 1921, 1923, and 1924. Incomplete results, Stewart noted, revealed 8,764 fatalities and 1,209,151 injuries during 1921; the comparable figures for 1923 were 9,862 and 1,496,197, and for 1924, 10,268 and 1,531,104 (coal mine and many interstate railroad accidents were not included). Estimates by the Bureau of Labor Statistics suggested that in any given year there were 2,453,418 industrial accidents. Of these, 21,232 were fatal, 1,728 resulted in total disability, and 105,629 in permanent partial disability. More than 227 million days of work were lost, with a commensurable loss in wages of over one billion dollars. Although Stewart thought that accidents were "steadily on the increase," he could produce no authoritative data to support his generalization, nor did he offer any incidence estimates.[38]

▼ ▼ ▼

The rise of an industrial economy often led to the use of new materials as well as accelerating the use of familiar ones. Some of the materials that played crucial roles in industrialization possessed toxic properties. Lead is an obvious example. Known since ancient times, lead had certain virtues because of its softness and plasticity. It was used in pipes and ceramics, and in the eighteenth and nineteenth centuries was even incorporated into the medical pharmacopoeia. By the late nineteenth century it had found many new uses in an economy receptive to novel technologies, thus leading to a dramatic increase in the mining and smelting of lead. In 1801 perhaps 1,000 tons of lead were produced from ore; a century later production had reached 371,000 tons.

Those involved in mining, producing, and using lead were at risk. Lead miners, noted Frederick Hoffman, suffered from miners' phthisis, although he conceded that it was difficult to differentiate between the true form of pulmonary tuberculosis (a bacillary disease) and nontuberculosis fibroid lung disease. From the mine lead went to the smelter, where the workforce was exposed to lead in purer form. The mineral found a wide market, and producers and users—miners, painters, solderers, printers, potters, brass workers, plumbers, and construction workers, as well as a larger public—were exposed to its toxic qualities. Hospital admissions for lead poisoning became more common toward the end of the nineteenth century.[39]

In 1873 Allan McLane Hamilton, a physician who also served as a health inspector for New York City, investigated manufacturing establishments where lead and arsenic were used, including foundries, pie plants, and factories printing wallpaper. His report to the city's Board of Health also covered dusty environments and working conditions. Although he could find no cases of paralysis resulting from lead poisoning, he did concede that lead colic was more common. The appearance of printers, he noted, was "bad." In the factories he visited "the men seem to be generally anemic, and the children brought up in these places are weak and puny." In printing plants and wallpaper factories the air was full of dust containing lead and arsenic, which entered the nose, ears, mouth, and eyes, causing irritations and ulcerous sores. Conjunctivitis, rhinitis, epistaxis, and bronchitis were common.[40]

Although the dangers of lead had long been known, few factories took precautions to protect their workforce. In her investigations of lead poisoning in the early twentieth century, Alice Hamilton—one of the pioneers in the study of industrial diseases—provided a graphic description of an old Philadelphia factory producing white lead. She found exceptionally dangerous conditions and tracked down twenty-seven cases of lead poisoning among employees. Her letter to the foreman proposing remedial measures provided a graphic description of the dangerous factory environment. "As long as your roller room has piles of white lead on the floor and in open trucks," she wrote,

> you will always be having lead poisoning. You see you will never be able to make your men careful under those circumstances, for they get so used to dust and untidiness, that they do not know it when they see it. Make a rule that the floor must be kept clean and all white lead covered up . . .
>
> There is one matter that I want to speak about: the widow of one of your fatal cases told me that her husband contracted lead poisoning very quickly because he was doing an unusually dangerous piece of work. He was packing barrels and he was induced by the promise of extra pay to ram down the white lead in the barrel so as to be able to pack in an extra quantity. I hope this is no longer done at Wetherill's.[41]

Changes in modes of production brought more and more workers into job environments that jeopardized their health and safety. In 1870 180,000 persons were employed in mining and 2,750,000 in manufacturing, the hand trades, and construction. Forty years later the figures were 1,050,000 and 10,530,000, respectively. Some hazardous occupations were eliminated by technological innovation. Nailmakers, who were prone to "nailmakers' consumption"—a variant of silicosis caused by the presence of the dust that resulted from the grinding process—were one example. But in many industries work-related diseases were on the increase even before the end of the nineteenth century.[42]

Diseases of the workplace took many forms. In a few cases the use of chemicals with toxic properties had a severe impact upon workers' health. Hatmaking is a case in point. Mercury began to be used as early as the seventeenth century to make rabbit and hare furs—which were less expensive than more desirable beaver fur—more malleable. When hatmaking shifted from artisans' workshops to more mechanized factories, the risk of mercury poisoning increased. The absence of safety precautions and poor ventilation only magnified the dangers of mercury. Exposure to mercury among hatters led to ulceration of the gums, loosening of the teeth, and tremors of the upper extremities.[43]

By the early twentieth century the use of benzol and other chemical solvents in the manufacture of such materials as tin, rubber, leather, paints, and explosives had become common. When World War I resulted in a decline in imports and an accelerated demand for such materials, a commensurate increase in the use of benzol and other solvents followed. After the war the existing surplus of benzol led other industries to develop new applications, and more and more workers came into contact with the chemical. Exposure to benzol often results in aplastic anemia, a disease that impairs the ability of the bone marrow to generate red blood cells and is often fatal. When the relationship between benzol and aplastic anemia became apparent in the early twentieth century, medical explanations tended to focus on the role of individual "susceptibility" and inadequate personnel management. Such ambiguities notwithstanding, it is clear that the increased use of such toxic substances was playing a more important role in workers' morbidity and mortality.[44]

▾   ▾   ▾

Small workshops and even homes presented occupational risks. At that time ventilation received little attention from architects or builders; the high cost of land in urban areas led to the construction of buildings that lacked adequate ventilation. The use of such structures in the burgeoning clothing and other industries posed two mutually reinforcing threats to health. First, the work environment created a variety of occupational hazards. More important, the concentration of people in crowded quarters magnified the prevalence of infectious diseases.

Lower Manhattan in the late nineteenth and early twentieth centuries was perhaps an extreme but representative example of the impact of economic and technological change on health. It was the most densely populated urban area in the United States at that time. In parts of the lower East Side inhabited by Jewish immigrants, 300,000 persons lived in one square mile. Immigrants from eastern and southern Europe migrated to America in large numbers and provided much of the labor for the city's rapidly growing manufacturing enterprises.

By World War I nearly 10 percent of the nation's manufactured goods were produced in New York City. Most urban areas experienced a comparable expansion.[45]

Some production took place in home workshops located in tenement housing, which had originated in the middle of the nineteenth century. "It is the one hopeless form of tenement construction," the Tenement House Commission noted in 1894.

> It cannot be well ventilated, it cannot be well lighted; it is not safe in case of fire. It is built on a lot 25 feet wide by 100 or less in depth, with apartments for four families in each story . . . The stairway, made in the centre of the house, and the necessary walls and partitions reduce the width of the middle rooms (which serve as bedrooms for at least two people each) to 9 feet each at the most, and a narrow light and air shaft . . . still further lessens the floor space of these middle rooms. Direct light is only possible for the rooms at the front and rear. The middle rooms must borrow what light they can from dark hallways, the shallow shafts, and the rear rooms. Their air must pass through other rooms or the tiny shafts, and cannot but be contaminated before it reaches them. A five-story house of this character contains apartments for eighteen or twenty families, a population frequently amounting to 100 people, and sometimes increased by boarders or lodgers to 150 or more.

Such conditions magnified occupational health risks.[46]

By the beginning of the twentieth century there were at least six industrial groups in which home work was prominent: clothing, fur and leather, textiles, food, tobacco, and paper products. Contemporary observers were divided in their evaluation of home work. In 1874 Roger Tracy and Nathaniel Emerson reported to the Board of Health on working conditions in the cigarmaking trade. Although both factories and homes could be ventilated, the need to conserve heat resulted in closed windows and doors; the result was poor air circulation. Tobacco leaves, they concluded, did not act as fomites (articles that spread pathogens) nor did cigarmaking aid in the dissemination of contagious disease. Nevertheless, they found some evidence that cigarmaking might promote infertility among women. Five years later Tracy suggested that miscarriages were common among women working with tobacco, and reported that a French physician had found nicotine in the amniotic fluid. In his classic study

of New York City slums, Jacob Riis wrote that cigar workers looked
sallow as a result of the "all-pervading smell of tobacco," but were
not less healthy than other indoor workers.[47]

The production of clothing, which was concentrated either in
home workshops or in small factories, was New York City's most important industry. The industry had expanded dramatically with the
beginnings of Jewish emigration from eastern Europe after 1880.
Many Jews possessed tailoring skills acquired in Europe, which stood
them in good stead in the United States. The majority labored in the
needle trades, which began to satisfy an unprecedented demand for
mass-produced clothing.[48]

In both home workshops and factories, crowding and lack of ventilation were exacerbated by long hours, low wages, repetitive work,
and physical settings that placed severe strains on workers. The bulk
of the work, according to Riis, was done in tenements to which statu-
tory codes did not apply. A ride on the elevated railroad, he added,
was revealing.

> Every open window of the big tenements, that stand like a continu-
> ous brick wall on both sides of the way, gives you a glimpse of one
> of these shops . . . Men and women bending over their machines, or
> ironing clothes at the window, half naked . . . Morning, noon, or
> night, it makes no difference . . . in a Ludlow Street tenement . . .
> [f]ive men and a woman, two young girls, not fifteen, and a boy . . .
> are at the machines sewing knickerbockers . . . The floor is littered
> ankle-deep with half-sewn garments . . . The faces, hands, and arms
> to the elbows of everyone in the room are black with the color of
> the cloth on which they are working.

"Sweated labor," according to an editorial in the New York *Medical
Record* in 1908, "is, therefore, to a certain extent, a menace to the
health of the entire community, for those who perform this description of labor, as a rule, work under unsanitary conditions and receive
quite inadequate wages. Further, homework is the worst paid of the
sweated industries, and is usually accomplished under circumstances
which render it not only dangerous to the health of the workers
themselves but a distinct source of danger to the public at large."[49]

Specialized trades such as furmaking were also located in old tenements lacking adequate ventilation or separate drying rooms. Nearly
three-quarters of furs were dyed with harmful chemicals, and dust

from furs constituted an additional hazard. When a New York State commission examined a sample of workers in the furrier trade, they found only about 11 percent to be in good health; the remainder suffered from respiratory problems and allergic reactions related to fur dust as well as to skin diseases from dyes. A federal study in 1913 that included a much larger sample of workers in the clothing trades generally concluded that rates for respiratory and digestive disorders, hearing impairment from workshop noise, and spinal curvatures were higher among this occupational group than in the general population.[50]

The experience of New York's immigrant Jewish population was similar to that of other ethnic groups arriving from southern and eastern Europe. A physician on the staff of the Massachusetts General Hospital in Boston who was appointed to inspect clothing workshops and factories in 1907 reported comparable conditions. In studying the finishing of pants—done largely by Italian women—he emphasized the overcrowded, ill-ventilated, and unsanitary conditions of the homes in which they worked. Such an environment, combined with inadequate nutrition, made them susceptible to various illnesses, particularly tuberculosis and other infectious diseases.[51]

Many trades were conducted in workshop and factory settings that ostensibly came under regulatory codes designed to modify working conditions that were inimical to the health and safety of workers. Inadequate enforcement diluted the effectiveness of such codes. More important, in the early twentieth century it was difficult to identify specific occupational hazards and to separate them from such general environmental factors as housing and behavior. Neither states nor the federal government possessed the administrative capacity to identify many hazards (which was and is extraordinarily difficult under any circumstances). Equally significant, occupational diseases often had an ambiguous character. Many did not manifest themselves immediately. Symptoms sometimes emerged years later, so that it was difficult to relate diseases to specific job experiences. Workers, particularly males, had few contacts with physicians who might have interpreted their symptoms as a function of their occupation. The fact that physicians were preoccupied with infectious diseases as well as their inability to treat them tended to enforce a feeling of skepticism about the redemptive powers of the profession. The masculine trait of "toughing it out" and a fear of unemployment led many workers to persevere on the job as long as possible. Geographic and job mobility, especially among the less skilled, also tended to mask some occupational risks.

Often etiological explanations for occupational diseases centered less on the job and more upon the behavior and living conditions of workers. Medical education largely ignored the category of occupational disease. That many physicians worked for companies ensured that they would not be receptive to any concept of disease that placed responsibility on their employers. Work-related health risks went unrecognized or else were interpreted in nonoccupational terms. Much the same was true of corporate owners and managers, many of whom remained indifferent to or ignorant about occupational disease hazards.[52]

What was the overall impact of occupation on the morbidity and mortality of workers in the late nineteenth and early twentieth centuries? The answer to this complex but fascinating question is far from clear. Part of the difficulty arises from the contemporary failure to recognize many occupational risks and to collect appropriate data. In his study of mortality from respiratory diseases in dusty trades in 1918, for example, Frederick Hoffman confined his analysis to inorganic dust, thus omitting mention of the clothing and textile industries. Moreover, occupational diseases rarely had a simple etiology; other cofactors—economic status, living conditions, personal behavior—played a role as well.

The diagnostic categories employed by physicians at the turn of the century simply exacerbated the problem presented by unreliable or inadequate morbidity and mortality data. Before the advent of the specific-germ theory of disease, for example, the category of consumption or phthisis was an integral part of medical classification systems. Its common symptoms were coughing, wheezing, spitting blood, and a generalized apathy. Indeed, the Greek term *phthisis* meant simply "wasting away." Phthisis also had multiple etiologies. It could reflect a dusty environment; it could arise in crowded urban slums; it could be rooted in abnormal personal behavior; and it could reflect climate, geography, and population density. Phthisis could be an acute illness that ran its course within weeks, or it could evolve into a chronic disease. Although pulmonary involvement was characteristic, the disease could affect any part of the body. In short, phthisis was a protean category.

After Robert Koch's discovery of the tubercle bacillus in 1882, phthisis was redefined as tuberculosis. Pulmonary disease was now a function of the presence of an invading organism that could be passed from person to person under appropriate conditions. The transformation of phthisis into tuberculosis had significant implications for medical theory and practice. European physicians in particular had investigated many occupational diseases related to the presence of dust in the workplace, and had produced an extensive literature dealing with industrial diseases. After 1880, however, most lung disorders were diagnosed as tuberculosis, and interest in the effects of dust and other contaminants diminished sharply. Morbidity and mortality data after the 1880s reflected a preoccupation with infectious disease and a lessening interest in the role of occupation. A well-known Swiss hygienist dismissed such "curiosities" as quartz lungs, coal lungs, and iron lungs, "all of which belong rather in a cabinet of curiosities than in industrial hygiene."[53]

Public health work underwent a corresponding transformation. In the mid-nineteenth century disease was interpreted in social and environmental terms. Physicians such as John Griscom, author of *The Sanitary Condition of the Laboring Population of New York* (1845), emphasized the need to improve personal and social hygiene, housing, living conditions, and sanitation and to assure clean water and pure food. By the end of the century public health enthusiasts had turned to laboratory science; they were preoccupied with the identification of specific pathogens and routes of transmission. Workers and unions were not in a position to challenge the dominance of the specific-germ theory of disease. Muckraking journalists and novelists writing in the first years of the twentieth century publicized the dangers of factory production, the employment of children, the inattention to sanitation, and high accident rates. With but a few exceptions, however, their accounts rested on impressions rather than on systematic analysis of data.[54]

It is virtually impossible to generalize about the role of industrial disease as a factor in total mortality at the turn of the century. Occupational death rates can never be separated from a variety of other intervening influences. Income, residential location, and social class all shape overall morbidity and mortality rates. Moreover, the data-collecting mechanisms that were in place between 1890 and 1910 left much to be desired. The causes of death on death certificates were (and are) unreliable, and the collection of mortality data included only a minority of the total population. Furthermore, the data dealing with the cause of death omitted occupation.[55]

In certain industries, notably mining, there is little doubt that dust diseases and accidents had a profound impact upon workers. But however important, mining was only one of many industrial occupations. In studying available but admittedly deficient data from the three federal censuses from 1890 to 1910, Paul Uselding found little evidence to support the allegation that those in industrial occupations had higher mortality rates than those in nonindustrial occupations or than their age-sex cohort in the general population. Assuming that manufacturing and mechanical employments were similar to industrial (factory) work, he found that those in the industrial category had a lower death rate than those in other occupations. When compared with that for all males, the mortality rate for manufacturing and mechanical workers was .87 for 1890, .95 for 1900, and 1.04 for 1910. The impact of the industrial work environment, he concluded, remained "an unresolved issue in the history of the American economy."[56]

Perhaps variability is the only term that can adequately describe the impact of occupational disease during the second half of the nineteenth and early twentieth centuries. The economic and technological changes that transformed mining after 1850 had a distinctly adverse impact upon workers; the same may have been true for some other occupations in which dust and toxic substances constituted a major hazard. Those who were employed in tenement workshops and factories, where crowding and inadequate ventilation were common, were at risk from a variety of infectious diseases. Changes in occupational structures, however, had positive consequences as well. Many of the gains that followed rising incomes balanced or exceeded health risks that were involved in occupational transformations. In some occupations, mechanization and technological innovation alleviated the physical burdens of labor and contributed to better health. Given this mix of consequences, it is virtually impossible to offer any definitive verdict on the impact of industrialization upon the health of workers.

CHAPTER 8

Stopping the Spread
of Infection

Florence Kelley, a leading social activist, observed in 1915 that in the past child deaths had been accepted with "resignation," and that mourning was the general response. "Today," she wrote in impassioned words, "we now know that every dying child accuses the community. For knowledge is available for keeping alive and well so nearly all, that we may justly be said to sin in the light of the new day when we let any die."[1]

Kelley's comments were a reflection of the marked transformation in the pattern of disease that became evident at the turn of the century. Infectious diseases were beginning a dramatic decline as the primary cause of mortality. By 1940 the infectious diseases that had made infancy and childhood the most dangerous stage of life were still prevalent, but they no longer posed a serious threat. As infant and child mortality declined, more Americans reached adulthood and survived to old age. Under these circumstances long-term diseases, including cardiovascular-renal diseases and malignancies, slowly became the major causes of mortality.

This change constituted what demographers have called the second epidemiological (or health) transition (the first being the change from a hunting-gathering to an agricultural society). This transition was to have vast consequences, for it altered the age structure of the population. In the nineteenth century the population was relatively young. In 1850 and 1900 the median ages were 18.9 and 22.9, respectively. The proportion of elderly people was, at least by contemporary standards, relatively low. In 1850 only 4 percent were aged 60 or over; a half-century later the figure was 6 percent. In 1995, by contrast, the median age was 34.3, and 17 percent of Americans were 60 or over (or 43.6 million out of a total population of 262.8 million).[2]

The dramatic decline in mortality from infectious diseases is often attributed to advances in medical science after 1900. The evidence to support this claim, however, is extraordinarily weak. Before 1940 the function of medicine was the diagnosis of disease; the therapeutic armamentarium to treat disease was, with a few exceptions, scanty. The introduction of antibiotic therapy, for example, came only during and after World War II. Yet by then infectious diseases were no longer significant causes of mortality. Why, then, did infectious diseases become less of a threat? The answer to this seemingly simple question poses a fascinating puzzle to scholars from many disciplines and backgrounds.

▼   ▼   ▼

By the end of the nineteenth century some of the infectious diseases that had appeared in epidemic and endemic form had declined or almost completely disappeared. Cholera, which reached the United States in 1832, 1849, and 1866, made its final appearance in attenuated form in 1873. Although Robert Koch did not identify the cholera vibrio until 1883, the earlier epidemiological work of John Snow provided persuasive evidence that the disease was transmitted by contaminated water. The demonstration that public health measures could prevent the spread of cholera helped weaken an ideology that had earlier attributed responsibility for the disease to immoral and dissolute behavior by urban ethnic minorities.[3]

Smallpox and yellow fever exhibited similar patterns. In seventeenth- and eighteenth-century Europe, endemic smallpox played a significant role in inhibiting population growth.[4] During the nineteenth century smallpox episodes diminished in both frequency and virulence. New York City had ten major epidemics between 1834 and 1875, but only two smaller ones in 1901 and 1902. The patterns in Baltimore and Milwaukee were similar. The last outbreaks occurred in Baltimore in 1881 and 1882, and were less severe than earlier ones. Milwaukee experienced outbreaks in 1872 and 1876, followed by a smaller one in 1894. Between 1854 and 1873 the mortality rate for smallpox in Massachusetts was 17 per 100,000, but declined to 0.8 between 1874 and 1893. In New Orleans, on the other hand, smallpox maintained a steady presence until the early twentieth century; between 1863 and 1883 nearly 6,500 residents died from this disease.[5]

The introduction of vaccination after 1800 and the continued use of inoculation undoubtedly contributed to the decline of epidemic smallpox by decreasing the number of susceptible individuals. Nevertheless, it is difficult to specify the precise roles of these procedures. The vaccine employed was variable in quality and sometimes failed to induce immunity. Even when effective, vaccination did not confer lifelong immunity, and revaccination had yet to be accepted by the public. Universal vaccination, moreover, remained an ideal that was never realized in practice; opposition to compulsory vaccination was present. A Buffalo public health official complained in the early 1880s that he had "experienced a great deal of opposition among the German people to vaccination. This seems strange, for it is very seldom you will ever find a person, born in Germany, who has not been vaccinated, as there it is compulsory. The moment they land on our free soil, they imbibe the spirit of freedom, especially as regards vaccination." Responding to criticism of the state board of health in Louisiana in the early 1880s for failing to take preventive action against smallpox, the secretary dismissed the idea of general compulsory vaccination as "visionary and impracticable." The people of Louisiana, he added, had not reached the appropriate "stage of civilization," and any attempt to impose the procedure "would probably meet the passive resistance of one-third of our people, the violent opposition of another third, and cheerful compliance by the small faction comprising the intelligent and law-abiding class." Opposition to vaccination reflected a fear that government was violating personal liberty as well as a well-founded concern with the safety of the procedure as then practiced.[6]

If vaccination and inoculation by themselves did not lead to the decline of smallpox, what did? There is scant evidence to suggest that changes in nutrition and the standard of living were significant, if only because mortality from smallpox is largely unrelated to nutritional status. To be sure, extreme nutritional deprivation (i.e., starvation) can increase vulnerability, but such deprivation was rare in America. A greater emphasis on surveillance and isolation of cases by public health authorities during the latter half of the nineteenth century may have limited the spread of the disease once an epidemic was under way. Recognition that the disease could be imported also led to somewhat greater vigilance by port officials. Smallpox virulence seemed to decline in England during the first half of the nineteenth century, but it is unclear if the same was true for America.

After 1896, however, a much milder form of smallpox—*Variola Minor*—appeared in the United States and largely replaced the more virulent *Variola Major*, which had predominated since the early seventeenth century. Although there is no satisfactory explanation for this development, it is clear that a sharp decline in the death rate from the disease followed. Before 1896 the case fatality rate was as high as 20 percent; thereafter the death rate from *Variola Minor* fell dramatically. In the peak years of 1920 and 1921 nearly 200,000 people were infected with the disease. Nevertheless, the case fatality rate for these two years was 0.43 and 0.55 percent, respectively. As late as 1930 there were over 30,000 cases, but the mortality rate was only 0.3 percent, and by midcentury the disease disappeared altogether. Vaccination, surveillance, and isolation of active cases undoubtedly helped to reduce the threat of a disease that in the seventeenth and eighteenth centuries had limited population growth. Nevertheless, diminished virulence probably also played an important role in the decline of mortality from smallpox.[7]

Yellow fever followed a similar pattern. After 1822 yellow fever was confined to southern seaports and to communities adjacent to inland waterways. New Orleans in particular bore the brunt of yellow fever epidemics; its semitropical climate and low-lying location provided ideal conditions for the replication of the mosquito that acted as the vector. The city experienced major outbreaks in 1858 and 1867, with death tolls of 4,854 and 3,107, respectively.[8] During the last three decades of the nineteenth century the frequency and intensity of yellow fever epidemics gradually diminished. The last major outbreak came in 1878. New Orleans and Memphis were hit hardest, but nearly two hundred communities in eight lower Mississippi states were also affected. About 120,000 people fell ill, and approximately 20,000 deaths were recorded. The severity of the epidemic aroused fears that yellow fever would once again become a recurrent menace. The Tennessee Board of Health observed that 1878

will be long remembered by the people of Tennessee as a year especially marked as one of disaster and death. The yellow fever was brought up the Mississippi River and fastened its deadly fangs upon the Western Division of our State, carrying dismay and death into almost every household. It did not stop here, but traveling with dread fatality on the lines of the railroad and river, it swept into the mountain city of Chattanooga, and into the various towns and cities of Kentucky. Nor were its ravages confined, as heretofore, to towns, but it scattered through all the villages and farms of West Tennessee, with a virulence and fatality heretofore unknown in the annals of this dread pestilential fever.[9]

Between 1879 and 1905, however, yellow fever appeared only six times in the United States, and there were slightly fewer than 2,000 fatalities. After 1905 there were no recorded cases of yellow fever within the continental United States.[10]

The decline and eventual disappearance of yellow fever from its last bastion in the Lower Mississippi Valley was not the result of any better understanding of either the mode of transmission or knowledge of the causative virus. Carlos Finley, a Cuban physician, had argued since 1881 that yellow fever was spread by mosquitoes. But nearly two decades passed before Walter Reed and others proved the mosquito hypothesis. Nevertheless, by the time Reed identified the role of the *Aedes aegypti* mosquito in transmitting the virus, the disease was already in decline.

The disappearance of yellow fever—much like the disappearance of several other epidemic diseases—reflected a process shaped less by conscious design than by serendipity. In places like New Orleans past outbreaks had immunized a large proportion of the population, and the subsequent decline of immigration diminished the pool of susceptible persons. The epidemic of 1878 created circumstances conducive to more government action. Quarantines, disinfection interventions, an emphasis on sanitary reform that led to the paving of streets and construction of sewers (thereby diminishing stagnant water pools), the decline in frequency of the disease in Havana (thus diminishing the odds of importing the disease from that port), and perhaps an apparent diminution in viral virulence during the nineteenth century all probably played a part. By the last outbreak in 1905, a better understanding of etiology and the growing role of the federal government combined to limit the severity of outbreaks through more effective mosquito suppression measures.[11]

Malaria—unlike cholera, smallpox, and yellow fever—proved a more persistent problem. Nevertheless, even before the turn of the century the geographic borders of the disease had reached its outermost limits and were beginning to shrink. By then malaria had largely disappeared from the Northeast and the Upper Mississippi Valley. It had also begun to decline in such states as Virginia and Kentucky. Between 1910 and 1920 the mortality rate in Kentucky fell from 10 to 1 per 100,000, and in Virginia from 3 in 1915 to 1 in 1920. Nevertheless, it remained one of the more important diseases in the South, and did not disappear until midcentury.[12]

The disappearance of malaria did not follow the introduction of any public health measures or novel medical therapies. Indeed, the fact that the disease established such a firm foothold in the United States at all was itself surprising; malaria, after all, was a tropical disease. Settlement patterns near waterways, disruption of drainage patterns, and agricultural practices, however, combined to create optimum conditions for the spread of the disease by providing mosquitoes with ideal breeding sites. In the South the *Anopheles quadrimaculatis* was the primary vector. This mosquito breeds in still water, prefers an alkaline pH, and has an affinity to live in buildings rather than the wild.

At the beginning of the Great Depression of the 1930s, the areas with high malarial morbidity and mortality rates included parts of South Carolina, Georgia, Florida and Alabama, the Mississippi Delta region, and the portion of the Red River Valley near the junction of Oklahoma, Arkansas, Louisiana, and Texas. In many of these places human environmental modifications proved crucial. The experience of the Mississippi Delta region is instructive. This area was devoted to cotton cultivation and provided an ideal environment for mosquito breeding because of the multiplicity of ponds of still water that followed the receding of river floods in the spring season. Agricultural laborers tended to live close to the fields, and thus provided a reservoir of infected and susceptible persons. Although the cultivation of rice and sugar took place in similar settings, malaria was much less common in these areas; field labor was done largely by machine, and the workforce generally resided in towns. Generally speaking, malaria had long since disappeared in more urban sites.[13]

Although drainage projects and the use of insecticides became more common after 1900, neither played decisive roles in the disappearance of the disease. Malaria tended to wax and wane during the first half of the twentieth century. Ernest C. Faust, a leading authority, identified four peak periods of malaria cycles: 1914–1918, 1920–1922, 1927–1929, and 1933–1935. Mortality was highest in the last cycle. After 1935 malaria morbidity and mortality began to decline, and by 1943 it had almost disappeared. Faust was unable to provide a persuasive explanation of the variations in the incidence and prevalence of malaria, although he indicated that improving economic conditions may have played an important role.[14]

More recently Margaret Humphreys has emphasized the critical role of population movements. During the 1930s people moved from urban areas with high unemployment rates and returned to abandoned shacks in the countryside; many of these were located adjacent to stagnant water. The migration of infected persons further assisted the spread of the disease. By the end of the decade, however, the situation was reversed; outmigration from the southern countryside was characteristic. New Deal agricultural legislation encouraged large-scale farming and mechanization, which in turn depopulated rural areas and hastened the growth of towns and cities outside the infective zone. As the number of infected persons declined, the ability of mosquitoes to spread malaria diminished correspondingly. The malaria parasite, in other words, depended on frontier conditions of poverty and proximity to water. As rural southern poverty diminished, the parasite disappeared.[15]

▾   ▾   ▾

Though reducing the prevalence of some infectious diseases, social and economic changes enhanced the virulence of others.[16] The experience of late nineteenth-century urban areas is illustrative. In 1860 no American city had yet reached 1 million in population; only two had more than half a million residents, and seven had between 100,000 and 500,000. By 1900 three cities exceeded the million mark, and thirty-five had between 100,000 and 500,000 residents. These figures in some ways underestimate the actual extent of urban growth as metropolitan areas overflowed their precise city limits. In 1880 New York City had a population of 1.9 million, yet the New York City Metropolitan Zone had more than 3.4 million.[17]

The growth of urban areas was generally accompanied by the construction of central water systems that relied on reservoirs outside their borders.[18] As water consumption increased commensurately, the problem of waste disposal became more acute. The ability of cesspools and privy vaults to handle organic wastes (including human excrement) was severely compromised, and they were unable to perform their function of infiltrating wastewater into the soil. The resulting runoff of polluted water in turn began to threaten public health. In 1895 the Baltimore commissioner of health noted that the city's privies were "the most dangerous enemies of our lives and happiness."

> The contents of these abominable receptacles have free access to the soil, and saturate the ground with liquid filth to such a degree, that specimens of sub-soil water taken from different depths, and in different sections, yield a large percentage of organic matters, the products of animal excretion.
>
> Many of them overflow, and the liquid contents flow into yards and gutters, emitting most offensive odors, which are a fruitful source of disease, operating indirectly in its production, and directly in lowering the vital stamina of the unfortunates compelled to breathe a polluted atmosphere.[19]

Although a variety of technologies were available (including separate systems for wastewater and surface water from rain and snow), most larger cities opted for sewer systems that combined wastewater and stormwater, which in turn were discharged into adjacent rivers and streams. This system of wastewater technology was based on the assumption that a process of dilution would alleviate any health risks from wastes that had the potential to threaten health. Although sanitary engineers were aware that raw sewage could present health hazards, few understood how far downstream the hazard extended. Indeed, before 1880 few communities thought it necessary to treat wastewater or sewage. By 1905 there were 3,756 miles of sanitary sewers and 847 miles of storm sewers, as compared with 14,857 miles of combined sewers. As late as 1910 less than a third of urban residents were supplied with treated water to prevent infectious diseases, and 88 percent of the wastewater of the population served by sewers was disposed of in waterways without treatment.[20]

Undertaken in the belief that health benefits would accrue, the construction of sewers paradoxically increased mortality from some water-borne diseases. Mortality from typhoid fever, for example, rose in many late nineteenth-century urban areas located on streams and lakes, particularly after they began to construct sewers. Between 1880 and 1890 sewer mileage in Philadelphia rose from 200 to 376. Mortality from typhoid fever increased during the same period, from 58.7 to 73.6 per 100,000. Washington, D.C., San Francisco, and Chicago manifested similar patterns. Downstream communities were often the hardest hit by their upstream neighbors' release of untreated wastes. Investigations by public health authorities in Baltimore found that contaminated city water was by far the most important source of infection. In 1900 the morbidity and mortality rates were 172 and 37, respectively; by 1910 they had risen to 330 and 41, but fell to 36 and 5 by 1920. To be sure, contaminated food and carriers played a role in the dissemination of typhoid, but at best they accounted for only a small proportion of cases.[21]

The failure to understand that discharges from sewers constituted a serious health menace reflected two nineteenth-century beliefs that shaped public policy: that dirt and filth were the basic causes of infectious diseases, and that running water purified itself. Hence public officials were primarily concerned with the discharge of industrial wastes. In 1876 an engineer commissioned by the Massachusetts Board of Health to examine the state's rivers concluded that the "fluid refuse from . . . factories . . . some of it very poisonous, produced in the processes of cleaning and preparing the manufactured article . . . forms the chief element in the pollution of these streams" and renders the water "not merely repulsive or suspicious, but more or less dangerous for family use."[22]

The advent of the specific-germ theory of disease following the work of Louis Pasteur, Robert Koch, and others in the 1870s and 1880s led to a recognition that contamination by infectious pathogens could exist even in the absence of particulate matter. Yet remedial measures were slow in coming. In the early 1890s William T. Sedgwick, head of the Department of Biology at the Massachusetts Institute of Technology and consulting biologist at the Lawrence Experiment Station of the Massachusetts Board of Health, clarified the etiology of typhoid fever and confirmed its relationship to sewage-polluted waterways. Reduction in the mortality rate from such waterborne diseases as typhoid, however, did not occur until after 1900. By then some urban areas had begun to make provision for filtration at the intake, while others developed distant and protected watersheds. (Sewage treatment at that time was not a viable option, given the prevailing state of technology.)[23]

Social and environmental change had the capability to alter the virulence of some diseases. Poliomyelitis is a case in point. Before the 1880s polio affected individuals but never appeared in epidemic form, nor was it an object of public concern. Descriptions of the disease existed in the medical literature, but relatively few persons, including physicians, were even aware of its existence. Poliomyelitis was and remains a much-misunderstood disease. The causative element—the poliovirus—is an enterovirus. There are three immunologically distinct forms, of which Type 1 is most common. Human beings are the only natural host, and infection occurs through direct contact and is highly contagious. Contrary to popular belief, polio is not synonymous with paralysis. Indeed, most cases are inapparent infections; the ratio of inapparent infections to clinically recognized cases exceeds 100:1, and the percentage of cases of paralysis is even lower. The poliovirus enters the mouth, and viral replication occurs in the oropharynx and intestinal tract. In these locations the virus is harmless; the characteristic symptoms include low fever, headache, sore throat, and malaise. Generally speaking, the production of specific antibodies inhibits viral spread; recovery occurs within two or three days, and the result is lasting immunity. If the virus reaches the spinal cord and brain, however, the consequences are devastating. The destruction of motor nerve cells leads to permanent paralysis, the extent of which is determined by the location of lesions in the central nervous system. When muscles used in breathing were affected, patients often died.

Probably of ancient lineage, polio aroused relatively little interest before the twentieth century. Before 1900 sanitation and hygiene, at least by modern standards, were relatively crude, and crowded homes were the rule rather than the exception. In such an environment, infants, particularly in urban areas, were exposed to all three types of the poliomyelitis virus early in life; by age 3 or 4 they had been infected with at least one strain. Early acquired immunity precluded the buildup of a large group of susceptibles, and epidemics were rare. In countries where sanitary arrangements were no longer primitive, exposure to the virus at an early age became less common. More children, therefore, reached the ages of 6 to 10 without having acquired immunity. Such populations were ripe for epidemics, and the rate of

the paralytic form rose dramatically because of the absence of residual maternal antibodies found in infants. Environmental factors thus
played a crucial role in the spread of the disease.[24] Paralytic polio, in
other words, was a disease directly associated with improved sanitation and housing. In even simpler terms, it was a disease associated
with cleanliness. The life of Franklin D. Roosevelt is an illustrative
case study, albeit an extreme one. Born into a wealthy household, he
had been raised in protected surroundings. Unlike children in congested urban environments, he had never been exposed to the
poliovirus. Hence he remained vulnerable and became paralyzed
when he contracted the disease in 1921.

The first polio epidemics occurred in rural areas of the Scandinavian countries during the last third of the nineteenth century. Because
travel to these areas by visitors was increasing, the large susceptible
population was exposed to the virus for the first time.[25] The fact that
the Scandinavian countries had made distinct strides in sanitation
and hygiene further reduced exposure in early life. Toward the close
of the nineteenth century polio epidemics began to occur elsewhere.
Western Europe experienced epidemics after 1880. In the United
States 26 cases were reported in the Boston area suburbs in 1893,
compared with 6 in 1888 and 1892 and 3 in 1889. The following
year the first large-scale epidemic appeared in the Rutland area of
Vermont; 132 persons were affected. Of this number, 119 developed
paralysis, 7 died before paralysis was noted, and 6 exhibited early
symptoms but were not paralyzed. Fifty-six recovered, and 30 suffered permanent paralysis; the death rate was 13.5 percent. The outbreak also anticipated a shift in age incidence; polio began emerging
as a disease of somewhat older children and young adults. Although
90 cases in 1894 were under the age of 3, 20 were between 9 and 12,
and 12 were over 15. The change in age distribution remained relatively constant during the first half of the twentieth century.

After 1894 similar though generally smaller outbreaks occurred in
other parts of the United States. In 1907 New York City had the largest epidemic ever recorded in the United States, with about 2,500
cases reported. Three years later a new peak was reached; nationally
there were 13.3 cases per 100,000 of population. Rural areas were
hardest hit; their case fatality rate was much higher than urban rates
(largely because urban areas had proportionately a smaller susceptible population). In addition, the 6-to-10 age group in rural areas had

higher attack rates than their urban counterparts. These rural-urban differences persisted over time. Two studies of an epidemic in 1944 found much higher rates in rural than in urban areas.[26]

In 1916 the Northeast suffered one of the most devastating polio epidemics ever recorded. Within the epidemic area the case rate was 28.5 per 100,000, more than three times the national rate in the previous seven years. New York City alone had 9,000 cases and slightly more than 2,400 deaths—an astonishing case fatality rate of 27 percent. Quite naturally the epidemic aroused terror in most households. A social worker reported that despite the summer weather,

> mothers are so afraid that most of them will not even let the children enter the streets, and some will not even have a window open. In one house the only window was not only shut, but the cracks were stuffed with rags so that "the disease" could not come in . . . I do not wonder they are afraid. I went to see one family about 4 P.M. Friday. The baby was not well and the doctor was coming. When I returned Monday morning there were three little hearses before the door; all her children had been swept away in that short time. The mothers are hiding their children rather than give them up [by sending them to a hospital].[27]

Although the specialty of virology did not yet exist, a study conducted by the U.S. Public Health Service and published in 1918 came to remarkably accurate conclusions. First, polio was a human infection passed from person to person. Second, the infection was far more prevalent than was apparent from the clinically recognized cases. Third, unrecognized carriers and mildly abortive cases that escaped diagnosis were the most important means of dissemination. Fourth, an epidemic of 1,000 to 3,000 recognized cases immunized the general population and led to a spontaneous decline in the epidemic as well as limiting the incidence rate in a subsequent outbreak. The report provided a wealth of documentation that illuminated many features of the disease. But its publication came at an inauspicious moment. The American people were preoccupied with World War I as well as the devastating influenza pandemic of 1918–19, that resulted in the deaths of hundreds of thousands. Consequently, the report had little impact, nor did it become the starting point for an investigation into the environmental factors that had transformed the epidemiology of polio.[28]

In terms of morbidity and mortality rates, poliomyelitis was never of major importance. But because it affected children, the disease captured the imagination of the American people during and after the Roosevelt presidency. Yet its appearance in epidemic form illustrates the manner in which beneficial environmental changes can have unforeseen deleterious consequences. Indeed, paralytic polio proved a threat to American soldiers serving in the Middle and Far East during World War II. Whereas the case rate among the native population was nil (largely because of crude sanitation), the corresponding rate among susceptible servicemen was high. Within about two weeks after the landing on the Philippine island of Leyte in late 1944, there were 47 cases of polio, of which 37 were paralytic. This pattern was repeated between 1943 and 1948 in such diverse countries as Japan, Burma, India, and Korea.[29] After the development of a vaccine in the mid-1950s, paralytic polio virtually disappeared.

▾   ▾   ▾

Despite epidemiological shifts, infectious diseases generally remained the major cause of mortality in the late nineteenth century. The majority of deaths in 1900 still fell into the infectious category. Of the fifteen leading causes of death, infectious diseases accounted for 56 percent of the total, chronic degenerative diseases for 37 percent, and accidents and suicide for 7 percent. Three infectious conditions—influenza and pneumonia, tuberculosis, and gastroenteritis—accounted for 31.4 percent of all deaths, whereas the comparable figure for three cardiovascular-renal conditions—heart diseases, cerebral hemorrhage, and chronic nephritis—was 18.4 percent.[30]

Of all age groups, infants and young children remained the most vulnerable. In this respect the situation differed little from earlier decades. Between 1850 and 1865 infants and children under the age of 5 accounted for about 67 percent of the total number of deaths in Boston. In Massachusetts in 1865 slightly over 20 percent of all of those born died in less than a year; in 1900 the figure was 19 percent. Mortality rates for children between the ages of 1 and 4 exhibited a similar pattern. In 1865 the death rate among this group was 68.6 per 1,000; by 1900 it had fallen only slightly, to 57.8.[31]

In reporting such death rates, Massachusetts was by no means unique. Between 1900 and 1904 national data from the Death Registration Area (created by the U.S. Bureau of the Census and designed to collect data on the age, sex, and cause of death) provided dramatic evidence that high mortality rates continued to prevail among the very young. The death rates for white males and females under age 1 were 154.7 and 124.8 per 1,000, respectively; the comparable figures for nonwhites (largely African Americans) were 342.5 and 285.7. The risk of dying was also high among those between 1 and 4. Indeed, child mortality rates in the United States in 1900 exceeded rates now prevalent in Asia and Latin America. Older children and adults were at less risk, but their death rates also remained high as compared with today's rates (although the differential narrowed with advancing age).[32]

High mortality rates among the very young reflected the continued significance of infectious diseases. Data from the Death Registration Area for 1899–1900 revealed that gastrointestinal diseases were responsible for 25 percent of all infant deaths and 14 percent of deaths among those between ages 1 and 4. A variety of respiratory diseases took a similar toll among these two groups (19.2 and 31.9 percent, respectively). Diseases associated with childhood (measles, scarlet fever, diphtheria, and whooping cough) accounted for 22.5 percent of all deaths in the 1-to-4 age group. Birth defects of one form or another were the only other significant factor in mortality, accounting for 26.7 percent of deaths among infants.[33]

To be sure, social class, race, ethnicity, occupation, geographic location, parenting practices (e.g., breast feeding), and other elements gave rise to differential mortality rates between groups. Nevertheless, these differences were relatively small; economically advantaged families were not much better off than those at the lower end of the economic ladder. Professionals—technical and medical—had child mortality rates not fundamentally different from those of the general population. The mortality of children of physicians, for example, was only 6 percent below the national average. Clerks and copyists, by contrast, had rates 8 percent below the national average, and children of teachers had rates equal to the average.[34]

What explains the continued significance of infectious diseases, particularly in one of the wealthiest nations? Could not American families in the late nineteenth century have acted in ways that might have reduced mortality among their very young, particularly at a time when the standard of living was rising (albeit unequally)? To ask such a question presupposes that Americans possessed both the knowledge and authority to lessen the impact of infectious disease. The fact of the matter is that understanding of many infectious diseases, whether of bacterial or viral origin, was either lacking or incomplete at the turn of the century. Moreover, the presence of a pathogen may be necessary to explain the presence of a particular disease, but it is rarely sufficient. Behavior, environment, host-pathogen relationships, and immune response are all important variables, and their interactions are complex and rarely clear-cut. Americans a century ago lacked both the knowledge and the means to take decisive action to limit infectious diseases.[35]

The medical history of the Spanish-American War of 1898 provides another example of the continued significance of infectious diseases. In the nation's past wars the overwhelming majority of fatalities had resulted from infectious diseases rather than from combat wounds. Indeed, after the Civil War the army collected a huge mass of data documenting the role of disease in that conflict. Yet the "lessons" learned from past experience were often ignored by military authorities. Military culture at the turn of the century was combat oriented. Line officers (who command) generally were indifferent or even hostile to recommendations by medical officers.

In the decades following the end of the Civil War, the American military underwent dramatic reductions. By 1875 the army had a peacetime force of only about 25,000, two-thirds of whom were engaged in efforts to ensure domination of the Indian population in the West. When war on Spain was declared in April 1898, military authorities were preoccupied with efforts to raise and equip a wartime army that would be ten times the size of its peacetime counterpart. At the war's outset the army had slightly over 28,000 men. By May the size had risen to 163,592, and the peak strength in August was over 272,000. The army was ill prepared to house such a large force, and its commanders were not disposed to accept advice about sanitation. Moreover, the army's rapid expansion overwhelmed its small Medical Department, which had to recruit a large number of physicians and surgeons from the civilian sector. Most were professionally qualified by the standards of that day, but were unprepared to deal with sanitary and disease prevention responsibilities on a large scale.

Although the first battle of the Spanish-American War took place in the Philippine Islands, the Cuban campaign involved far more personnel and accounted for 91 percent of the casualties. Battle-related deaths and wounds, however, were far less significant than the ravages of infectious diseases. The Cuban campaign was fought during the summer months, and malaria, typhoid fever, dysentery, and heat proved to be the most formidable foes. Before the outbreak of hostilities the death rate was 0.21; in August 1898 it peaked at 6.14, largely as a result of infectious diseases.

Health conditions in army camps, most of which were located in the American South, also took a heavy toll. In many typhoid reached epidemic proportions. The largest, Camp George H. Thomas in Georgia, housed the I and III Corps, each averaging about 40,000 men. By early summer crude sanitary conditions had led to a major outbreak of typhoid fever. The soil of the adjacent woods was covered with excrement because the geology of the region made it difficult to dig proper latrines. Flies from the woods contaminated the food supply, and a two-week rainfall caused sinks to overflow, thus contaminating the water supply. Intense crowding facilitated the spread of the epidemic, and lack of adequate hospital and isolation facilities exacerbated the situation. Conditions at other military installations, though not as extreme as those at Camp Thomas, exhibited similar characteristics. Aggregate data once again revealed that infectious disease was the major cause of mortality during the Spanish-American War. There were 2,910 deaths, of which 2,565 were the result of disease rather than combat.[36]

Although infectious diseases continued to take their greatest toll on infants and young children in the general population, their impact on the adult population was by no means insignificant. The two leading causes of death in 1900, for example, were respiratory disorders (influenza and pneumonia) and tuberculosis, with mortality rates of 202.2 and 194.4 per 100,000, respectively. Yet other infectious diseases that did not result in death played important roles in health patterns. Some give rise to lasting chronic conditions that resulted in ill health and eventually diminished longevity. Two examples were hookworm and some venereal diseases.

Hookworm was endemic in warm, moist areas. It was imported into the American South in the seventeenth century by Europeans engaged in the slave trade. African slaves carried the parasite, which had little difficulty in adapting itself to a region whose climate and soil provided ideal conditions. It thrived during the colonial period along the Atlantic seaboard and was carried to cotton country in the interior in the early nineteenth century.

The hookworm parasite usually enters the human host through the tender skin between the toes of people who walk barefoot. Hookworm rarely kills, but it leaves its victims feeling weak and listless, and increases their vulnerability. The disease was subsequently identified in the popular press as the "germ of laziness." It was a disease associated with poverty and poor sanitation. A sufficient supply of iron provided greater resistance, but diets that were less than satisfactory—particularly among poor rural farmers—increased susceptibility to the clinical form of the disease. Although a cure was developed in the late nineteenth century, reinfection was so pervasive that even the massive campaign undertaken by the Rockefeller Sanitary Commission for the Eradication of Hookworm in 1909 could not eliminate the disease. Prevention required that individuals wear shoes and use sanitary outhouses. The elimination of hookworm in the early twentieth century involved both the creation of public health agencies capable of launching effective campaigns to induce behavioral changes and a standard of living that provided an adequate diet and shoes.[37]

Like hookworm, venereal diseases shared many of the attributes of long-duration diseases. The two most readily identifiable ones at the turn of the century were syphilis and gonorrhea. Both are highly contagious. By the nineteenth century syphilis had emerged as a three-stage disease. In the incubation or primary stage, a chancre appears around the genital organ. In the secondary stage (beginning anywhere from six weeks to six months after infection), skin eruptions and a variety of other symptoms appear as the spirochete invades the body. A period of latency follows that may last for a brief period or as much as decades. In this stage the organism bores into the bone marrow, lymph glands, and other vital organs. In some instances the pathogen and host coexist peacefully. But in many cases the disease enters the tertiary stage, during which the cardiovascular and central nervous system are affected. In this stage the disease may take a variety of forms, the most devastating of which is paresis, or general paralysis of the insane. The invasion of the brain by the spirochete results in dramatic neurological and behavioral symptoms, paralysis, and eventually death. Congenital syphilis can be transmitted from the mother to the fetus and give rise to serious health problems in the child.

Gonorrhea, like syphilis, is a bacterial infection with long-term consequences. It too can be transmitted to the fetus and may result in a series of ailments, including urethral strictures, peritonitis, meningitis, pericarditis, and arthritis. Female sterility follows the disease's obstruction of the Fallopian tubes. In 1900 one physician estimated that about 12 percent of all marriages were sterile; of these at least two-thirds were the result of gonococcal infection.[38]

Syphilitic and gonococcal infections were by no means uncommon even though estimates of their prevalence are problematic. Military officials were especially preoccupied with venereal disease. During the Civil War the average yearly rate of cases was 82 per 1,000. Admission rates for venereal disease in the army in 1909 were about 200 per 1,000. Other estimates were even higher. By the early twentieth century American mental hospitals were receiving substantial numbers of paretic patients. From 1911 to 1919 about 20 percent of all male first admissions to New York State mental hospitals (the largest public hospital system, accommodating about 20 percent of the nation's institutionalized population) were cases of general paresis (the rate for women was about one-third that of men).[39]

Unlike acute infections, venereal diseases had consequences that made them similar to polio and other long-duration diseases. A classic study of neurosyphilitic patients published in 1917 provided a description of an individual admitted on two occasions to a Massachusetts mental hospital between 1904 and 1906. In 1904 his speech was "somewhat defective," his handwriting "had lost appreciably in legibility," his memory was "decidedly imperfect," and his judgment of space and time was "imperfect." During his second stay and not long before his death the patient "was at first restless, sleepless, profane, imperfectly oriented for time . . . A few weeks later he became stuporous and confused . . . Death was preceded by a semi-comatose condition."[40]

Other diseases, though statistically of less significance, also took a toll. Many of those who survived the health hazards of infancy and childhood died in later life from cardiovascular-renal diseases and malignant neoplasms. This is not to suggest that the incidence of these diseases was rising, for such was not necessarily the case. Age-corrected data for mortality from cancer, for example, showed only a modest rise in incidence in the early twentieth century. The increase in the number of deaths from cancer was largely a function of population growth and the commensurate rise in the number of adults in the upper age groups.[41]

Morbidity and mortality from chronic degenerative disease were related in part to the age distribution of the population. Other noninfectious diseases reflected local social, economic, and environmental conditions. An excellent example is pellagra, a disease that came to public attention at the turn of the century.

Pellagra, like scurvy and beriberi, is a vitamin deficiency disease, although it was not recognized as such at the beginning of the twentieth century. It is marked by symmetrical skin lesions, including a butterfly-shaped design across the nose, and is often accompanied by gastrointestinal disorders. People with pellagra tend to be listless. The mind can also be affected; confusion, hallucinations, and delusions of persecution are common. Those with the disease have high suicide rates. Pellagra follows an irregular course. In some cases the symptoms appear around December, peak in the spring, and sometimes disappear in the late summer and fall. Some cases are chronic; in other cases death occurs quickly. The underlying cause is a deficiency of niacin (nicotinic acid), a member of the vitamin B complex group.

In nineteenth-century Europe pellagra was linked to people who subsisted on a diet in which maize was the basic staple. It was rediscovered in the United States shortly after the turn of the century by southern physicians, who found large numbers of cases in the region's mental hospitals. Subsequent research showed that the disease was concentrated in the South and was especially prevalent in cotton mill communities, which had expanded in the post–Civil War decades. Southerners began to invest heavily in textiles and drew upon poor whites as their primary source of labor. Identification of the disease was followed by realization that large numbers of people were affected. In 1907 fewer than 1,000 cases were reported; by 1911 there were more than 7,000. Mortality ran as high as 40 percent or more. Although evidence on the nature and etiology of pellagra was fragmentary, explanations were abundant. Some insisted that pellagra was an infectious disease; others located its cause in spoiled corn; some associated the disease with Italian immigrants; some argued that it was a water-borne disease disseminated by insects or animals;

and some attributed it to heredity. Medical therapies were equally eclectic.

In 1914 the U.S. Public Health Service appointed Dr. Joseph Goldberger to head its ongoing investigations of the disease. From that point on his name was forever linked with pellagra. Within weeks Goldberger made an intuitive leap; he suggested that the disease was related to the monotonous "three-M" diet of the South—meat (fatback), meal, and molasses. In a series of classic epidemiologic studies, he and his colleagues demonstrated that pellagra was neither infectious nor related to poor sanitation. In investigating institutional populations, including orphanages, mental hospitals, and prison farms, he demonstrated that a varied diet could either prevent or cure pellagra. Moreover, the more closely he studied the disease, the more cases he found. Pellagra, he and Edgar Sydenstricker noted in 1915, was a disease associated with poverty. Two-thirds of all cases were found among children aged 2 to 15. The disease proved remarkably sensitive to changing economic conditions. As agricultural prices and income declined during the 1920s, morbidity and mortality from pellagra rose. By the early 1930s the Public Health Service estimated that there were more than 200,000 cases a year. "The disease may occur anywhere and in anyone, but it is the poor man who is the chief sufferer from it," Goldberger wrote in 1927. "This explains why hard times, especially when accompanied by rising food prices, are likely to be followed by an increase in the disease."[42]

In 1937 Conrad A. Elvehjem and his associates at the University of Wisconsin discovered that nicotinic acid cured black tongue, which was the canine version of pellagra. The disappearance of pellagra, however, was ultimately associated with basic social and economic changes that transformed the South and ultimately reshaped dietary patterns. During World War II high employment and mobilization of the armed forces provided fiscal resources that permitted more nutritious diets. The enrichment of bread and flour with vitamins (including nicotinic acid) as a wartime measure also made a major contribution. After the war the rapid urbanization of the South and the decline of the one-crop system of agriculture completed the transformation of the southern diet by sharply increasing the availability of a variety of foods, thus eliminating the conditions responsible for pellagra.[43]

▼ ▼ ▼

Somewhere around the turn of the century infectious diseases declined precipitously as the major cause of mortality. Infants, children,
and adults continued to contract infections, but in general their lives
were no longer at risk to the degree that they had been before.

Beginning in 1915 the Bureau of the Census organized the Birth
Registration Area, thus making available comprehensive data on infant mortality. At that time the mortality rate for infants had already
fallen to 100 per 1,000 live births. The trend continued downward
on a reasonably straight line, and accelerated after 1937. By 1940 the
death rate was 47 and fell still further, albeit unevenly, after World
War II. The decline was not equal throughout the United States; the
mountain and southern states had higher rates than the northeast,
north-central, and Pacific regions. Rates were higher for males, children of foreign-born women, and African Americans. The decline in
mortality was also evident in the 1-to-4-year age group. A comparable trend occurred in all age groups, although its magnitude was considerably smaller.[44]

The seeming decline of infectious diseases had a profound impact.
Between 1900 and 1940 life expectancy at birth rose from 47.3 to
62.9, a result of the fall in infant and child mortality. Life expectancy
at age 20 and above also rose, although the magnitude of the gain
was far less. During the twentieth century the number of people who
survived into the sixth and seventh decade of life rose, as did the median age of the population.[45]

What drove the epidemiological transition that began in the late
nineteenth century and was largely completed by the 1940s, by which
time chronic degenerative diseases had replaced acute infectious diseases as the major cause of mortality? Scholars from many disciplines
have offered a variety of answers. Some have emphasized the crucial
role of nutrition and a rising standard of living; others have focused
on broad environmental transformations; some have pointed to
changes in public health practices; and others have emphasized the
importance of stable governments able to impose appropriate sanitary regulations. Indeed, comparative studies revealed that this shift
in the causes of mortality was not limited to the United States, but occurred in many other countries at roughly the same time (though not
necessarily at the same rate).[46]

Whatever the explanation for the epidemiologic transition, there is general agreement that strictly medical therapies did not play a significant role. Before World War II the medical armamentarium to deal with infectious diseases was sparse. To be sure, some effective medical interventions were available, including smallpox vaccination and diphtheria antitoxin. Yet even in these cases it is not entirely clear that the reduction in mortality from these diseases was due solely to their use. In general, physicians lacked therapies to deal with infections, including gastrointestinal disorders, tuberculosis, respiratory diseases, and most diseases associated with childhood. In a study of the first edition of R. L. Cecil's textbook on medicine published in 1927, Paul Beeson found that most of the recommended therapies before World War II were subsequently shown to be largely ineffectual. Evaluating the role of medicine in the decline of mortality from infectious diseases, John B. and Sonja M. McKinlay noted that the ten major infectious diseases that had accounted for approximately a third of all deaths at the turn of the century were insignificant causes of mortality by 1940. The introduction of effective therapies (e.g., antibiotics) and vaccines occurred after 1940, and by that time mortality from the major infectious diseases had fallen dramatically. Moreover, medical expenditures before 1940 were relatively modest; the share of the gross domestic product spent on health care did not begin to rise until after World War II. "*In general,*" the McKinlays concluded,

> *medical measures (both chemotherapeutic and prophylactic) appear to have contributed little to the overall decline in mortality in the United States since about 1900—having in many instances been introduced several decades after a marked decline had already set in and having no detectable influence in most instances . . . it is estimated that at most 3.5 percent of the total decline in mortality since 1900 could be ascribed to medical measures introduced for the [infectious] diseases considered here.*[47]

The claim that specific medical treatments played an insignificant role in the reduction of mortality from infectious diseases is true. Yet such an argument rests on an overly narrow definition of medical intervention that assumes a one-on-one patient-physician interaction. In reality, medicine, broadly defined, included a broad range of public health activities relating to sanitation, pure water, housing, quarantine, and general preventive measures. Accurate diagnoses of infectious diseases—even if unrelated to specific treatments—affected the provision of care, which influenced outcomes. Similarly, the rise of nursing had significant influence on infant and childrearing practices. Any effort to understand the roots of the epidemiological transition, therefore, requires an understanding of medicine broadly rather than narrowly conceived.[48]

A monolithic explanation of the epidemiological transition is inherently attractive because of its simplicity and lack of nuances. Yet available empirical data render such an interpretation suspect. Recent scholarship has revealed sharp differences among geographic regions as well as among urban areas. The infectious diseases that were the major contributors to mortality, to be sure, declined during the same period. It does not necessarily follow, however, that common causes were responsible. In fact an examination of the changing disease environment in the late nineteenth and early twentieth centuries suggests that the decline in mortality from specific infectious diseases may have had varied rather than common causes.

Without doubt gastrointestinal (i.e., diarrheal) diseases remained the major cause of mortality among infants and young children in the late nineteenth century. In 1870 the mortality rate from these diseases in Philadelphia among the 1-to-4 age group was 41.4 per 1,000; thirty years later it had fallen to a still relatively high level of 21.6. For infants the rates were much higher. Data from selected northern and western cities for 1900 reveal that the infant mortality rate for diarrheal diseases was 41.7 per 1,000. Between 1902 and 1910 about 30 percent of all infant deaths in New York City were from gastrointestinal disorders. In his pioneering study of eight cities in the early twentieth century, Robert M. Woodbury found that about a third of all infant deaths were caused by gastrointestinal disorders. Most of these deaths resulted from "improper feeding." Breast-fed infants, by contrast, had much higher survival rates. Although there were sharp variations in urban and regional death rates from diarrheal diseases, there is no doubt that these were the leading cause of death among infants and children. Mortality tended to peak in the warmer months and decline in cold weather. The indeterminate state of knowledge at the time precluded effective interventions. Those professionals who saw infant and child mortality as pressing problems could never decide whether sanitary reform or parental education was a more appropriate strategy to deal with diarrheal diseases. There was only a vague recognition that dehydration and the ensuing systemic shock represented the greatest dangers.[49]

Somewhere toward the close of the nineteenth century mortality from diarrheal diseases began to fall among infants and children. By 1930 the rate among the 1-to-4 age group in Philadelphia was 5.4 per 1,000. Decreasing death rates from diarrheal diseases accounted for about 16 percent of the mortality decline in that city between 1870 and 1930. Changes in the reporting of causes of death make it difficult to provide precise national data on mortality from diarrheal diseases, but it is clear that by 1940 gastrointestinal disorders no longer presented major threats to infants and young children.[50]

In the mid-nineteenth century physicians and social activists attributed high infant death rates to urban poverty, filth, and overcrowded housing. Toward the end of the century infant mortality began to be reconceptualized. Older concepts persisted but were modified by newer ideas. In the first edition of his classic textbook on diseases of infancy and childhood in 1897, L. Emmett Holt observed that infant mortality was on the rise. The increase, he suggested, was due "to many causes—overcrowding, neglect, and unhygienic surroundings. But more important than all is artificial feeding as at present ignorantly practised." The focus on infant feeding practices helped to direct medical attention to the digestive and nutritional disorders of infancy. In 1915 John Howland and William Marriott noted that high fatality rates among infants with severe diarrhea were connected to the state of acidosis (reduced alkalinity of the blood and body tissues) that the disorder produced. Slowly but surely the conviction grew that infant deaths were preventable by public health interventions and changes in parental behavior.[51]

The decline in mortality from gastrointestinal disorders was due largely to preventive rather than therapeutic interventions. Figures like Holt promoted breast feeding. In 1900 most mothers probably breast fed for the first six months, but the practice was clearly declining. Cow's milk served as the principal source of nutrients for those who were artificially fed. At the turn of the century, however, the milk supply in the United States was seriously contaminated with pathogens, including the tubercle, typhoid, diphtheria, and streptococci bacilli, as well as others capable of causing enteric disorders. Examining fifty-eight samples of milk in 1901, Baltimore inspectors found between 100,000 and 21 million bacteria per cubic centimeter; only eleven samples were under 1 million when 500,000 was the standard for a warning. Those involved in the production and distribution of milk, they concluded, "fail to keep the cows clean, they fail to keep the stables clean daily, they fail in personal cleanliness, and fail in milk handling. They know nothing about bacteria and care less."[52]

By the early twentieth century there was increasing emphasis on the pasteurization and sterilization of milk, bottles, and nipples. Local health codes mandated that milk be pasteurized and sold in sealed containers. A growing preoccupation with cleanliness, isolation of sick siblings, home visitations by nurses and social workers to educate mothers about the importance of appropriate infant rearing practices, and the establishment of infant welfare and milk stations also contributed to the decline.[53]

Nowhere was the role of behavioral factors better illustrated than in the mortality experiences of children born of French-Canadian and Jewish immigrants in 1911–1915 in eastern cities. The infant mortality rate from gastrointestinal disorders among Jews was 10.5 per 1,000, as compared with 25.2 among native whites and 64.2 among French Canadians. Dissimilar breast-feeding rates accounted for only part of the difference. The Jewish advantage in infant and child survival was probably the result of culture-related childcare practices, including feeding, hygiene, and family size. The prohibition against serving meat and milk together may also have conferred an advantage, given the impure state of the milk supply and the absence of effective refrigeration. Jews also purchased much of their food from street vendors, who generally did not keep unsold food for any length of time (as compared with ordinary grocery stores). By limiting the size of their families, they increased per-capita income and devoted more attention to the care of fewer children. In 1911 Maurice Fishberg noted that "the smaller number of children born [among Jews] has as a concomitant a smaller infant mortality, and also gives the parents an opportunity to raise their offspring on a more desirable standard." Child-centered homes, low rates of labor force participation by mothers, low birthrates, lengthier periods of breast feeding, and certain religious practices such as an emphasis on ritual hand washing probably gave Jews a decided advantage in terms of infant survival. French-Canadian mothers, by contrast, tended to return to work and thus had briefer periods of breast feeding. Moreover, they had larger families, shorter birth intervals, and a lower quality of childcare.[54]

The decline in mortality from gastrointestinal disorders was by no means unique. Most of the so-called diseases of childhood manifested similar patterns. Whooping cough, measles, scarlet fever, and diphtheria—all of which had taken a heavy toll among children in the nineteenth century—began to fall as a cause of mortality even though prevalence rates often remained high. By 1940 these diseases no longer posed a serious threat to life. Survival rates among children were correspondingly enhanced. Mortality rates in the 1-to-4-year group fell from 19.8 per 1,000 in 1900 to 2.9 in 1940. The pattern among those aged 5 to 14 was similar: 3.9 in 1900 and 1.0 in 1940.[55]

The decline in mortality from infectious diseases associated with childhood admits of no simple explanation. The case of diphtheria is something of an exception, largely because effective interventions became available in the 1890s. During the second half of the nineteenth century mortality from this disease followed an irregular course. In 1898 Arthur Newsholme, a distinguished English epidemiologist, claimed that the disease had declined in many urban areas during the previous two decades. Some American data supported his claim. In Baltimore, for example, the incidence and mortality rate peaked about 1880 and then declined fairly rapidly. The mortality reduction in New York City was somewhat less pronounced. In 1880 2,303 deaths from diphtheria were recorded. In 1885 and 1890 there was a decline to 2,179 and 1,839, respectively, followed by a slight increase to 1,987 in 1895. During these same years New York City's population increased from 1.2 to nearly 1.8 million. Philadelphia, on the other hand, experienced an increase in mortality from diphtheria between 1870 and 1900.[56]

For much of the nineteenth century physicians were unable to distinguish between diphtheria and pseudo-membranous throat inflammations probably associated with some form of streptococci. In 1884, however, Friedrich Loeffler identified the pathogen that was responsible for the disease *(corynebacterium diphtheria)*.[57] This bacillus had three biotypes: *mitis, intermedius,* and *gravis.* The latter two had high fatality rates; the former was relatively mild. In the early 1890s Dr. William H. Park of the New York City Board of Health identified the role of asymptomatic carriers and developed a simple means of culturing the organism to assist in diagnosis. Nevertheless, the only means of dealing with the disease were isolation and disinfection, both of which proved disruptive to people who worked and lived in crowded tenement houses.

By 1894 an antitoxin with therapeutic qualities had been developed, and two decades later an effective means of immunizing children became available with the introduction of the toxin-antitoxin. Yet the precise role played by both in reducing mortality from diphtheria is ambiguous. Comparative data from European nations indicate that mortality had begun to fall before 1894. Moreover, there is some evidence that the emergence of a dominant strain of *mitis* reduced the virulence of the disease. Antitoxin serum may therefore have merely assisted a natural decline of the disease already under way. During the 1920s the New York City Health Department launched an educational campaign directed at all ethnic and racial groups in the hope of creating an awareness of diphtheria. The goal was to provide access to treatment and a preventive vaccine even among those lacking the ability to pay. These immunization campaigns probably led to the eventual disappearance of the disease by World War II.[58]

The case of diphtheria is atypical because of the availability of a therapy and a means of immunization. The decline in mortality from other diseases associated with childhood had different origins, if only because effective treatments or preventive vaccines were unavailable. Measles is a case in point. It was a serious disease that appeared in both epidemic and endemic form. In urban areas high attack rates in an epidemic year were followed by lower rates because of the reduced pool of susceptible children. Between 1858 and 1923 mortality from measles in Providence, Rhode Island, exceeded 20 per 100,000 in eleven years, remained under 10 for thirty-one years, and peaked in 1887 at 74. A study published in 1930 indicated that perhaps 95 percent of urban children had been infected by the measles virus by age 15. In the late nineteenth century mortality from measles began to decline even though incidence rates increased. Whether the increase in incidence was real or due to better reporting cannot be determined.[59]

Why did measles mortality decline? The stability of the virus makes it unlikely that mutations decreased virulence. External factors, therefore, probably played the key roles. Some have suggested that improved nutrition among children diminished mortality, while others emphasized the importance of overcrowding and implicitly the impact of its lessening. In fact, the decline in measles mortality may have been due to the interaction of several factors. By the late nineteenth century parents of sick children with communicable diseases were more likely to isolate them and thus inhibit the spread of the disease to other siblings. There is evidence that greater attention to the care of sick children was a significant factor. Indeed, most deaths from measles were due not to the disease itself, but to respiratory complications, particularly bronchopneumonia. In 1925, for example, the Census Bureau reported that 2,404 deaths were due to measles; but 2,261 (94.1 percent) were complicated by another disease, and in 1,462 cases (60.8 percent) bronchopneumonia was the complicating condition. Improved housing may have also diminished overcrowding and provided more effective ventilation.[60]

In some respects the decline in mortality from pertussis (whooping cough) bears some resemblance to the trend for measles. Whooping cough results from infection by a gram-negative bacillus (*bordella pertussis*) unable to survive outside its human host. Deaths from this disease were generally confined to infants and children under the age of 4. The disease peaked toward the end of the nineteenth century and then declined steadily. Like measles, death followed respiratory complications. Of 6,948 deaths in 1925 attributed to whooping cough, 5,546 (80 percent) were complicated by another disease, and in half the deaths the contributory cause was bronchopneumonia. The decline in mortality from pertussis remains something of a mystery. One possibility is that greater resistance to the disease developed in cities, which had suffered most; the experience of London and Scottish cities in the late nineteenth century lends weight to this interpretation. Higher levels of care may also have minimized respiratory complications.[61]

Other infectious diseases present equally puzzling problems. Many of the efforts to illuminate the decline in mortality from infectious diseases assume that human interventions—medical, social, behavioral, environmental—played key roles. Yet there is a distinct probability that changes in virulence can follow genetic changes in the invading pathogen, creating new epidemiological patterns. Like all other forms of life, bacteria and viruses evolve over time, and the complex ways in which they react with their human hosts may give rise to variable virulence.

Scarlet fever and rheumatic fever—both related to the Group A streptococcal strains—are examples of diseases whose virulence diminished over time. Scarlet fever has as its main features a sore throat and bright red rash. The infection often led to complications and death. Mortality rates for the disease in twenty-one American cities peaked in the early 1890s and then gradually declined. The infection was essentially one of childhood. A study by the Metropolitan Life Insurance Company of policyholders aged 1 to 14 found that the death rate fell about 72.5 percent between 1911 and 1935. Charles V. Chapin offered two explanations for this decline: high mortality rates eliminated the more virulent strains of the pathogen, and the growing practice of isolating serious cases prevented the spread of the more severe type. Whatever the reasons, it was evident that declining mortality from scarlet fever reflected diminished virulence of the invading pathogen.[62]

The example of rheumatic fever is somewhat different. Like scarlet fever, the disease is associated with the Group A streptococcus. It assumed its modern form in the early nineteenth century, peaked toward the end of the century, and declined in both prevalence and severity thereafter. During the nineteenth century its symptoms became more severe. Many individuals became invalids because rheumatic fever led to arthritis and chorea (an involuntary movement disorder). Others died because of inflamed heart tissues; initially the pericardium (tissues surrounding the heart) and subsequently the endocardium (heart valves) were affected. In the twentieth century the disease became less virulent; a more benign myocarditis (inflammation of the heart muscle) became characteristic. In the nineteenth century rheumatic fever was a disease of children and young adults. In the twentieth century rheumatic fever became a long-duration disease; those afflicted with rheumatic myocarditis could live past the age of 50. An epidemiological study in 1927 of rheumatic fever, erysipelas, and scarlet fever—all streptococcus-related illnesses—found that both incidence and mortality rates had fallen during the previous two decades despite the absence of effective therapies. The residual impact of the disease, however, was significant. At about the same time John R. Paul estimated that there were 840,000 cases of rheumatic heart disease, active and inactive, in a population of 100 million.[63]

After World War II molecular biologists began to unravel some of the mysteries of rheumatic fever. They found that exposure to the pathogen created antibodies that cross-reacted with heart tissue. In his history of rheumatic fever, Peter English suggests that the streptococcus of the eighteenth century contained components that cross-reacted only with human joints (thus causing arthritis); during the nineteenth century new molecular components transformed the pathogen so that human antibodies cross-reacted with heart tissue. The pathogens that cause disease thus constitute an independent variable; their interaction with human hosts may explain changes in virulence that created new epidemiological patterns. "Because of the role of hemolytic streptococcal infection in the etiology of rheumatic fever," notes Benedict E. Massell (a leading figure in research on the disease), "changes in incidence and severity of rheumatic fever must be closely linked to changes in incidence and rheumatogenicity (and virulence) of the streptococcus."[64]

To suggest that changes in bacterial virulence played perhaps the major role in transforming epidemiological patterns is not to argue that social factors were unimportant. Rates of rheumatic heart disease may have been related to residential crowding. A study of rheumatic fever in Baltimore, for example, found the highest rates among middle-class rather than lower-class African-American families. As their economic situation improved, upwardly mobile families moved out of the ghetto and into dwellings that often offered more space in the social areas of living and dining rooms, while sacrificing space in bedrooms. Since droplet infection was greatest in a narrow radius around an infected source, the result was higher rates of rheumatic fever and heart disease. Other studies confirmed the importance of household density in the etiology of infectious diseases. Both social and biological elements, therefore, played crucial roles in changing incidence and prevalence patterns.[65]

▼   ▼   ▼

Like infants and children, adults benefited from the decline in mortality from infectious diseases. Their gains, however, were more modest. Most had survived the diseases of early life. To be sure, some of the chronic health problems experienced in later life had roots in childhood encounters with infectious diseases. Yet those who survived into adulthood faced a somewhat diminished risk of dying from infectious diseases that traditionally had taken a heavy toll in lives. There were, of course, exceptions to this trend. Maternal mortality from the mid-nineteenth century until the 1930s remained more or less constant; puerperal sepsis and septic abortion still accounted for about half of all deaths. Indeed, maternal mortality rates in the United States remained among the highest among comparable developed nations until World War II.[66]

Of all the infectious diseases, tuberculosis was among most important causes of adult deaths before 1900. Much of the data dealing with the incidence and prevalence of this disease are probably exaggerated, for it was often confused with other pulmonary and respiratory disorders. Even after identification of the tubercle bacillus in 1882, differential diagnoses were unreliable. Nevertheless, there is little doubt that tuberculosis in one form or another was one of the major causes of mortality among adults; its ravages were often compared with those of the Black Plague in Europe in the fifteenth century. Tuberculosis, wrote an early twentieth-century journalist,

> is a Plague is disguise. Its ravages are insidious, slow. They have never yet roused a people to great, sweeping action. The Black Plague in London is ever remembered with horror. It lived one year; it killed fifty thousand. The Plague Consumption kills this year in Europe over a million; and this has been going on not for one year but for centuries. It is the Plague of all plagues—both in age and in power—insidious, steady, unceasing.[67]

Somewhere toward the end of the nineteenth century mortality from tuberculosis began to fall, and by the beginning of World War II the disease was no longer a major threat to health. In the mid-nineteenth century the estimated death rate from all forms of tuberculosis was over 400 per 100,000. In 1900 the death rate from all forms of tuberculosis in the original Death Registration Area was 194; the disease accounted for about 10 or 11 percent of all deaths. By 1945 the rate had declined to 39.9. Between 1900 and 1940 population increased from 76 to 132 million, whereas the number of deaths from tuberculosis fell from 154,000 to 64,000.[68]

As tuberculosis mortality declined, there was a shift in incidence by age. In 1900 three out of four deaths from this disease were among persons under 45 years of age; the death rate was highest in the 25–34 category (294). The rate in the over-45 group was slightly lower, though rising with age and reaching 256 in the 65–74 cohort. By

1950 42 percent of deaths were among those under 45; their death rate was 13, as compared with 46 in the over 45 group. A wide disparity existed between whites and nonwhites (largely African-American). In 1910 the mortality rate for the two groups was 146 and 446, respectively. Thirty years later there was a dramatic reduction in the death rate for both, but the differential persisted (37 and 128).[69]

The decline of tuberculosis morbidity and mortality is much easier to describe than to explain. There is general agreement that the varied treatments for tuberculosis prior to the introduction of drug therapy after World War II were largely ineffective. The BCG vaccine, developed in France in the 1920s, was widely employed in Europe and Canada. In the United States, on the other hand, it was rejected because it rendered the tuberculin skin test useless. The American medical profession also believed that social and environmental factors— poverty, malnutrition, slum housing—played the major role in the etiology of tuberculosis, and that its control required their alleviation. Yet its members were in no position to change the structure of American society.[70]

The answer to the puzzling problem of why mortality from tuberculosis declined is by no means self-evident. The biology of the tubercle bacillus is extraordinarily complex, and the mechanisms that shape human susceptibility and resistance are equally murky. Nor is it possible to determine whether the virulence of the pathogen has changed over time. The inability of biology to explain changing epidemiological patterns has therefore led scholars to focus on the role of external elements that mediated the host-pathogen relationship. In the early 1930s Edgar Sydenstricker, a distinguished epidemiologist, prepared a study on the relationship of health and the environment for the President's Research Committee on Social Trends that resulted in the publication of the classic and influential *Recent Social Trends in the United States* in 1933. Sydenstricker's comments reflected prevailing sentiments. "In no disease, as far as we know," he wrote,

are so many social and economic conditions involved as in tuberculosis . . . it has been thoroughly established that improvement of the standard of living is essential in its prophylaxis. In fact, all efforts to combat the disease are concerned with the economic condition of the affected family and its position in the social scale . . . The provision of proper diet, freedom from worry, rest, fresh air and sunlight, and "good" housing . . . are regarded as essentials in the cure of the disease as well as in its prevention.[71]

An explanation that links the decline of tuberculosis to changes in the standard of living is inherently attractive. Yet the data to support such an interpretation are at best weak. The disease, for example, was found in middle- and upper-class households where deprivation was absent. Comparative data from countries as different as Ireland and Norway revealed that a rise in the level of wages had been accompanied with a rise in tuberculosis mortality. In New York City housing became increasingly crowded between 1880 and 1900, whereas deaths from the disease were declining. In Ireland, by contrast, improvement in housing occurred at the same time that mortality from tuberculosis was rising.[72]

In the early twentieth century Arthur Newsholme, who served as medical officer for health for Brighton, in England, while exploring epidemiological problems, turned his attention from diphtheria to tuberculosis. In a series of articles and a book published in 1908, he advanced the proposition that the decline of mortality from tuberculosis in England was the result of the segregation of infected persons in institutions, particularly workhouse infirmaries. The real decline in mortality began about 1870, when the number of beds (especially in infirmaries) increased rapidly (the only interruption in this trend occurred during World War I). The exponential decline in mortality from tuberculosis, Newsholme concluded, occurred because the identification of persons with pulmonary tuberculosis and their segregation during the infective stage limited their ability to spread the infection. At Brighton about one-fifth of all consumptives were in infirmaries. Taking into account their average length-of-stay and their period of infectivity, Newsholme calculated that their segregation prevented the spread of about 2 percent of total infection. Aggregate data supported his conclusion; from 1871 to 1905 the average annual decline of tuberculosis mortality was precisely in this range.[73]

Whether Newsholme's explanation was applicable to the United States is more problematic. Lawrence Flick, a physician who played a prominent role in the antituberculosis movement, also believed that institutionalization was the critical variable in explaining the decline in mortality from the disease in Philadelphia, but the statistics he employed to support his claim were suspect. Other local and state data are at best ambiguous. In 1889 pathologists at the New York City Health Department reported that the risk of spreading the bacillus could be minimized by disinfection of hospital rooms and sanitary disposal of sputum. Four years later the department made tuberculosis a reportable disease and established a special institution for consumptives. From 1913 through 1916 the city created three additional hospitals with substantial bed capacity. Indeed, both New York and Massachusetts led in the movement to establish special tuberculosis hospitals. Other states followed, and during the 1920s the number of special hospitals devoted to the care of consumptives expanded rapidly. In 1925 there were 466 such institutions, with more than 49,000 beds, and a decade later the number of beds had almost doubled. From 1915 to 1934 the proportion of tuberculosis cases that were hospitalized rose from 4 to 25 percent.[74] That identification of cases and hospitalization played important roles in reducing the spread of the disease seems clear. Yet the decline in mortality began well before the creation of such an extensive system of tuberculosis hospitals, suggesting that other factors were also significant.

The Metropolitan Life Insurance Company, which conducted a vigorous antituberculosis campaign, concluded that identification of cases and appropriate treatment (including isolation in sanatoriums) played a major role in the reduction in morbidity and mortality. Because of its successes in treating active cases from 1913 to 1945 at its own sanatorium at Mount McGregor, near Saratoga Springs, New York, it decided to provide resources for a demonstration project.[75] Framingham, Massachusetts, was selected as the site for the study, which was conducted by the National Association for the Study and Prevention of Tuberculosis from 1917 through 1923. The project was designed to control tuberculosis morbidity and mortality, although data were also collected on dozens of other illnesses and conditions (including bad teeth, enlarged tonsils, and respiratory infections). Nearly two-thirds of the population of Framingham received complete physical examinations. In the first year 96 individuals were diagnosed with tuberculosis, of whom 25 were listed as incipient, 17 as advanced, and 54 as arrested. Of these, 10 were treated at a sanatorium. The results of the Framingham Demonstration appeared to validate the effectiveness of intensive community action. Mortality dropped from 121 per 100,000 in the predemonstration decade to 38 in 1923 (a decline of 68 percent). During the same period the combined rate for seven control towns fell from 126 to 85 per 100,000 (a decline of 32 percent).[76]

The project appeared so successful that the city of Syracuse, New York, with the support of the Milbank Memorial Fund, launched a communitywide project in 1923 that was designed to demonstrate the value of an advanced public health program. The tuberculosis control program attempted to reduce opportunities for infection by the pasteurization of milk and the control of human sources of infection. Case finding, clinic and nursing services, sanatorium care, and such treatments as pneumothorax (forcing air into the chest in order to compress the lung and limit its movement) and surgery to immobilize the lung seemed to have clear benefits. Since 1900 the death rate from tuberculosis in Syracuse had been slightly below that of New York State as a whole. During the demonstration project mortality—which had been declining since the turn of the century—continued to fall, but at the same pace as that throughout the state.[77]

Neither the Framingham nor the Syracuse project, however, provided data that conclusively explained the mortality decline from tuberculosis. The hallmark of both projects was community mobilization and publicity; there were virtually no specific interventions that might explain the decline of tuberculosis mortality. Indeed, the Framingham results might have very well reflected closer attention to epidemiological trends in that community than in the control towns. Writing in 1937, Wade Hampton Frost (a faculty member of the Johns Hopkins School of Health and Hygiene and a key figure in the creation of modern epidemiology) rejected the hypothesis that measures undertaken during the last half-century had reduced infection. His data also disproved the claim that childhood exposure to tuberculosis with disease conferred adult immunity. Nor was there evidence that the tubercle bacillus had undergone evolutionary change that diminished virulence. Frost rather emphasized "progressively increasing human resistance, due to the influence of selective mortality and to environmental improvements . . . tending to raise what may be called nonspecific resistance." The eradication of the disease, he insisted, did not require isolation of all active cases, but "only that the rate of transmission be held permanently below the level at which a given number of infection spreading (i.e., open) cases succeed in establishing an equivalent number to carry on the succession." In other words, as the number of infectious hosts was reduced, the disease would be set on the road to extinction.[78]

Despite numerous explanations, the reason for the decline in tuberculosis morbidity and mortality remains somewhat unclear. Some have suggested that the fall in the birthrate was an important element; reduced family size led to better nutrition and less crowded housing. A study of New York City covering 1949–1951 found that prevalence rates were highest where housing was "grossly dilapidated." Some areas, on the other hand, deviated from this pattern. In parts of the city tuberculosis rates were low even though housing was poor; elsewhere high rates were present where homes and apartments "were in good condition." Certain occupations were conducive to the spread of tuberculosis. Moreover, the relationship of tuberculosis mortality with differentials in education was quite pronounced. In 1960 mortality from tuberculosis for white males aged 25–64 with less than eight years of schooling was 8.79 times that of men with one or more years of college even though for all causes of death the ratio was only 1.48 to 1. Whatever the reasons, the risks to health and life posed by tuberculosis markedly diminished during the first half of the twentieth century.[79]

The reduction in mortality from infectious disease carried over into military life. From the American Revolution to the Spanish-American War, the overwhelming majority of deaths were the result of disease rather than battlefield wounds. World War I proved a turning point in the annals of American military warfare. During that war there were approximately the same number of deaths from disease as from battle injuries and wounds. But if deaths from the influenza pandemic of 1918–19 (a worldwide pandemic that killed millions) are omitted, the declining role of infectious diseases as a cause of mortality becomes readily apparent. Indeed, influenza and other respiratory disorders accounted for about 80 percent of the deaths from disease. Although conditions of military life undoubtedly magnified their effects, these respiratory diseases would probably still have taken a high toll. Many diseases that in past wars resulted in fatalities had more favorable outcomes from 1917 through 1919. To be sure, the Medical Department of the Army was better prepared in terms of hygienic and sanitary practices. Nevertheless, effective therapies for the most part were still lacking. Yet with the exception of influenza and other respiratory disorders, morbidity and mortality rates in the military were not fundamentally different from those among the general population.[80]

That infectious diseases played a declining role in morbidity and mortality after 1900 is quite clear. The origins of this epidemiological transition, however, remain controversial. Economist Robert W. Fogel, who studied the mortality decline, concluded that the "principal mechanisms for the escape from high mortality and poor health were the elimination of chronic malnutrition, the advances in public health, the improvement of housing, the reduced consumption of toxic substances, and advances in medical technology." Yet he also conceded that the "relative importance of each of these factors in the escape is still a matter of controversy."[81]

If the causes of the epidemiological or health transition remain somewhat obscure, its consequences are clearer. In general, the reduction of mortality from infectious diseases at the end of the nineteenth century set the stage for progressive improvements in health in the twentieth. Infectious diseases not only threatened the lives of infants and children but had long-term consequences for health status in later life. Indeed, there is some (though inconclusive) evidence that some of the long-duration diseases that are associated with aging may have roots in exposure to infectious diseases in infancy and childhood. Those who were born after 1900 had a better chance not only of surviving the vicissitudes of infancy and childhood, but of postponing the burden imposed by the diseases that are associated with advancing age. In many respects, therefore, the history of health in the twentieth century would be very different from its history in the preceding millennia.

CHAPTER 9

The Discovery of
Chronic Illness

"The problem of chronic disease will not be downed," wrote George H. Bigelow and Herbert L. Lombard in a pioneering study published in 1933.

> Increasingly great numbers of people are ill, crippled and dying from chronic disease . . . There is hardly a family in Massachusetts without immediate experience with cancer, heart disease, or rheumatism . . . not only do chronic diseases make up two-thirds of all deaths in Massachusetts, whereas fifty years ago they were but one-third, but also from the duration as noted on the death returns there is a marked increase in the length of the chronic disease that kills.[1]

For much of human history, by contrast, death was associated with the infectious diseases that took such a heavy toll among infants and children. Beginning in the late nineteenth century the reduction in mortality from infectious diseases among the young permitted more people to reach adulthood and live longer. Under these circumstances it is not surprising that long-duration illnesses—notably cardiovascular-renal diseases and a variety of neoplasms—became more prominent factors in morbidity and mortality patterns. These diseases tended to be associated with advancing age; the longer individuals lived, the greater the risk of becoming ill or dying from them. In one sense the increasing prominence of long-duration diseases was in part a reflection of the fact that more and more people were enjoying greater longevity.

To point to the growing significance of long-duration illnesses in the twentieth century, however, is not to suggest their unimportance before 1900. In the nineteenth century high death rates among the very young tended to mask the presence of chronic illnesses and disabilities among both young and older adults. Mortality remained the measure of health, and long-duration illnesses and a variety of disabilities among a significant proportion of the population were often overlooked.

The transition to new morbidity and mortality patterns was by no means clear-cut. Infectious diseases, to be sure, declined as the major cause of mortality, but they did not disappear. Yet health indicators began to move on an upward gradient, although the improvement was not linear. Mortality rates among infants and children fell dramatically, thus increasing life expectancy at birth. But the longevity gains associated with the decline in mortality among the young were not shared by those over the age of 50, all of whom had been born before 1900.

The growing association of mortality and advancing age was accompanied by the "discovery" of the importance of chronic or long-duration diseases and disability. Indeed, the very definition of health underwent a fundamental transformation. After 1900 morbidity rather than mortality became the measure of health. The result was to heighten interest not only in long-duration illnesses and disabilities that affected younger and older adults, but in the role of home, industrial, and automobile accidents, all of which posed risks to health and life. Changing perceptions of health and disease, to be sure, were not accompanied by significant institutional or policy changes before 1940. Nevertheless, they played a vital part in hastening the fundamental changes that transformed health practices and policies during the second half of the twentieth century.

▼ ▼ ▼

Before 1900 Americans were preoccupied mainly with acute infectious disease. Aside from their impact on mortality, such diseases were eminently visible. The symptomatic manifestations of diphtheria, smallpox, measles, and enteric disorders—to cite only the more obvious—were dramatic. That infants and children were at higher risk of dying from these diseases than any other age group served to magnify their significance. Chronic diseases, by contrast, were often more difficult to identify. Indeed, the federal census focused on the causes of mortality rather than the prevalence of morbidity. The census of 1880 was typical. The data indicated that eight of the ten leading causes of death were the result of infections; the remaining two were diseases of the nervous system and diseases of the digestive system (which accounted for 32 percent of total mortality).[2] The use of the latter two diagnoses—which may have included infections—was indicative of the growing tendency to explain disease in terms of invading pathogens. By that time bacteriologists and other medical scientists had had considerable success in identifying the role of specific pathogens in the etiology of some diseases. Such successes reinforced interest in acute infectious diseases, and deflected concern from chronic diseases that appeared to be noninfectious. Moreover, very few physicians possessed the ability to identify many chronic illnesses. Finally, long-duration illnesses presented novel social and economic problems. How would society provide resources for the care of individuals with chronic health problems or who were incapacitated by the infirmities associated with advanced age?

Equally significant was the fact that there was relatively little interest in disability. Disability, of course, is a generic term that has many different facets. Some disabilities were genetic; some were congenital; others were a consequence of occupation or accidents; and still others were associated with illness or old age. In fact in the late nineteenth century the concept of disability was virtually nonexistent. The federal censuses of those decades used a limited definition with three categories: "Defective, Dependent, and Delinquent." The first was composed of insane persons, idiots, and blind and deaf-mute persons. The second consisted of paupers, and the third was made up of criminals. According to the census of 1880 nearly 92,000 persons were insane, 77,000 were idiots, 49,000 were blind, and 34,000 were deaf-mutes. Slightly more than 67,000 paupers were in almshouses, and nearly 22,000 were receiving some form of "outdoor" assistance (although census officials conceded that the latter statistic was virtually worthless).[3]

Only severe and chronic mental illnesses drew public attention. Those who fell into this category were often incapacitated and thus had to rely on others for their survival. They constituted one of the largest dependent groups in the country. Although it is difficult to determine whether rates of mental illnesses changed during the nineteenth and twentieth centuries, the number of individuals diagnosed as such clearly increased. In the early nineteenth century states began to assume responsibility for their care and undertook the construction of a large public mental hospital system. The costs of caring for the mentally ill remained the single largest item in most state budgets during the second half of the nineteenth as well as the early twentieth century. In 1880 half of those identified as mentally ill were found in public mental hospitals. Of the nearly 77,000 categorized as "idiots," by contrast, 87 percent lived at home.[4]

Chronic illnesses may have been less visible, but they were by no means insignificant. Chronic diseases, though often unrecognized, clearly played a major role in the lives of many Americans. Ironically, rural areas, which had lower mortality rates than urban areas, had higher levels of chronic disease and impairments, particularly in the rural South for males and females and in the rural West for females. Although the reasons for higher morbidity rates in rural areas remain obscure, Cheryl Elman and George C. Myers have recently speculated that such rates might have been the outcome of earlier episodes of infectious disease and "exposures to historical natural conditions and conditions generated by human action, such as war and mass migration."[5]

Data from pension records of Union Army Civil War veterans offer further confirmation of the importance of chronic illness. Begun in 1862 to assist soldiers who had become severely disabled, the system by 1890 had become a universal disability and old-age pension program for veterans (as well as their dependents) regardless of the origin of the disability. By 1907 all veterans aged 65 and over were covered by a program that was the largest of its kind prior to the passage of the Social Security Act of 1935 (perhaps 25 percent of all those aged 65 and over were enrolled). In 1902 there about 1 million pensioners, and the amount allocated for this program accounted for nearly 30 percent of all federal expenditures.[6]

Individuals applying for pensions under this program underwent some sort of medical examination. A sample of these records for men aged 50–64 in 1900 is illuminating. At the time of their military service during the Civil War they were probably healthier than the population as a whole. Yet prevalence rates of chronic conditions in later life were high: 23.7 percent suffered from decreased breath or adventitious sounds, 48.2 percent had joint problems, 40.4 percent had back problems, 30 percent had an irregular pulse, 29.1 percent had heart murmurs, and 19.2 percent had valvular heart disease. A decade later rates for chronic conditions among the 65-and-over group were even higher. Musculoskeletal disorders were found among 68.4 percent of the sample, digestive disorders among 84 percent, genitourinary problems among 27.3 percent, circulatory conditions among 90.1 percent, and respiratory disorders among 42.2 percent. Only 2.2 percent had a neoplasm, although the widespread inability to diagnose this category renders this low figure suspect.[7]

Recognition of the growing significance of long-duration diseases was slow in developing. The modern hospital, which came into existence toward the end of the nineteenth century, generally dealt with acute rather than long-duration diseases. Though ultimately becoming the centerpiece of the nation's health care system, its preoccupation in its formative years with acute cases delayed recognition of the significance of long-duration illnesses.[8]

Cancer (a generic term for a multiplicity of diseases), which in the twentieth century became the "Dread Disease," aroused relatively little interest in the nineteenth century. It did not occur in epidemic form, nor did it for the most part affect children and young people. Cancer appeared to be a random disease associated with older persons. Public discussions were rare, and newspapers and magazines all but ignored the disease. Only when Ulysses S. Grant, the nation's most revered war hero and former president, became ill with squamous-cell carcinoma in the winter of 1885, did newspapers begin daily coverage that ceased only after his death that summer. More often than not the stories reflected journalistic imagination rather than fact. Recognizing that little could be done, Grant was far more stoic and analytical than journalists. "I can feel plainly," he wrote to his physician about a month before his death,

> that my system is preparing for dissolution in one of three ways: one by hemorrhage; one by strangulation; and the third by exhaustion . . . With an increase in daily food, I have fallen off in weight and strength very rapidly in the past two weeks. There cannot be hope of going far beyond this period. All my physicians, or any number of them can do for me now, is to make my burden of pain as light as possible. I do not want any physician but yourself, but I tell you, so that if you are unwilling to have me go without consultation with other professional men, you can send for them. I dread them, how-

ever, knowing that it means another desperate effort to save me, and more suffering.[9]

Following Grant's death, discussions of cancer virtually disappeared from public view, largely because it did not appear to affect many individuals.

▼ ▼ ▼

In the early decades of the twentieth century the decline in infant and child mortality became more visible. In 1900 the death rate for those under 1 year of age was 162.4 per 1,000; the comparable figure for the 1-through-4-year-old group was 19.8. By 1920 these rates had dropped to 92.3 and 9.9, respectively, and expectation of life at birth during these years rose correspondingly. Between 1900 and 1930 death rates in the states included in the Death Registration Area in 1900 fell in all age groups but was most pronounced among younger individuals. The gain beyond age 55 was small, but between ages 10 and 35 mortality was halved; at ages 5 to 10 it declined by 60 percent; and among children under 5 the reduction was 66 percent.[10] As morbidity and mortality slowly became associated with age rather than with infancy and childhood, the longstanding preoccupation with acute infectious diseases was replaced by a growing concern with chronic disease and, to a lesser extent, with disability.

Epidemiological change, however important, was not the only reason for the heightened public awareness of chronic illness. During the early decades of the twentieth century data-gathering capacities began to grow. The collection of national data on morbidity and mortality, even if not reliable, offered some indication of trends. The U.S. Census Bureau slowly expanded the birth and death registration areas; by 1927 the latter included over 91 percent of the population. The bureau and the U.S. Public Health Service also began to conduct surveys of health and illness. Selected state and local departments of health expanded their data-gathering capabilities. The activities of the New York State Department of Health, for example, paralleled those of federal agencies. Private organizations, notably the Metropolitan Life Insurance Company, also created units that not only collected and analyzed health statistics but conducted sickness surveys. Such data were vital for the establishment of actuarial rates as well as for the formulation of preventive strategies designed to defer morbidity and mortality. Community studies of the incidence of illness became more common. In late 1921 more than 1,800 households in Hagerstown, Maryland, were observed for up to twenty-eight months. Each family was visited at two-month intervals and all diseases and accidents recorded. In 1923 the Milbank Memorial Fund agreed to support a demonstration project in Syracuse, New York. Though designed to show that increased expenditures could improve public health, the project also provided detailed morbidity data. Private and public organizations undertook surveys of physicians in an effort to determine venereal disease rates, while others focused on the health of children and the incidence of blindness.[11]

Before the twentieth century the mortality rate was the measure of health. Although sickness—both acute and chronic—was prevalent, the absence of data and the inability to diagnose many diseases created a situation in which the focus was on mortality. The decline in mortality among the young and the growing sophistication of both diagnostic techniques and data-collection capabilities, however, combined to transform the very meaning of health. Mortality rates remained an important measure of health, but lifetime morbidity assumed an equal position. "It has come to be recognized," wrote Margaret L. Stecker, a member of the Research Staff of the National Industrial Conference Board in 1919, "that the death rate cannot be accepted as the final standard of measurement for health. Any community with relatively few deaths may still contain a large number of individuals who are so disabled physically or mentally as to be useless, indeed, even burdensome, to the groups of which they are a part." Morbidity, admittedly, was much more difficult to measure than mortality, given the absence of a generally accepted standard of normality. Nevertheless, the developing knowledge "that most diseases are, within reasonable limits, not only curable but preventable" made accurate knowledge of the incidence of sickness mandatory. Stecker's optimistic claims about curability and prevention were illusory, but her assertion that the mortality rate was not an accurate measure of health mirrored a growing recognition of the distinction between mortality and morbidity. "The assumption that *mortality* in the general population," wrote two Public Health Service figures in the midst of the depression of the 1930s, "is an accurate index of *sickness* in the families of the unemployed is still less tenable. Recent morbidity studies have shown that the important causes of death are *not* the most frequent causes of illness."[12]

The decline in mortality from infectious diseases that became evident in the early decades of the twentieth century was a source of satisfaction and pride to most Americans. Yet appearances could be deceptive. The influenza pandemic that began in the spring of 1918 demonstrated that infectious epidemic diseases could still take a heavy toll.

Influenza is an ancient viral disease that may have originated with the domestication of such animals as pigs, which served as reservoir hosts. Before the twentieth century influenza epidemics tended to be confined to the hemispheres of origins. But the development of railroads and steamships, which transported both humans and the virus, made possible the dissemination of influenza throughout the world. The first worldwide pandemic occurred in 1889–90. Europe, which had a total population of about 360 million, had a mortality rate of 0.75 to 1 per 1,000 (or between 270,000 and 360,000 deaths). Most influenza outbreaks were characterized by high morbidity and low mortality. Aged persons and those with severe chronic diseases were most vulnerable, and death in most cases followed secondary bacterial infections.[13]

The pandemic of 1918–19 was more devastating. The disease appeared in the spring of 1918 and quickly assumed a lethal form. Perhaps 20 or 30 million perished throughout the world, and probably ten times that number became ill. In the United States at least a quarter of the population was infected, and in the military an even higher proportion became ill. The navy estimated that 40 percent of its personnel had flu in 1918. Crowded conditions both in military camps and on ships undoubtedly facilitated the spread of the virus.[14]

What made the pandemic of 1918–19 unique was a sharply elevated mortality rate. In an average year about 125,000 Americans would have perished from influenza and pneumonic complications. During the pandemic the actual number of deaths was in the range of 675,000. Almost as many American military personnel died of influenza and pneumonia (44,000) as were killed in battle (50,000). Equally significant, young people were at much higher risk of dying. In Connecticut—a typical state—56 percent of all deaths were found in the 20—39 age group. Nationally adults between ages 25 and 29 had the highest excess death rate, whereas those above age 70 had a death rate equal to the rate of 1914. A navy medical officer noted that most of his service's flu victims "were robust, young men when attacked and the number of these well-developed and well-nourished bodies at necropsy [postmortem examination] made a sad spectacle beyond description."[15]

Virtually all preventive and interventionist measures proved futile. Some cities enacted laws requiring the wearing of face masks; others forbade public gatherings. Yet San Francisco—a city that utilized virtually every known preventive measure and adopted stringent enforcement measures—had over 50,000 cases and 3,500 deaths, of which two-thirds were between the ages of 20 and 40. Entire neighborhoods were devastated. The experience of other cities was not fundamentally different. One area, the visiting nurse superintendent in Chicago reported,

> was a hotbed of influenza and pneumonia. People watched at the window, at the doors, then beckoned us to come in, although our gowns and masks frightened some. On one of the coldest, rainiest days which we had, the nurse met on the sidewalk in front of a home, an 8-year-old boy, barefoot and in his nightdress. She quickly saw that he was delirious and coaxing him back into the house, she found his father sitting beside the stove, his head in his hands, two children in one bed, the mother and a two weeks old baby in another . . . He had been up all night and day caring for the wife and children, all with temperatures above 104°. The nurse sent for the doctor, administered to the woman, bathed all the patients and sent the youngest child to the hospital, where he died a few days later. Four of our families lost both mothers and fathers.[16]

The pandemic, however deadly, quickly receded from public attention, in part because the nation was preoccupied with World War I. Although annual influenza outbreaks recurred throughout the century, none approached the 1918–19 pandemic in lethalness.[17] Samples of the virus prevalent in 1918 were subsequently recovered from lung tissues from flu victims that were preserved at the Armed Forces Institute of Pathology. Although scientists determined the sequence of an essential gene—the hemagglutinin—they have yet to understand why it proved so deadly.[18]

During and after the 1920s mounting data demonstrated that

chronic illnesses—previously overshadowed by acute infectious diseases—were both more prevalent and increasing in significance.
Chronic diseases and disabilities admittedly had their greatest impact
on adults and older individuals, but they were not absent even among
younger groups. Data collected from 1915 through 1917 by the Metropolitan Life Insurance Company are illustrative. The data were derived from seven community sickness surveys that included more
than 500,000 of its 13 million policyholders. The company found a
rate of sickness (including injuries) so serious as to be disabling of
18.8 per 1,000 exposed. Disability that had lasted for one year or
more at the time of the survey ranged from 18.5 to 50.1 percent of
those who were sick. If these rates are extrapolated to include the total industrial population, perhaps 2.25 percent of wage earners were
constantly so sick as to be incapacitated for the ordinary pursuits of
life. The major causes of disability included violence, rheumatism (a
catchall category for aches and pains not otherwise defined), and
influenza and other epidemic diseases. Although chronic diseases
were replacing infectious diseases as the major causes of mortality,
acute diseases (often infectious) accounted for the bulk of sickness.[19]

The experiences of World War I played a role in calling attention to
the significance of chronic conditions. During that conflict physical
examinations were administered to several million potential draftees;
the result was a wealth of information on the health of young males.
Some of the defects that disqualified men for military service, of
course, proved no handicap in civilian life. Yet in the aggregate the
proportion of "defects" seemed troubling. Twenty-six percent were
found to have some defect but were not rejected, and an additional
21 percent were rejected as unfit. Such findings were undoubtedly exaggerated because of the criteria employed to establish fitness. Twelve
percent, for example, were listed as having "weak feet," 5.8 percent
had a venereal disease, and 5 percent were underweight. Nevertheless, the results of these examinations reinforced a growing realization that chronic and disabling illnesses were by no means limited to
the elderly.[20]

After World War I studies of chronic illness began to proliferate.
Massachusetts undertook one of the most ambitious studies of
chronic disease ever attempted; the result was the collection of a mass
of data. In 1926 the legislature enacted a resolution committing the
state to a program of cancer control. The following year the Depart-

ment of Public Health began to gather data dealing with total sickness. In 1929 it inaugurated a three-year study of chronic disease that involved house-to-house canvasses in fifty-one cities and towns. In the first year all age groups were included in the survey; during the second and third years only individuals over the age of 40 were included. Eventually the combined surveys included 75,000 records. Much of the data that were collected were admittedly of dubious quality, although they shed light on professional and public perceptions of disease. Some of the questions in the survey, for example, dealt with possible etiology at a time when the causes of many chronic diseases were (and still remain) unknown. Yet the study highlighted the growing concern with chronic disease and disability.

Chronic disease, according to George H. Bigelow (the department's commissioner) and Herbert L. Lombard (director of the Division of Adult Hygiene), was now of major significance. Their findings, they insisted, required the development of a multifaceted program that included the following elements: general education about the importance of personal hygiene and early detection; a determined effort to ensure the availability of appropriate therapy; an emphasis on the postgraduate education of physicians to alleviate a sense of hopelessness and the dissemination of therapeutic knowledge; and a more important role for public health officers and state government.[21]

The rising incidence of chronic disease, according to Bigelow and Lombard, had multiple causes. The gradual aging of the population was a critical variable that was an outgrowth of several demographic trends. The imposition of restrictionist immigration laws in the early 1920s had reduced the migration of younger persons from abroad. At the same time the decline in the birthrate was more rapid than the decline in the death rate. Slowly but surely, therefore, the mean and median age of the population began to increase. Chronic diseases then assumed a larger significance, since they had a major impact upon older persons. At the time of the survey, chronic diseases in Massachusetts accounted for 66 percent of all deaths; a half-century earlier the rate was only 33 percent.[22]

The human and economic costs of chronic disease, the two officials noted, were considerable. Unlike acute infectious diseases, chronic diseases were of long duration and involved pain as well as disability. The average untreated case of cancer survived for twenty-one months; those with heart diseases survived for seven to nine years;

and persons with "rheumatism" (which included neuritis and arthritis) lived fourteen years or more. Lost wages alone amounted to 40 million dollars per year, which was equal to the total cost of state government for the same period. The amount expended for care, the services provided by private philanthropy or government, the loss of income to family members providing care, and other indirect costs were probably equal to the total of lost wages.[23]

In the past chronic disease rates had been understated—since they were aggregated from hospital and death records—and therefore did not count those who had not been hospitalized. The three-year survey of households, by contrast, found a much higher prevalence of chronic disease. About half a million persons out of a total population of 4.25 million suffered from a chronic illness. Of this number, 45 percent were partially disabled and 5 percent totally disabled. Rheumatism (a term preferred over arthritis), heart disease, and arteriosclerosis accounted for somewhat more than half of all cases of chronic illness in Massachusetts. Morbidity was also inversely related to economic status; poor people were at much higher risk. Indeed, chronic illness was a significant factor in public welfare expenditures. The importance of chronic diseases was also reflected in the changing causes of mortality. Between 1850 and 1920 the death rate from infections (including tuberculosis) fell by 600 percent. During that same period the combined death rates for cancer, diabetes, heart disease, and nephritis increased more than sevenfold.[24]

In the same year that the Bigelow and Lombard study appeared, Mary C. Jarrett (one of the most important social workers of her generation) published an even more detailed analysis of chronic illness in New York City. Chronic illness, she noted, conjured up an image of incurable maladies among the aged. Yet such illnesses affected individuals of all ages: infants injured at birth or born with congenital defects; children who were victims of poor hygiene or infections and had residual health problems for the remainder of their lives; handicapped people; persons disabled by disease or accident; and the aged, whose life was "ending in the feebleness of natural senescence." Indeed, of the 20,700 persons incapacitated by chronic illness and found in the care of the city's medical and social agencies, only 20 percent were 70 years of age or older; considerably more than half were under 45. Children under 16 constituted a third of the whole number, and nearly a fourth of these children were under 6 years of age.[25]

Although Jarrett's study was based largely on data derived from a census of 218 welfare and medical agencies and correctional institutions, she estimated that 700,000 New Yorkers (approximately 10 percent of the population) suffered from chronic diseases, of whom 64,000 were wholly disabled. There were perhaps 20,000 crippled children, some of whom had congenital defects and others who were the victims of paralytic polio. Such infectious diseases as rheumatic fever and encephalitis created lifelong health problems, as did diabetes and chronic asthma. Adults (in the census of the chronically ill under the care of medical and social agencies) between the ages of 16 and 40 suffered from a variety of ailments. Heart disease was the leading cause of illness, but orthopedic diseases, encephalitis, and narcotic addiction were also significant. Among middle-aged people between 40 and 60 neurological disorders were most frequent in the younger group and cardiac and circulatory diseases most important in the older. Cancer and rheumatism each accounted for 10 percent of total morbidity.[26]

Jarrett noted that the indifference of the medical profession as well as the general public to chronic illness had its origin either in misunderstandings or in lack of information. The belief that chronic diseases were peculiar to the aged was one such misconception. The discovery of the bacterial origin of communicable diseases, while having distinct benefits, nevertheless "threw into greater obscurity the unknown origins of chronic diseases." Another factor contributing to medical indifference was that chronic disease, much more so than acute disease, required knowledge of social conditions in the their treatment. "The prevention of chronic disease is the most pressing public health problem of today," Jarrett wrote. "Only a beginning has been made so far in a few communities toward organized efforts for the study and control of the chronic diseases."[27]

The Massachusetts and New York City studies of chronic illness were by no means idiosyncratic or unique. By then morbidity, whether acute or chronic, aroused as much interest as mortality had before 1900. Indeed, the growing faith in the importance of medical care was accompanied by a debate on how to finance and organize medical services. Knowledge about the incidence and prevalence of

sickness began to assume a more central role in the debate over policy. The Committee on the Costs of Medical Care, which was created
in 1927 "to study the economic aspects of the prevention and care of
sickness," insisted that any plan to reorganize medical services had to
take morbidity data into account.[28]

During the early decades of the twentieth century such federal
agencies as the Census Bureau and the Public Health Service expanded their data-collecting capabilities. The Public Health Service in
particular went beyond the mere collection of data. From 1916
through 1918 it surveyed health conditions in South Carolina cotton
mill villages in an effort to prove the dietary etiology of pellagra;
from 1921 through 1924 it studied in detail the population of
Hagerstown, Maryland; in cooperation with the Committee on the
Costs of Medical Care it surveyed 9,000 families in 130 communities
nationwide; and in 1933 its Health and Depression Studies collected
data on 11,500 wage-earning families in eight large cities and two
groups of coalmining and cotton-mill villages. None of these studies,
however, attempted to estimate the prevalence of chronic illness and
disability *in the general population*.

In the early 1930s massive unemployment forced the federal government to take a far more active role in the development of relief
policies. The debate that followed dealt not only with the unemployed but also with those individuals with chronic illness and disabilities who were unable to work and unable to pay for the costs of
care. The Social Security Act of 1935 included several provisions that
provided assistance to disabled individuals. The development of a
comprehensive policy, however, required specific knowledge about
the extent of chronic illness and disability in the general population.
In 1935, therefore, the Public Health Service, which had dramatically
expanded the scope of its studies during the previous fifteen years,
launched the most ambitious survey of health ever undertaken up to
that time. The National Health Survey of 1935–36 covered 703,092
households in eighty-three cities, and provided data on more than 2.5
million persons (or 3.6 percent of the urban population). An additional 36,801 households comprising over 140,000 persons were
canvassed in primarily rural counties. The communities included constituted a fairly representative sample of the nation as whole. The survey was designed to ascertain the incidence and prevalence of illness
that caused disabilities lasting a week or more, serious physical im-

pairments, and chronic diseases that were not necessarily disabling. The result was a dramatic and revealing portrait of the pervasiveness of chronic disease and disability.[29]

The findings of the National Health Survey proved surprising. Nearly a fifth of the population had a chronic disease or impairment (defined by the study as any permanent handicap "resulting from disease, accident, or congenital defect") whether disabling or non-disabling. Low-income groups were at higher risk for illnesses that resulted in disability for a week or more. Disability was a major element in forcing families to rely on some form of assistance. Families on relief had a much larger proportion of members who were unemployed because of chronic disability. In the age 15–64 category, families on relief had ten times the number of unemployed members who suffered from some chronic disability as families having incomes of 3,000 to 5,000 dollars. Chronic illness and disability, in other words, led to unemployment and dependency. Nor were chronic diseases and permanent physical impairments concentrated among the aged. About 7.9 percent of those with chronic illnesses were children under the age of 15; 8.4 percent were between 15 and 25; 35.1 percent were in the 25–44 age group; 33 percent were between 45 and 64; and 15.6 percent were found among those 65 years of age and over. Indeed, over half of those permanently disabled, and nearly 30 percent of those who died from chronic disease, were under 55 years of age. Chronic diseases were not only pervasive, but contributed to the ranks of the disabled.[30]

Extrapolated to the entire population of about 129 million, the data suggested that chronic disease and disability was "A National Problem."[31] Overall 16.2 million men and women in the productive ages of 20 through 64 and living at home had one or more handicapping chronic disease or serious physical or mental impairment. About half a million persons were in mental or tuberculosis hospitals. An additional 5.2 million had one or more acute illness that disabled them for one week to three months during the year.[32]

Two percent of the population had a permanent orthopedic impairment that partially or completely crippled, deformed, or paralyzed them. Of the 2.6 million in this category, 210,000 were under the age of 15, 1.9 million fell into the 15–64 age group, and the remainder were over the age of 64. About one-third of these impairments were the result of job-related accidents, one-sixth were due to accidents in the home, and about 10 percent resulted from automobile accidents. More than one-third of orthopedic impairments resulted from disease (of which two-thirds were the result of apoplexy, polio, and arthritis).[33]

Before 1900 there was little appreciation that accidents were an important determinant of health and longevity. Yet by the late nineteenth century accidents, notably in the extractive and in some manufacturing industries, were taking a heavy toll. Faith in science and technology and concern with efficiency began to transform public perceptions, and the belief that accidents were preventable rather than inevitable slowly emerged. In 1913 the National Safety Council was established to promote industrial safety. Many industrial leaders had come to the realization that accidents were not necessarily the fault of workers and that the introduction of safety measures could enhance efficiency and productivity. Between 1914 and 1940 industrial mortality and morbidity from accidents declined from the peak reached early in the century.[34]

Awareness of home and public accidents increased in the interwar years, but never approached the preoccupation with industrial safety. Part of the difficulty was the absence of reliable national data. The Bureau of the Census began publishing data on mortality from accidents in 1935, but had not collected information on accidents that did not result in death. From 1935 through 1938 the average annual mortality from accidents was slightly over 102,000. About 10 percent of deaths from accidents occurred in industry, 23 percent in homes, 48 percent in public settings, and 19 percent were unspecified as to place of origins. Of the 49,272 who perished from accidents in public settings, 70 percent (34,256) died in automobile accidents.[35]

The National Health Survey, by contrast, collected a mass of data on accidents that did not result in deaths but often led to disability. Before that time the only statistics on nonfatal home accidents were compiled from records of safety organizations, which were not necessarily representative of the total population. The findings of the survey proved sobering. The total rate for all accidents that resulted in disability for a week or more was 16 per 1,000 persons, of which 29 percent occurred in the home, 24 percent on the job, 20 percent in automobiles, 21 percent in other public accidents, and 6 percent were of unspecified origin. Many accidents, moreover, led to orthopedic impairments. The rate for home accidents that resulted in loss of members and crippled or paralyzed members was 2.88 per 1,000 persons, a figure that represented the permanent effects of injury over the attained lifetime of living individuals in the surveyed population.[36]

The study also gave special attention to the problem of blindness. In the urban population surveyed, the rate of blindness in one or both eyes was 40.9 per 1,000. Approximately one-sixth of the cases of total blindness and one-half of those blind in one eye were the result of accidents; the remainder were probably due to disease, congenital causes, or causes characteristic of infancy. Age was a significant factor; more than a quarter of those blind in both eyes were over 75 years of age, and two-thirds were over 55.[37]

With the exception of Joseph Schereschewsky's study of the health of New York City garment workers in 1914, the involvement of the Public Health Service in studying occupational diseases was minimal. Indeed, Schereschewsky (who played an important role in cancer research and therapy during the years before his death in 1940) had relied on comprehensive physical examinations that proved effective in identifying well-established infectious diseases but could not deal with subtle workplace hazards such as carbon monoxide poisoning from gas-heated pressing irons.[38] In its canvass of families, the National Health Survey collected data on injuries and disabling morbidity in several industries. But these data in general were not analyzed with a view to isolating the manner in which the workplace environment created risks to the health of workers.[39]

A pioneering effort, the National Health Survey nevertheless had serious methodological shortcomings. House-to-house canvassing identified some but not all chronic diseases that resulted in disability. The absence of physical examinations and the limitations inherent in the questionnaire rendered its findings at best incomplete. The prevalence of serious mental diseases found in the survey, for example, underestimated the true situation. If survey data had been adjusted for underenumeration and if the nearly 500,000 persons in mental hospitals had been included, the prevalence rate of 9 per 1,000 would have had to be adjusted upward to about 15. Moreover, the survey did not enumerate venereal diseases, which often led to chronic health problems.[40]

That chronic illness and disability were serious problems was obvious. In a 1948 summary that drew upon the National Health Survey and other sources, Howard A. Rusk and Eugene Taylor found that more than 2.25 million Americans had orthopedic impairments, of whom 341,000 were incapacitated. Selective Service data for 1941–1945 revealed that 4.8 million men were rejected for military service. About a quarter had disqualifying musculoskeletal, or neurological defects, and nearly 7 percent had cardiovascular problems. There were perhaps 900,000 amputees in the mid-1940s; each year an additional 75,000 people fell into this category. In 1933 there were about 368,000 crippled children and 175,000 who suffered from cerebral palsy. The acoustically and visually handicapped constituted another large group. Conceding that reliable statistics and data were incomplete, Rusk and Taylor insisted that "the totals are tremendous," and that only a small proportion were benefiting from rehabilitation even though the needs of these individuals "could be met more effectively."[41]

The American health care system, however, remained focused on rather traditional goals: increasing the number of professionals and hospitals providing acute care; expanding efforts to control infectious diseases; finding ways to deal with the consequences of workplace injuries and acute occupational illnesses; and creating a system that would enable all social classes to pay for expensive hospital stays for acute conditions. Such a system reflected the late nineteenth- and early twentieth-century belief that acute infectious diseases represented the greatest threat to health and well-being and could be alleviated by a finite amount of time and money. Chronic disease and disability, by contrast, were problems presumably confined to low-income groups and could be addressed by expanding state mental hospitals, city and county hospitals and sanatoria, and workmen's compensation. Indeed, the debate over compulsory health insurance in the 1920s centered as much on income replacement during illness as on access to medical care.[42]

The data on the high prevalence of chronic illness and disability were largely ignored before World War II. To a relatively small group, however, the new epidemiological patterns required fundamental changes in the American health care system. George H. Bigelow, who had overseen the study of cancer and chronic illness in Massachusetts in the late 1920s and early 1930s, insisted that the "outstanding sickness and health problem of the present day is the control of chronic diseases of the middle-aged." His views were echoed by such figures as Sigmund S. Goldwater, commissioner of health and then commissioner of hospitals in New York City; Louis I. Dublin, the noted statistician of the Metropolitan Life Insurance Company; Alan Gregg, of the Rockefeller Foundation; Alfred E. Cohn, of the Rockefeller Institute for Medical Research; and Ernst P. Boas, of Montefiore Hospital in New York City.[43]

In 1940 Boas attempted to broaden public appreciation of the growing importance of chronic disease and the absence of an "orderly program for combating its disastrous consequences." "Chronic diseases," he observed, "create not only medical problems, they are a major cause of social insecurity; their malign influence permeates into all phases of our living, causing indigency and unemployment, disrupting families, and jeopardizing the welfare of children . . . There is no realization that they are ever present and inescapable, that they occur at all ages, that if we are spared them in our youth they will almost inevitably overtake us in our older years." Most families had at least one member stricken by such illness as heart disease, rheumatism, cancer, or diabetes. The human and economic consequences to families required a radical rethinking of the roles of both society and the medical profession. Cure, he insisted, was an unrealistic goal. Chronic illness and disability required a comprehensive approach that placed a premium on management and care.[44]

Three years before the appearance of Boas' book, Dublin and Alfred J. Lotka published a lengthy analysis of the mortality experiences of his company's industrial policyholders that provided dramatic evidence of changing patterns. They pointed to the decline in mortality from infectious diseases among infants, children, and young adults, which they attributed to sanitary and public health interventions. The result was a major shift in the causes of mortality. In 1911 heart disease and cancer had accounted for 16.6 percent of total mortality; a quarter of a century later the share had leapt to 30.4. "In combating diseases characteristic of midlife and after," Dublin and Lotka conceded, "we have had at most only moderate success." Their data and analysis suggested that the distinction between acute infectious and chronic diseases was in some ways spurious. The rank-order position of influenza and pneumonia as the most important causes of death between 1911 and 1935, for example, remained unchanged. Yet they took their highest toll among those in the 45-and-older age group. Elderly persons with other chronic health patterns were more vulnerable to infectious respiratory disorders. Moreover, occupation was also a factor in pneumonia mortality. The data indicated that three occupational hazards played a role, namely, dust, extreme heat, and sudden temperature variations or exposure to the weather. The pneumonia death rate was also related to class; unskilled workers were much more at risk than those above them in the occupational and income hierarchy.[45]

A decade later Dublin and Richard J. Vane noted that the longevity of industrial workers who were insured by their company had improved markedly. In 1948 the workers' expectation of life at age 20 was only one year less than that of their counterparts in the general population, as compared with a difference of nearly six years in 1911–12. Yet Dublin and Vane conceded that knowledge about occupational morbidity and mortality was at best fragmentary. Much could be done, they concluded,

> to reduce further the mortality of industrial workers . . . A complete study of occupational mortality would answer many questions for which there is now no answer. What has been the over-all effect on mortality from tuberculosis and other causes of the measures instituted to control the hazard of silica dust among granite cutters, tunnel and subway workers, sandblasters, and other workers exposed to this hazard? What are the effects, if any, on the mortality from specific causes among workers exposed to inorganic dusts not containing free silica or asbestos? Has mortality from pneumonia among iron and steel and foundry workers been markedly reduced by the use of new drugs? What, if any, are the effects on mortality of exposure to radiations among workers in the field of nuclear fission? Are there other classes of workers exposed to unsuspected dangers to life, such as the chromate workers, who quite recently were discovered to have a very high mortality from cancer of the lungs?[46]

Dublin and Vane's concern with occupational hazards was understandable. The goal of the Metropolitan Life Insurance Company (of which Dublin was a vice-president) was to compress morbidity and thus postpone mortality. To this end it devoted considerable resources and time in analyzing statistical data in order to identify those behaviors and environments that could diminish risk and thus avoid sicknesses which concluded in death. Most business firms, by contrast, were preoccupied with efforts to reduce accidents. They were less concerned with, if not overtly hostile to, the idea that the workplace could pose threats to the health of workers. Consequently, the category of occupational and industrial disease remained sharply circumscribed before World War II. The National Health Survey, as we have seen, virtually ignored the subject even though its data had the potential to identify occupational health risks. Similarly, the Public Health Service collected data on the health of workers but rarely associated those data with workplace settings.[47]

Yet workplace threats to health were by no means uncommon. Industries in which dusty environments prevailed continued to pose the greatest danger to the health of workers. Underground coal mining remained the most dangerous occupation. Between 1913 and 1933 1,307 men perished in Colorado coal mines alone (626 from falls of rock and coal, 276 in explosions, 207 in haulage accidents, and 65 by electricity and machinery). The total for the United States as a whole during this period was 45,525, a fatality rate of nearly 3 per 1,000 employed. During the 1930s alone 13,203 miners lost their lives in accidents, and 657,544 sustained nonfatal injuries. The dangers of accidents, however, were dwarfed by the extraordinarily high prevalence of what subsequently became known as black lung disease, which incapacitated or killed far more miners.[48]

Industrial changes also led to the introduction of materials that posed new dangers. The widespread use of steam engines created a need for various kinds of seals and packings. Initially leather or hemp was employed, but they deteriorated rapidly. Heat loss was another problem. The early insulating substances, including hairfelt and wool, often failed under high temperatures because their extreme dryness magnified the risk of fires. The introduction of asbestos in the late nineteenth century seemed to overcome the hazards of earlier materials. Its relative indestructibility, strength, and fireproof nature made it an ideal insulator as well as an important component in building materials. With a plentiful supply from Canadian mines, asbestos use in the United States expanded dramatically. By 1930 asbestos consumption reached 190,000 metric tons. A little more than a decade later about 19,000 workers were employed in the asbestos industry, and many more worked with finished products.

Asbestos proved to be an extraordinarily hazardous substance. Disability and death occur as much as twenty years after exposure. Inhalation of asbestos dust and fibers, as subsequent research revealed, causes asbestosis, lung cancer, and mesothelioma. Those who worked in the building trades and particularly shipbuilding were at risk, but even the general public was unknowingly exposed (at sharply reduced levels) because of its use in buildings. Evidence about the dangers posed by the use of this mineral was available both before and during the 1930s and 1940s, but was either suppressed or ignored. Consequently, reliable data on disability and mortality rates are absent. Whatever the precise numbers, it is clear that asbestos-related diseases added to the health burdens of many workers.[49]

Working conditions in other extractive industries, construction, and manufacturing contributed significantly to ill health among workers. Employees in southern textile mills were exposed to high levels of cotton dust. Yet for a variety of reasons byssinosis was not recognized as a serious occupational disease until the 1960s. A similar situation prevailed among workers involved in the mining of lead or processes in which this mineral was widely used. The growing use of such coal-tar distillates as benzene (a solvent that found wide application) and other chemicals added to health hazards.

Two disasters dramatically illustrated the risks faced by workers. The first involved a relatively small group of women (probably numbering no more than 2,000) who painted watch dials with paint that had luminous qualities because of the addition of radium and its isotope mesothorium. During World War I the paint was applied to military instruments. After the war sales of luminous watches soared. The consequences quickly became clear at the United States Radium Corporation in New Jersey, which employed 250 women in its dial-painting unit. Exposure to radium led to jaw necrosis, aplastic anemia, and osteogenic sarcomas. By the early 1920s the first illnesses and deaths occurred. Although most workers survived, the number of occupationally related deaths among this group was far in excess of the expected death rate.[50]

The second disaster—perhaps the worst in American history—involved the construction of the Hawk's Nest Tunnel at Gauly, West Virginia, in the early 1930s. The tunnel was built to divert water from a river to a hydroelectric plant owned by Union Carbide. Close to 5,000 workers were employed; perhaps 3,000 worked either full or part time inside the tunnel. The rock had a high silica content, and the contractor virtually ignored all safety procedures. Testimony before a congressional committee in 1936 provided a dramatic portrait of working conditions.

The dust was so thick in the tunnel that the atmosphere resembled a patch of dense fog. It was estimated on the witness stand in the courtroom in Fayetteville, where suits against the builders of the tunnel were tried, that workmen in the tunnel could see only 10 to 15 feet ahead of them at times . . . [Workers] said that although the tunnel was thoroughly lighted, the dinkey engine ran into cars on the track because the brakeman and dinkey runner could not see them . . . Dust got into the men's hair, on their faces, in their eyebrows; their clothing was thick with it. Raymond Jackson described how men blew dust off themselves with compressed air in the tunnel; if they did not they came out of the tunnel white, he said. One worker told how dust settled on top of the drinking water.

The official statistics were sobering; 476 workers perished and 1,500 were disabled. An unofficial but more sophisticated analysis found that within five years after its completion, the Hawk's Nest Tunnel claimed more than 700 lives from silicosis.[51] Construction of the Hoover Dam on the Colorado River and other public projects also proved costly in terms of health and lives.

That occupation was a significant variable in shaping morbidity and mortality patterns is obvious. The unwillingness to recognize the role of the workplace in the etiology of many diseases, however, makes it difficult, if not impossible, to provide accurate statistical data. Both the Public Health Service and the U.S. Department of Labor, to be sure, undertook field research that led to reports dealing with the dangers of lead, phosphorous, dust, carbon monoxide, and some specific trades. In general, their modest recommendations and conclusions did relatively little to create an awareness of occupational risks. Employer resistance to the very concept of industrial diseases and the absorption of workers with wages, hours of work, and job security (particularly during the Great Depression) precluded careful evaluation of workplace health risks. In his fictional portrayal of the tragic Triangle Waist Company fire in the New York City garment industry in 1911, Sholem Asch provided a commentary on prevailing attitudes.

More than one hundred and fifty girls had lost their lives in the fire. They were buried at mass funerals; the Jewish girls in Jewish cemeteries, the Christian girls in Christian cemeteries. The survivors soon began to search for work in other factories. The wave of excitement and anger that swept through the city and all through the country didn't last very long. A commission was appointed to investigate fire hazards in the state's garment factories. Some bills were introduced into the Assembly. There were heated debates; some measures were adopted, others were defeated. When it was all over, everything in the needle industries remained the same.[52]

▾ ▾ ▾

The increase in life expectancy at birth that followed the decline in mortality from infectious diseases among the young was not necessarily matched by comparable gains among other age cohorts. Between 1900 and 1930 life expectancy at birth for males and females increased by 10.86 and 11.54 years, respectively. These gains continued through age 30, but at a sharply reduced rate. The gains at age 40 and beyond were relatively modest. During this same period males at age 40 gained only .91 and females 1.77 years.[53]

Why did adults fail to share in the health gains experienced by their younger counterparts during the first third of the twentieth century? Any answer to this complex question requires that a differentiation be made between mortality and morbidity. That mortality among the young declined dramatically is obvious. But mortality is not a synonym for morbidity even though they are closely related. Individuals who survived infancy and childhood could have high rates of sickness and disability that would limit their longevity. This was as true for the early twentieth century as it was for earlier centuries.

Those who reached the age of 40 and beyond in 1930 had been born before 1900. Virtually all had survived those infectious diseases that were responsible for high mortality among the young. Their immune systems proved capable of producing disease-specific antibodies that generally provided either lifelong or partial immunity against specific infection-causing pathogens. But if their immunologic response was beneficial, other consequences were harmful. Some infectious diseases, for example, caused lasting tissue damage at various sites in the body and thus promoted morbidity in later life. Having survived the vicissitudes of infancy and childhood, they had to cope with the residual effects of early life infections.[54]

Americans born between 1870 and 1900 and who survived infancy and youth often had high rates of exposure to such infectious diseases as rheumatic and scarlet fever, influenza, tuberculosis, syphilis, and gonorrhea, to cite only a few. Many of these diseases had the potential to cause lasting tissue damage in different parts of the body. Tuberculosis, even when controlled, sometimes created long-term pulmonary problems. Influenza was associated with encephalitis and myocarditis. Syphilis and gonorrhea led to a myriad of complications, including sterility, bacteremia, cardiac problems, and central nervous system disorders. Frequently the consequences of such infections did not manifest themselves until years after the initial infection.

The widespread prevalence of "rheumatism"—a category employed by the National Health Survey—was indicative of the presence of chronic conditions that possibly were related to infectious diseases in early life. Rheumatic fever was one such example. It had its highest incidence in childhood and early life, and often left residual heart damage. In 1930 slightly less than 1 percent of a population of 100 million had suffered serious and permanent heart damage from the disease. Physicians associated with schools found that between 1 and 2 percent of all school-age children had cardiac damage with varying degrees of handicap. Although deaths from rheumatic fever among the 6–19 age group declined, those who had had the disease were more likely to face serious cardiac problems later in life.[55]

Early twentieth-century autopsy findings provided some evidence —admittedly impressionistic—that early life infectious diseases may have resulted in lesions that played a role in later years. William Ophüls, who was involved in more than 3,000 autopsies in San Francisco hospitals during the first quarter of the twentieth century, found that lesions associated with early life infections were quite common. He collected evidence that included disease histories as well as age at death, class, race, and sex. Though dealing with an unrepresentative population, he employed part of his data to investigate whether arterial disease in adulthood might be traced to earlier infectious diseases. Taking into account the age distribution of observed damage, he compared individuals with a history of infectious diseases with those who did not. Ophüls found that aging alone could not explain the differences between the two groups; the former had far greater arterial and aortal damage. "The development of arteriosclerosis," he concluded, "is closely connected with injury to the arteries from various infections." Rheumatic chronic septic infections in particular seemed "to play the most important role." Moreover, arterial lesions reached "their full development after the active infectious process has long subsided."[56]

The conditions of life in the late nineteenth and early twentieth century, particularly in densely populated urban areas, were conducive to the dissemination of infectious diseases in early life. Crowding, unhygienic conditions both within households and in the general environment, behavioral and occupational patterns that compounded risks, for example, all played a role in the prevalence of infectious diseases. To be sure, mortality from such diseases began to fall. Yet their presence may have had an impact on those who had high rates of infection in early life but survived to adulthood. Even as adults, however, such persons continued to be exposed to infections. The thesis that early life infections can result in damage to organs—the consequences of which do not become apparent until later life—remains unproven. Yet it is clear that specific infections did have long-term consequences. Rheumatic fever, of course, is a classic example. Atherosclerosis—a condition characterized by the deposit of plaque in medium and large arteries that ultimately may produce critical stenosis, thrombosis, and aneurism—is perhaps another example. Recent research has raised the possibility that *Chlamydia pneumoniae,* which causes pharyngitis, bronchitis, and pneumonitis, largely in older children and young adults, may be related to the appearance of atherosclerosis in later life.[57]

The health of Americans in the early decades of the twentieth century, therefore, presents something of a paradox. Infants and children were the clear beneficiaries; their chances of surviving to adulthood improved dramatically. For their parents and other adults born before the turn of the century, the gains in longevity and health were less impressive. They may have been fortunate enough to survive the vicissitudes of early life, but they had to contend with a variety of long-duration illnesses and disabilities that limited their life expectancy. As successive generations born after 1900 reached maturity, they would—unlike their parents—benefit from the ensuing compression of morbidity that would increase age-specific life expectancy and thereby give rise to a much older population.

CHAPTER 10

No Final Victory

"What is the nature of the world we are bequeathing to the youngsters who will inherit the twentieth century?" Robert W. Fogel–a Nobel laureate in economics–recently asked. His response was extraordinarily optimistic. "On the material side," he observed,

> it is clearly a richer and healthier world than that inherited by my parents, who were born in 1898. Not only is life expectancy thirty years longer today than it was a century ago, but it is still increasing . . .
>
> Lifelong good health for our grandchildren is a reasonable expectation, partly because the average age for the onset of chronic diseases will be delayed by ten or more years, partly because of the increasing effectiveness of medical interventions for those who incur chronic diseases, and partly because an increasing proportion of the population will never become severely disabled.

Such optimism is widespread. Molecular medicine, according to William B. Schwartz, has the potential "to attack disease processes at their subcellular origins . . . and usher in a new era of vastly more effective care." It is not unlikely, he adds, that children born in the mid-twenty-first century "could enjoy a life expectancy of 130 years or more and be free of the major chronic illnesses that now plague the aging."[1]

Confident predictions for a healthier future reflect developments since World War II. During these decades Americans experienced dramatic changes in health and longevity. Infant mortality, which seemed to have reached a plateau in the two decades following the war, subsequently resumed its decline. The generations born after 1900 also shared in the mortality reduction as the very concept of "old" continued to be pushed further up in the life cycle. Indeed, health indicators reached all-time highs in the closing decades of the twentieth century even as there were significant changes in the causes of mortality.

Improved longevity, paradoxically, was accompanied by fears and anxiety about the future. An increasingly sophisticated diagnostic and imaging technology, aggressive marketing of drugs and other substances, a proliferation of epidemiological studies purporting to identify numerous dangers to health, and exploitation of these findings by the media—all combined to create concern that impersonal forces were having a detrimental impact on health.

▼   ▼   ▼

During World War II the introduction of antibacterial drugs, the replacement of blood, plasma, and fluids, and the increasing effectiveness of surgery heightened postwar health expectations, thereby reinforcing the faith that further medical progress would preserve and lengthen life. "The seemingly infinite productive capacity of the nation during the war, enhanced by the brilliant success of scientists in the application of their knowledge of atomic energy through the Manhattan Project," Dr. Julius B. Richmond noted, "fortified the expectation that no result was unattainable if the resources were adequate."[2]

The dream of a health utopia was fueled by dramatic social, economic, and scientific changes. A steadily rising standard of living mitigated some environmental features that in the past had an adverse impact on health. After 1945 biomedical research played a major role in transforming medical practice. The ability of medicine to intervene in many hitherto intractable disease processes–perhaps best symbolized by the introduction of antibiotic drugs and chemotherapies for certain cancers–made it possible to manage many illnesses and to ease disabilities that in the past incapacitated individuals. There were also striking changes in health policy generally. Employer-paid health insurance expanded rapidly. Equally significant was the growing role of the national government in shaping health policy. Federal support for biomedical research expanded dramatically after 1945; the Hill-

Burton Act of 1946 provided funds for hospital construction; from the mid-1960s on, Medicare and Medicaid provided coverage for the aged and the indigent; and the growth of entitlement programs offered resources to the disabled.

All these developments created an impression of irresistible progress. Sickness and disability were no longer perceived as inevitable consequences of life; they represented problems to be conquered by scientific and medical advance. The spread of the gospel of health was facilitated not only by the press but by television. The message conveyed was simple: disease could be conquered if sufficient resources were devoted to research and health care. Scientific discovery, according to members of President Harry S Truman's Scientific Research Board, was "the basis for our progress against poverty and disease." "The challenge of our times," they added, "is to advance as rapidly as possible the understanding of diseases that still resist the skills of science, to find new and better ways of dealing with diseases for which some therapies are known, and to put this new knowledge effectively to work."[3]

In the half-century following World War II Americans made health care one of their highest priorities. Between 1929 and 1950 health care expenditures rose modestly, from 3.65 to 12.66 billion dollars (3.5 to 4.1 percent of the gross domestic product, or GDP). By 1998 such expenditures reached nearly 1,149 trillion dollars (or close to 14 percent of GDP). Between 1960 and 1998 per-capita health expenditures leaped from $141 to $3,912.[4] Technology played an increasingly central role in medical practice. Sophisticated imaging and laboratory equipment assisted in diagnosis, vaccines inhibited infections, and new drugs facilitated the management of many chronic conditions. Other innovations made possible such dramatic procedures as open-heart surgery, kidney dialysis, and organ transplantation.[5]

Health indicators appeared to confirm the value of medical science. In the postwar decades mortality rates continued the decline that had begun at the end of the nineteenth century, though not necessarily in a linear path. Infant mortality, for example, fell from about 100 per 1,000 live births in 1915 to 29.2 in 1950. Over the next two decades the rate of decline dropped, leading to predictions that an irreducible minimum had been reached. Yet between 1970 and 1998 the rate fell from 20 to 7.2. From an international perspective, the decline in American infant mortality rates was less impressive. In 1960 the

United States ranked eleventh out of thirty-five developed nations; by 1996 its rank had fallen to twenty-sixth.[6]

What accounted for the checkered history of infant mortality? The decline in the early twentieth century followed a recognition of the importance of such simple preventive measures as pure milk, water, and food, as well as hygienic measures that promoted cleanliness and ensured better care during episodes of sickness. Between 1900 and 1935 infant mortality declined approximately 3 percent per year. In the succeeding fifteen years the rate of decline rose to 4.7 percent, but then dropped to 1 percent in the next decade and a half.[7]

During the halcyon days of the 1960s concern with stagnant infant mortality rates resurfaced. By then the pattern of infant mortality had changed. In 1900 infant mortality remained high in all groups even though there were some differences. In 1960, by contrast, a large proportion of such deaths were found among disadvantaged groups having a much higher proportion of low-birthweight or premature infants. The relatively high rates of infant mortality in the United States, as compared with other industrial nations, reflected a higher percentage of low-birthweight infants. The subsequent decline in infant mortality in the United States was probably due to the passage of state and federal laws that provided greater funding for prenatal and maternity care for poor women who previously had lacked access to such services, to changes in medical technology, and to entitlement programs that provided resources for the poor.[8]

Life expectancy exhibited somewhat similar characteristics. Between 1940 and 1998 life expectancy at birth rose from 62.9 to 76.7. The pattern of change, however, was again not entirely linear. Between 1940 and 1954 the yearly decline in the death rate was 2 percent; between 1954 and 1968 it fell to 0.4 percent; and from 1968 to 1977 it rose to 1.6 percent. Between 1985 and 1997 the death rate declined an additional 12 percent. Part of the increase in life expectancy reflected the decline in mortality in the early years after birth. But the gains at the upper end of the age scale were equally impressive. Moreover, those born in the twentieth century enjoyed a distinct health advantage over their nineteenth-century predecessors. At age 65, for example, life expectancy increased from 13.9 years in 1950 to 17.8 in 1998. Those who survived to the age of 75 could expect on average to live an additional 13 years.[9]

Aggregate average data, of course, conceal as much as they reveal.

The reduction of infant mortality and the increase in life expectancy were by no means equally distributed. Although all groups had rising health indicators, sharp differences persisted between them. African-American infant mortality fell, but rates remained more than twice as high as those of whites. Similarly, mortality differences reflected the influence of such variables as occupation, education, income, marital status, nativity, and geographic location.

Because infant mortality data are aggregated by race rather than by socioeconomic class, it is difficult to sort out the relative importance of class and race in mediating African-American infant and child mortality rates.[10] A study analyzing the National Mortality Follow-back Survey and the National Health Interview Survey for 1986 (dealing only with adult mortality) concluded that class rather than race was a major determinant of mortality. Employing data from the former, the authors concluded that "the differences in overall mortality according to race were eliminated after adjustment for income, marital status, and household size." Two studies of prostate and breast cancer involving white and African-American men and women reached similar conclusions. In the initial analysis of mortality risk, African Americans appeared at higher risk. But when socioeconomic status was held constant, the influence of race disappeared. Other studies came to similar conclusions; African-American mortality patterns were heterogeneous rather than homogeneous. In one study white residents in Detroit fared as poorly as residents of certain African-American areas; in other areas Caribbean blacks enjoyed a substantial advantage over southern-born blacks. In addition to socioeconomic status, mortality differences may be influenced by a variety of other factors, including delays in diagnoses because of beliefs of patients, access to care, and types of physician-patient relationships.[11]

Shifting mortality patterns had a dramatic impact. Before 1900 death was associated with infancy and childhood. The emotional trauma of parents must have been profound. However extreme, the experiences of Charles and Caroline Kautz in Philadelphia were not totally atypical. Married for more than fifteen years, they had six children, including three sons and three daughters ranging in age from two to twelve. Toward the end of 1880 smallpox appeared in epidemic form. Between late November and mid-December the epidemic took the lives of five of their children, and only the oldest daughter survived. Although the responses of the parents were not recorded, the effect of such losses must have been wrenching. When the seven-year-old son of Mary Putnam Jacobi and Abraham Jacobi–two influential and famous physicians—died of diphtheria in 1883, the former revealed her inner pain in a letter written to a friend:

> But I never should feel that any knowledge now gained or even any lives saved, would be in any way a compensation for Ernst. I have rather a secret morbid longing to hear of everyone losing a first born son as they did in Egypt and had the death list every day to pick out the cases of seven and eight years. I feel sometimes as if the whole world must stand and [look] at me for my inability to [save] this lovely child. This feeling of self contempt perhaps in one way helps me to bear this terrible loss.[12]

A century later the situation was quite different. Of about 2.34 million deaths in 1998, 33,622 were under the age of 5, whereas 1.75 million were 65 or older.[13] That death at any age causes sorrow is incontrovertible. Yet most people do not mourn as deeply when an aged parent, relative, or friend dies.

▼   ▼   ▼

During the twentieth century there was a profound shift. Long-duration illnesses replaced acute infectious diseases as the causes of death, and involved mainly older Americans. In 1998 diseases of the heart accounted for 31 percent of all deaths, malignant neoplasms for 23.2 percent, and cerebrovascular diseases for 6.8 percent. Of the fifteen leading causes of death, pneumonia and influenza (3.9 percent) were the only ones that fell, at least directly, into the infectious group, and they took their great toll among those individuals suffering from a variety of other serious health problems. The remainder included such varied categories as chronic obstructive pulmonary diseases (4.8 percent), automobile accidents (4.2 percent), and diabetes mellitus (3.9 percent).[14]

The most striking feature of the leading causes of mortality was their relationship to age. Diseases of the heart (which included a variety of subcategories), for example, took an increasingly higher toll among the various age groups. In 1998 the age-adjusted mortality rate was 8.3 per 100,000 for the 25–34 age group, 30.5 for the 35–44 group, 101.4 for the 45–54 group, 286.9 for the 55–64, and 735.5 for the 65–74 group. Malignant neoplasms manifested a similar pattern. From birth to age 14 the mortality rate was slightly over 2. It then rose gradually to 11.3 in the 25–34 age group. The greatest increases were in the next four age groups: 38.2, 132.3, 383.8, and 841.3 in the 65–74 category.[15]

That age is an important factor in mortality from long-duration illnesses is obvious. Yet age by itself cannot explain the changes in their incidence and prevalence. In fact there were important if not clearly understood changes in their patterns over time. Two examples illustrate this generalization–diseases of the heart and cancer.

In the early twentieth century there was a steady rise in age-specific mortality from heart diseases among all age groups.[16] Between 1900 and 1920 the death rate remained more or less stable. About 1920 an upward trend began that continued unabated for thirty years. The rates for those with coronary heart disease peaked in the 1960s. Beginning about 1950, age-specific death rates for all major cardiovascular-renal diseases began to fall; somewhere in the mid-1960s the same trend set in for coronary heart disease. Between 1950 and 1998 the age-adjusted mortality rate for all heart diseases fell from 307.2 to 126.6 per 100,000. Virtually every age group shared in the decline. The aging of the population was not a factor in the increase in mortality from heart disease, if only because a larger proportion of people within each age group perished from heart disease in 1950 than in 1900. The increase in mortality from heart disease occurred in all advanced industrial societies.[17]

The decline in cardiovascular mortality had a significant effect upon life expectancy. Between 1962 and 1982 the death rate from all cardiovascular diseases dropped about 36 percent. By 1982 this translated into 500,000 fewer deaths than would have occurred had the 1963 rates remained constant. The improvement in cardiovascular mortality (a category that accounted for nearly half of all deaths) was an important component in the increase in life expectancy during these years.[18]

What explains the irregular trend of mortality from heart disease in the twentieth century? The answer to this seemingly obvious question is anything but simple. As late as the 1950s many researchers and clinicians believed that what is now known as coronary heart disease (CHD) was a chronic degenerative disease related to aging and could not be influenced by specific preventive measures. The Commission on Chronic Illness, created in the 1950s to study the problems of chronic disease, illness, and dependency, noted that the "causes of the most significant cardiovascular diseases—rheumatic fever, arteriosclerosis, and hypertension—are known only in part . . . In the present state of our knowledge, then, prevention of cardiovascular disease is largely confined to the prevention of complications." Atherosclerosis (coronary artery disease), it conceded, "is not preventable at the present time."[19]

During and after the 1960s the focus shifted to risk factors as crucial elements in the etiology of cardiovascular disorders. A series of community epidemiological studies, some of which began in the 1940s, transformed the manner in which CHD was understood. Ancel Key's cross-cultural studies, which began in the 1940s, related dietary habits, serum cholesterol, and CHD risk. The famous Framingham study, begun in 1948, enrolled more than 5,000 residents free of CHD in the early 1950s and tracked them for years. It was followed by other investigations, including the Alameda County study in California. Taken as a group, these studies rejected the degenerative hypothesis and substituted the claim that CHD was related to a series of behaviors peculiar to the industrialized world. Such an interpretation gave meaning to CHD in the sense that it identified those who were presumably at greatest risk and suggested ways of decreasing that risk. The mystery and randomness that had previously characterized explanations of CHD were superseded by the claim that individuals were at increased risk for the disease if they ate high-fat foods, smoked, were overweight, or were physically inactive. That such a theory emerged in the postwar decades is understandable. Risk factors reflected a belief that each individual was responsible for health as well as a faith that medical science and epidemiology could illuminate the behavioral etiology of CHD. Many chronic diseases, including CHD, various forms of cancer, diabetes, and other conditions, Lester Breslow noted in 1960, reflected the availability of rich and abundant foods, alcohol, smoking, less physical activity, and other "good things" associated with the modern industrialized world.[20]

In summing up their findings of the Alameda study, Lisa F. Berkman and Breslow concluded that health and disease "arise mainly from the circumstances of living."

> Rural communities with poor sanitation located in areas heavily infested by parasites, mosquitoes, and other disease agents and vec-

tors are afflicted with one pattern of health, disease, and mortality. Urban communities starting on the path of industrialization but affected by crowding, inadequate food, and poor sanitation have another pattern. Modern metropolitan communities with advanced industrialization and reasonably good sanitation, but low physical demand coupled with access to plenty of fatty foods, alcohol, and cigarettes, have still a third kind of health, disease, and mortality pattern . . . In the latter part of the twentieth century, their [infectious diseases] place has been taken by coronary and other cardiovascular diseases, lung cancer, and other forms of noninfectious respiratory disease.[21]

But the emphasis on risk factors as major elements in the etiology of CHD is not entirely persuasive. If a causative factor is responsible for atherosclerosis, a latency period of perhaps twenty years must be subtracted from the time when the mortality curve initially began its rise. Such was not the case for the risk factors that were subsequently linked with CHD mortality, which began to rise in the early twentieth century. Dietary change came after World War II. If the more recent switch from saturated to unsaturated fats and the decrease in serum cholesterol played a role in the last quarter of the twentieth century in declining CHD mortality, why did this not occur as well during the 1930s, when most Americans could not afford rich diets? Death rates for heart disease in general did not follow dietary changes.[22] Similarly, cigarette smoking–whose health effects generally take several decades to appear–first began in the 1920s, when the increase in mortality from CHD was already under way. Much the same holds true for the claim that diminished physical activity was a crucial factor. Like cigarette smoking, the use of automobiles was not common until the 1920s, and during the depression of the 1930s remained a luxury. Life for most Americans became more sedentary toward the end of the twentieth century. Yet during these decades mortality from CHD was declining. In a careful analysis of the major variables associated with CHD, Reuel A. Stallones observed that "hypertension does not fit the trend of the mortality from ischemic heart disease at all; physical activity fits only the rising curve, serum cholesterol fits only the falling curve and only cigarette smoking fits both. In no case is the fit as precise as one would like."[23]

Comparative data from other countries also fail to sustain the claim that risk factors such as high-fat diets explain CHD mortality.

Throughout southern Europe, for example, heart disease death rates have steadily declined while animal fat consumption has steadily risen because of increasing affluence. Some epidemiologists, as a matter of fact, have suggested that national differences may reflect the availability and consumption of fresh produce year round. Scotland and Finland have high rates of CHD; its citizens eat high-fat diets but consume relatively little in the way of fresh vegetables and fruits. Mediterranean populations, by contrast, consume large amounts of fresh produce year round. To University of Cambridge epidemiologist John Powles, the antifat movement was founded on the notion that "something bad had to have an evil cause, and you got a heart attack because you did something wrong, which was eating too much of a bad thing, rather than not having enough of a good thing."[24]

Risk factors are at best associations and do not necessarily explain the epidemiological patterns in time and space. Changing disease concepts, moreover, complicate the problem of measuring variations in incidence and prevalence. Advances in diagnostic technology, for example, have led to overestimation of the prevalence of many diseases and increased interventions of dubious benefit. Sophisticated imaging and laboratory technologies have determined that about a third of adults have evidence of papillary carcinoma of the thyroid, 40 percent of women in their forties may have ductal carcinoma in situ of the breast, and 50 percent of men in their sixties have adenocarcinoma of the prostate. Yet most of these individuals will not develop clinical forms of the disease, and treatment in such cases can result in harm.[25] Moreover, numerous epidemiological studies are severely limited by methodological inadequacies, and often fail to shed light on pathological mechanisms. A survey of the literature, Alvan R. Feinstein observed, found that "56 different cause-effect relationships had conflicting evidence in which the results of at least one epidemiologic study were contradicted by the results of another. About 40 more conflicting relationships would have been added if the review had included studies of disputed associations between individual sex hormones and individual birth defects."[26] The decline of rheumatic heart disease offers a contrasting example. Risk factors and even antibiotic therapy played minor roles at best in its disappearance, which probably followed the lessened virulence of the Group A streptococcus.

Yet the hold of the risk-factor hypothesis remains powerful. In discussing declining cardiovascular mortality, William B. Kannel and Thomas J. Thom conceded that "no one has yet established a convincing fit of trends for any risk factor with cardiovascular mortality trends." Nor was it possible to "directly associate specific improvements in cardiovascular disease prevention and treatment with the mortality decline." Conceding that the influences of altered behaviors, medical treatment, and prevention were "incomplete, indirect, and equivocal," they nevertheless suggested that they had "indeed contributed to the decline in mortality."[27]

The risk-factor theory is by no means the only explanation of the rise of CHD after 1900. In England David Barker was puzzled by the fact that CHD was a common cause of death among men who had low-risk characteristics. He ultimately pioneered the concept that fetal undernutrition during critical periods of development *in utero* and during infancy led to permanent damage that increased susceptibility to CHD and other chronic illnesses in adult life. He found that areas with the highest rates of neonatal mortality in the early twentieth century also had the highest rates of low birthweights. Barker then suggested that impaired fetal growth among those who had survived infancy predisposed them to CHD in later life. Low-birthweight infants, moreover, were at increased risk for hypertension, lung disease, and high cholesterol. The search for the causes of "Western" diseases, Barker noted, focused on the adult environment and ignored the childhood environment. He attributed the emphasis on the adult environment in part to the fact that most environmental models had their origin in the epidemiological studies dealing with the effects of cigarette smoking. Coronary heart diseases, he suggested, "may turn out to be the effect of the intrauterine or early postnatal environment."[28] The theory that adult disease may have fetal origins is intriguing, but the mechanism and supportive evidence are not at this time persuasive.

Recent research on CHD has also begun to focus on the possible role of infections. It has long been known that individuals with atherosclerosis and its clinical complications of unstable angina, myocardial infarction, and stroke have elevated markers of inflammation. Whether or not chronic inflammation is a cause or a result of atherosclerosis remains unknown. Nevertheless, there are some indications that certain chronic infections caused by *Chlamydia pneumoniae* and cytomegalovirus (as well as other infectious agents) may be etiologi-

cal factors. Potential mechanisms may include vessel wall contamination, which could result either in direct damage or in indirect damage
by initiating an immunologic response. Chronic infection may also
assist in the development or destabilization of atherosclerotic
plaques. It may be a coincidence, but the decline in atherosclerosis-
related deaths corresponded with the introduction of antibiotic therapy after 1945. Whether infections play a role in the etiology of CHD
remains a controversial issue.[29]

That CHD may be related to infections is not as novel as first appears. Until the 1980s peptic and duodenal ulcers were attributed to
gastric acidity, stress, smoking, alcoholic consumption, and genetic
predispositions even though in 1946 it was successfully treated at
Mount Sinai and the New York Hospital by an antibiotic (aureomy-
cin). But for unknown reasons–perhaps because of the prevailing paradigm that peptic ulcer was a noninfectious disease—a successful empirical treatment never entered clinical practice. In the 1980s the
Helicobacter pylori bacterium was identified as one of the causal elements. Though initially disregarded by clinicians, this finding ultimately led to a partial reconceptualization of peptic and duodenal ulcer and to the use of antibiotic as well as traditional therapies.
Whether research on CHD will follow a similar path is as yet unclear.
At present it is possible to diagnose and manage CHD by such means
as bypass surgery, angioplasty, stents, and drugs. In general these
medical technologies improve the quality of life even if they do not
for the most part extend it. The etiology of CHD, however, remains
shrouded in mystery.[30] In noting the decline in heart disease mortality,
Lewis Thomas admitted:

> No one seems to know why this happened, which is not in itself sur-
> prising since no one really knows for sure what the underlying
> mechanism responsible for coronary disease is. In the circumstance,
> everyone is free to provide one's own theory, depending on one's
> opinion about the mechanism. You can claim, if you like, that there
> has been enough reduction in the dietary intake of saturated fat, na-
> tionwide, to make the difference, although I think you'd have a
> hard time proving it. Or, if you prefer, you can attribute it to the ep-
> idemic of jogging, but I think that the fall in incidence of coronary
> disease had already begun before jogging became a national mania.
> Or, if you are among those who believe that an excessively competi-

tive personality strongly influences the incidence of this disease, you might assert that more of us have become calmer and less combative since the 1950s, and I suppose you could back up the claim by simply listing the huge numbers of new mental-health professionals, counselors, lifestyle authorities, and various health gurus who have appeared in our midst in recent years. But I doubt it, just as I doubt their effectiveness in calming us all down.[31]

Like diseases of the heart, cancer presents enigmas. In 1900 malignant neoplasms accounted for perhaps 3.7 percent of all deaths and ranked sixth as a cause of mortality. The proportion of deaths from cancer began a gradual rise, and by 1940 was ranked second and accounted for 11.2 percent of mortality. In 1960, 1980, and 1998 the shares were 15.6, 21, and 23 percent, respectively. Of 2.34 million deaths in 1998, about 541,000 were from malignant neoplasms.[32]

Rates of cancer mortality, however, have remained relatively stable. In 1950 the rate was 125.2 per 100,000. Over the next half-century there were slight fluctuations, but in 1998 the rate was essentially the same (123.6), despite the development of a myriad of therapies. As in the case of heart disease, mortality from cancer was related to age. Between birth and age 24 the rate in 1998 ranged from 2.1 for those under 1 year to 4.6 in the 15–24 group. There were gradual rises in the 25–34 (11.3) and 35–44 (38.2) groups, and accelerating rates in the next four age groups (132.3, 383.8, 841.3, and 1326.3, respectively). The increase in the number of cancer deaths was in part a reflection of the fact that far more individuals survived infancy and youth and lived a relatively long life.[33]

Statistical data, however, reveal little about a disease that has aroused profound fears and anxieties. Cancer, of course, is not a new disease; it has been found in mummies. But despite its ancient lineage, it has remained somewhat of a mystery. For precisely this reason, paradoxically, competing theories about its nature and etiology were plentiful in the early twentieth century. Some argued that it was a contagious disease caused by germs; some insisted that it was inherited; some thought it related to the rise of industrial civilization; some suggested that it was caused by emotional or mental stress; and others believed that various forms of irritation predisposed tissue to cancerous growth. The seeming inability of physicians to treat most forms of cancer also led to a proliferation of therapies. In 1913 the

American Society for the Control of Cancer (later the American Cancer Society) was created to educate the public about the importance of early detection and surgery. Nearly a quarter of a century later a congressional act created the National Cancer Institute, which after World War II enjoyed phenomenal growth. Indeed, by the late 1960s a powerful lobby had declared "war" on cancer, leading to the passage of the "war on cancer" act of 1971.[34]

As research into the mysteries of cancer proliferated after 1945, so did explanations. There were, of course, precedents to draw upon. In 1775 Percivall Pott noted that young English chimney sweeps often developed scrotal cancer, which he attributed to inflammation caused by soot. In 1910 Peyton Rous demonstrated that chicken sarcoma could be reproduced by a filterable virus. The major emphasis in postwar America, however, was on the effect of carcinogens, including radiation, air pollution, occupation, food additives, exposure to sunlight, and various chemicals. At the same time risk-factor explanations that emphasized diet and smoking proliferated.[35] The therapeutic armamentarium also multiplied, and surgical intervention was augmented by chemotherapy and new forms of radiation that were effective against certain types of cancers.

The expressions of hope that were so prevalent in the latter part of the twentieth century were accompanied, ironically enough, by rising fears. Indeed, cancer became a metaphor to explain innumerable individual and societal problems. "When it comes to cancer," noted an editorial by a leading medical writer in the prestigious *New England Journal of Medicine* in 1975, "American society is far from rational. We are possessed with fear . . . cancerphobia has expanded into a demonism in which the evil spirit is ever present, but furtively viewed and spoken of obliquely. American cancerphobia, in brief, is a disease as serious to society as cancer is to the individual–and morally more devastating."[36]

What is cancer? As in the case of many other long-duration illnesses, it is much easier to describe its pathology than its etiology. Cancerous cells are undifferentiated and concerned only with their own growth and hence disregard the needs of the organism. Unlike normal cells, which are limited to a fixed number of divisions, cancer cells can divide for an unlimited number of generations. Often they break away and seed new colonies at distant sites; these metastases add to the damage. Ultimately the organism perishes as organ functions are destroyed. Recent work in molecular biology has begun to unravel some of the mysteries of cancer. The mammalian genome contains tumor-suppressor genes as well as proto-oncogenes. The latter are essentially accelerators and the former brakes in cell growth. Excessive cell growth can result from a defect in either. A genetic accident–either random or induced by a carcinogen–transforms their function and distorts the normal process of cell growth and differentiation.[37]

Contrary to popular belief, the genesis of cancer is often a slow process; years if not decades can pass before the disease becomes symptomatic. The example of colorectal cancer (which ranks as the second most common cause of cancer death) is instructive. The natural progression of the disease is slow, often taking between twenty and forty years. At the outset epithelial cells lining the bowel wall proliferate excessively. In the second stage they thicken. Subsequently these thickenings protrude into the cavity of the colon, resulting in small polyps. These growths are not life threatening, but later some evolve into true malignant cells, obstruct the colonic tube, invade the underlying muscle wall, and eventually metastasize to other parts of the body. Recent research has revealed that each stage is accompanied by a genetic change. Early polyps follow the loss of a tumor-suppressor gene. The appearance of mature colorectal carcinomas is dependent on several genetic changes plus mutant forms of another gene.[38]

Unlike those for coronary heart disease, cancer mortality rates seem to have remained relatively stable during the past century.[39] Yet the overall cancer mortality rate is not necessarily an accurate barometer. Rates for specific cancers have changed dramatically over time. Moreover, there are considerable variations in mortality based on sex, ethnicity, race, class, age, and geographic location.[40] Such variations make it extraordinarily difficult to provide definitive statements about the etiology of what may be very different kinds of diseases even though they are all subsumed under a single general category.

Between 1930 and 1965 age-adjusted mortality rates from all cancers increased among white and African-American males and nonwhite females, but declined among white females. The greatest increase was among African-American males. A number manifested a consistent decline, including cancer of the bone, stomach, uterus, and cervix. Pancreatic cancer, particularly among those 45 or older, showed a decided increase, as did cancers of the urinary organs, kidney, ovaries, and intestines, but especially the lung. Cancer of the prostate declined for those under 65 and remained stable or increased for those over 65. Breast cancer mortality among women remained more or less stable while increasing among African-American females. The data on race and neoplasms, however, did not take socioeconomic class into account, thus limiting their usefulness.[41]

Many of the trends of cancer mortality remained more or less constant during the last third of the twentieth century. Lung cancer was a notable exception. Between 1960–1962 and 1990–1992 mortality from lung cancer among males increased 85 percent, from 40.2 to 74.4 per 100,000; after 1992 a slight decline became evident. Female rates leaped from 6.0 to 32.3, an increase of 438 percent. Indeed, overall mortality from cancer would have shown a slight decline had it not been for the increase in lung cancer. Although mortality from melanoma of the skin and multiple myeloma also showed large percentage increases, the number of cases was relatively small.[42]

What accounts for the stability of overall cancer mortality as well as changes in the rates for particular neoplasms? As in the case of CHD, the answer is by no means self-evident. There is general agreement that certain cancers have external causes. Lung cancer, for example, is clearly related to smoking even though other cofactors may play a role. In general, lung cancer was not significant in the early twentieth century, when tobacco consumption was low. In 1880, for example, the average cigarette smoker consumed .047 pound of unstemmed tobacco (before the removal of stems). There was a gradual rise in usage; as late as 1914 consumption was .82 pound. Shortly thereafter consumption began a steady rise; the first peak in usage came in 1953, when the average cigarette smoker over the age of 14 consumed 10.46 pounds, or 3,558 cigarettes, per annum. In 1979 the average smoker age 18 and over consumed 33.5 cigarettes per day.[43]

By 1930 mortality from lung cancer had begun a steep rise that would not be reversed for more than half a century. In 1992 nearly 521,000 individuals died from malignant neoplasms; lung cancer accounted for 28 percent of these deaths. After World War II epidemiological data and pathological evidence began to confirm the association between smoking and lung cancer even though the precise mechanism was unknown.[44] That other substances and behaviors are involved in specific cancers is also clear. Asbestos, certain industrial chemicals, prolonged exposure to sunlight, and ionizing radiation all have carcinogenic qualities, although the numbers of people exposed are far smaller than the number of cigarette smokers.

The etiology of most cancers and of changes in prevalence and mortality rates, however, remains unclear. Consider the case of gastric cancer. Before World War II gastric cancer was the leading cause of cancer mortality in males and the third in females. But by 1930 a decline in mortality appeared that persisted for the rest of the century. In 1960 it had fallen to sixth place, and in 1992 it ranked ninth. Between 1962 and 1992 the number of deaths fell from 19,378 to 13,630 even though population had increased. Other industrialized nations experienced a comparable decline, although there were considerable variations in rates.[45]

What is the reason for this dramatic decline? There is no evidence that new treatments played a role; surgery remained the only option and was effective only if the tumor was confined to the mucosa (lining) and submucosa. Nor was there any change in survival rates after diagnosis. Since the decline in mortality from gastric cancer was international, those who have studied the disease assume that the major etiologic influences were environmental rather than genetic, and that changes in referral, diagnosis, and treatment played no role. Of all environmental factors, diet was the focus of most attention. High-carbohydrate diets, nitrates and nitrites, and salt were implicated as potential etiologic factors, whereas the consumption of vegetables and fruits (and therefore an increased intake of vitamins C, E, and A) was associated with decreased risk. Yet the persistence of wide variations in mortality rates and diets among countries renders such explanations problematic at best. More significantly, the decline in mortality antedated dietary change, which in any case would have taken at least two decades to make its influence felt. Like the decline in mortality from CHD, the decline in mortality from gastric cancer remains a puzzle that epidemiological studies have failed to explain.[46]

In fact the etiology of most cancers remains largely unknown. Nevertheless, environmental explanations dominate both popular and professional beliefs. The striking relationship between smoking and lung cancer, as well as evidence that exposure to a relatively small number of chemicals and radiation can also result in malignancies, fostered the emergence of an explanatory model that emphasized an environmental and behavioral etiology for most cancers. Yet the evidence to demonstrate such linkages in many cases was hardly persuasive.

Richard Doll, who played a significant role in illuminating the risks

of smoking, extended the environmental interpretation of cancer etiology in dramatic fashion. Cancer, he and a colleague wrote in 1981,
"is largely a preventable disease." More than two-thirds (and perhaps more) of all cancers were due to smoking and diet, while occupational hazards, alcohol, food additives, sexual behavior, pollution,
industrial products, and medical technology played very minor roles.
Doll gathered comparative data that revealed differential incidence
rates for specific cancers in various countries. Only diet, he insisted,
could explain such differences. More recently Graham A. Colditz has
argued that with "population-wide increases in levels of physical activity and folate intake, and with reductions in alcohol intake, adult
weight gain and obesity, red meat consumption, and smoking, up to
70% of colon cancer could be avoided."[47]

The effort to link cancer to diet, carcinogens, and behavior–which
has been central to the campaign to prevent and control the disease–
has been rooted largely in belief and hope rather than fact. Smoking
is the one notable exception. Other *proven* carcinogens such as asbestos and high-level radiation hazards other than solar ultraviolet rays
affected relatively few individuals. The myriad epidemiological studies of the relationship of diet and behavior to the genesis of cancer–
which tended to give results that were constantly changing and usually contradictory–have generally been based on questionable methodologies.[48]

Prevention of cancer in the latter half of the twentieth century remained an elusive but persistently popular goal. Prevention, after all,
supported values that placed a premium on individual responsibility
for one's own health and well-being.[49] The alternative–that the etiology of cancer was endogenous and not necessarily amenable to individual volition–was hardly an attractive explanation. It is entirely
plausible, for example, that cancer is closely related to aging and genetic mutations, which together impair the ability of the immune system to identify and attack malignant cells and thus permit them to
multiply. If there is at present no way to arrest the aging process, then
cancer mortality may be inevitable. Moreover, some of the genetic
mutations that eventually lead to cancer may occur randomly, and
thus cannot be prevented.

There is also little evidence that overall cancer mortality has been
appreciably reduced either by screening to detect the disease in its
early stages or by a variety of medical therapies.[50] The result has been

an intensified interest in prevention. John C. Bailer III and Elaine M. Smith, who tracked cancer mortality over several decades, emphasized the failure to find effective therapies. "Age-adjusted mortality rates," they noted in 1986, "have shown a slow and steady increase over several decades, and there is no evidence of a recent downward trend. In this clinical sense we are losing the war against cancer." A decade later Bailer and Heather L. Gornick found little improvement even though there had been changes in the incidence and mortality rates of specific malignancies. Indeed, the death rate in 1994 was 2.7 percent higher than in 1982, the last year covered in the 1986 article. In 1986 Bailer and Smith wrote that thirty-five years of intensive effort to focus on improving treatment "must be judged a qualified failure." Twelve years later Bailer and Gornick saw "little reason to change that conclusion." "The best of modern medicine, they concluded, "has much to offer to virtually every patient with cancer, for palliation if not always for cure . . . The problem is the lack of substantial improvement over what treatment could already accomplish some decades ago. A national commitment to the prevention of cancer, largely replacing reliance on hopes for universal cures, is now the way to go."[51]

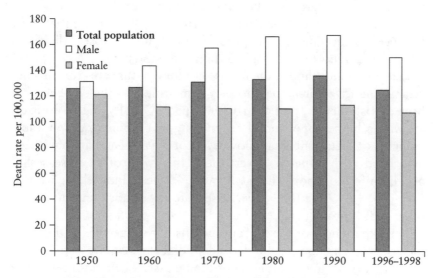

Age-adjusted cancer mortality rates by gender, 1950–1998

Diseases of the heart and malignant neoplasms were not the only long-duration diseases that played a role in shaping health indicators. Cerebrovascular diseases, chronic pulmonary obstructive diseases, diabetes mellitus, severe and chronic mental diseases, and many others too numerous to mention played much smaller direct roles in mortality but were nevertheless responsible for a considerable share of morbidity.

Diabetes mellitus, for example, was the eighth leading cause of death in 1998, accounting for 3 percent of total mortality. There are two forms, affecting different populations. Type I (insulin-dependent) diabetes appears at an early age. Type II (non-insulin-dependent) diabetes is found among people over the age of 30. The prevalence of Type I (which is more readily identifiable) was estimated to be about 1.1 per 1,000 among those under the age of 17. Though accounting for a small proportion of total mortality, Type II diabetes affects large numbers of people, accounting for more than 90 percent of diabetes mortality. Nor does the disease exist in isolation; it is closely related to heart and kidney disease and blindness and is a leading cause of amputation.

From 1965 to 1975 the share of known diabetics in the population increased from 1.5 to 2.3 percent. Moreover, the prevalence increased by age; the rate in the age 60–74 group was more than twice that of the 40–59 group. Whether the incidence of the disease was increasing, however, is problematic. There is some evidence that there has been a decline in the proportion of undiagnosed diabetics. Changing diagnostic criteria also complicate the picture.

Like CHD and cancer, the precise etiology of diabetes remains unclear. Genetic factors appear to play some role, but the emphasis has been on risk factors, particularly for Type II. Obesity, high-caloric diets with a high proportion of fat and simple carbohydrates and low amounts of dietary fiber, and low levels of physical activity have been associated with Type II. Nevertheless, this form of the disease has also been found among those who are not obese. Individuals with either Type I or Type II have decreased life expectancy and numerous other health problems.[52]

The experiences of the Navajo Indians are suggestive of the complexity posed by non-insulin-dependent diabetes. As late as the 1960s they had a very low prevalence of the disease. Their traditional diet was high in fiber and complex carbohydrates and low in simple sugars, fat, and calories. Beginning in the 1930s, overgrazing and soil erosion prompted the federal government to mandate a substantial reduction in the number of their livestock. Thereafter the Navajos relied increasingly on prepared foods. Their intake of fiber and complex carbohydrates decreased while that of fat and simple sugar increased. Dietary changes were accompanied by lower activity levels, and obesity became more common. By 1980 the diabetes-associated death rate was 40 percent higher than the national average. Using the experiences of the Navajos to explain the prevalence of Type II diabetes in other populations, however, is problematic. It is unclear, as David Weatherall has observed, why the disease is so common among American Indians, as well as Melanesians and Polynesians. Indeed, "it has become apparent that there are probably several other types of diabetes, some of which are also confined to certain racial groups."[53]

Though not a significant direct cause of mortality, serious and chronic mental illnesses affect large numbers of people. Accurate epidemiological data are hard to come by, in part because concepts of mental disorder are so fluid. Nevertheless, 1990 estimates of serious mental illnesses among persons aged 18 and older ranged from 7 to 13 million. The disabilities of people with severe and persistent disorders frequently exceed those with chronic physical conditions. Schizophrenia–the most serious mental disorder–often results in nearly total disability. Studies of depressive symptoms indicate that they can be more debilitating than diabetes, arthritis, gastrointestinal disorders, and back problems in terms of physical and social functioning. Unlike many illnesses that are concentrated in older age groups, serious mental disorders are distributed throughout the adult population. As with many other long-duration illnesses, their etiology remains unknown.[54]

Heart disease, cancer, diabetes, and other chronic degenerative or long-duration illnesses, many of which are associated with age, are also associated with high rates of disability. Not all disabilities, to be sure, result from illnesses; developmental and injury-related disabilities are not necessarily the consequence of disease. Many long-lasting pathologies—including osteoarthritis, cancer, heart disease, and diabetes—increase the risk of disability. Indeed, 1990 estimates of disability indicated that 35 million Americans, or one in seven, had a physical or mental impairment that hampered their daily activities, and perhaps 9 million were unable to work, attend school, or maintain a household.[55]

Physicians could diagnose many of the clinical symptoms associated with long-duration illnesses and provide palliative therapies that improved the quality of life if not longevity. Yet efforts to explain the long-term trends of these and other diseases generally lacked a solid evidentiary foundation. Epidemiological studies, however valuable, shed little or no light upon complex physiological mechanisms. Hence etiological explanations tended to be based more on opinion than on empirical evidence. That more Americans at the end of the twentieth century were living longer and in most cases healthier lives than their early twentieth-century predecessors was obvious. But the precise reasons for the changes in mortality and morbidity rates (and therefore life expectancy) remained murky.[56]

▼ ▼ ▼

The preoccupation with cancer, heart disease, and other long-duration illnesses during the second half of the twentieth century sometimes overshadowed other threats to health. After World War II, for example, the introduction of antibiotic therapy fostered a belief that infectious diseases–historically the major elements in mortality–would no longer play as decisive a role in either mortality or morbidity. The development of vaccines to prevent many early life diseases added to this belief. Infectious diseases might cause transient discomfort, but would never again become major threats to health or life.

The belief that infectious diseases no longer posed serious threats, however, rested on a slippery foundation. Antibiotic therapy, for example, was effective only against bacterial infections. Predictions about its efficacy, moreover, failed to take into account the evolution of resistant strains. Toward the end of the twentieth century, for example, multidrug-resistant strains of the tubercle bacillus had emerged.[57] More important, many infectious diseases were of viral origin, against which antibiotic therapy was ineffective. Consequently, infectious diseases continued to play a significant direct role in morbidity and perhaps an equally important if indirect role in mortality.

The history of influenza is illuminating. After the pandemic of 1918–19 the disease followed an irregular but cyclic pattern. From the 1950s through the 1970s epidemics with much higher than usual mortality appeared at roughly ten-year intervals. In "normal" years influenza (and pneumonia) accounted for 3 or 4 percent of total mortality. The pandemics of 1957 and 1968 were marked by sharply elevated mortality rates. In 1957 there were 70,000 more deaths than expected, and in 1968 34,000. The highest attack rates occurred among school children, who played a significant role in the spread of the virus; the highest mortality rates were among the elderly. Vaccination against the influenza virus between epidemics conferred only partial immunity because of its rapid mutation.[58]

Despite sophisticated surveillance systems, it was virtually impossible to predict either the severity or the appearance of an influenza pandemic. The reason is not complex. Influenza viruses constantly circulated among avian species and were periodically transmitted to other species, where genetic reassortment took place, thus transforming their virulence. The abortive influenza epidemic of 1976 demonstrated the limits of medical prediction. In that year a young soldier at Fort Dix, New Jersey, died of a strain of influenza virus antigenically related to the strain implicated in the 1918–19 pandemic. This particular strain had been absent from the United States since 1930. Consequently, the entire population of the United States under the age of 50 appeared to be susceptible. The scientific community was itself divided on a course of action. For a variety of complex reasons, President Gerald Ford and the Congress agreed on legislation providing for universal vaccination. Not only did the pandemic fail to materialize, but the effort to vaccinate an entire nation encountered a myriad of unforeseen problems. Moreover, the vaccine employed proved responsible for a significant increase in cases of Guillain-Barré syndrome, a paralytic disorder that can sometimes be fatal.[59]

The spread of influenza, like that of many other infectious diseases, was to a significant extent shaped by human factors. Crowding, the increased density of susceptible hosts, the domestication of animals, and the movement of people all played roles in the dissemination of influenza throughout the world, and few of these are amenable to human control. "Given the existence in the aquatic bird reservoir of all known influenza A subtypes," one authority has written, "we must accept the fact that influenza is not an eradicable disease. Prevention and control are the only realistic goals."[60]

In the biological world a huge variety of both viral and bacterial organisms (most of which are relatively benign) coexist. It is hardly surprising, therefore, that some pathogenic organisms continue to survive in susceptible human host populations. The dissemination of these pathogens is often shaped by the organization, technology, and behavior of human beings. Moreover, the means of dissemination may be related to virulence levels. Rapid dissemination through the population, for example, may increase virulence. Pathogens sometimes lose viability in the external environment. Those that pass quickly from one host to another, by contrast, often retain high virulence levels.[61] Two examples—Legionnaires' disease and diseases that tend to be related to sexual behavior—demonstrate the validity of some of these generalizations.

Soon after the Pennsylvania American Legion held its annual convention at Philadelphia's Bellevue-Stratford Hotel in July 1976, several members came down with a severe pneumonia. Ultimately 182 fell ill, 147 were hospitalized, and 29 died. Not until the following January was the cause of the disease identified–a previously unknown rod-shaped pathogen now called *Legionella pneumophila*. Since the bacterium had unusual staining characteristics, it had remained unknown, and deaths had been ascribed to other causes. It was subsequently determined that Legionnaires' disease accounted for 1 to 8 percent of all pneumonias and about 4 percent of lethal hospital pneumonias.

The pathogen's natural habitat is lakes and rivers. In the case of the Philadelphia outbreak, however, the source was aerosolized organisms from evaporative condensers in the hotel's air conditioning system. There was no evidence that the disease was transmitted from person to person. Retrospective immunologic and epidemiologic studies indicated that the pathogen had been responsible for some previously unexplained epidemics. In Philadelphia the outbreak of Legionnaires' disease was related to the modernization of an old hotel and the introduction of central air conditioning. The episode illuminated the difficulty, if not the impossibility, of predicting the manner in which pathogens are spread and the ensuing outbreak of infectious disease.[62]

Sexually transmitted diseases (STDs) are numerous. Some are of bacterial origin, some of viral. At present there are at least twenty-five known infectious organisms that are transmitted primarily through sexual contact, and secondarily through parenteral routes (e.g., blood transfusions, intravenous drugs administered by contaminated needles). Women and adolescents are disproportionately affected.

Before World War II syphilis and gonorrhea were the most feared venereal diseases. Even as late as 1970, a study of venereal disease by the American Public Health Association focused on syphilis and gonorrhea, with only a small section devoted to a few "minor" venereal diseases. The introduction of antibiotic therapy after 1945 tended to dissipate public fear. Rates for both syphilis and gonorrhea peaked during World War II and then began to decline, largely because of success in identification and treatment (but partly because of a diminution in case finding activity). Nevertheless, annual incidence rates remained high. In 1994 there were as many as 800,000 new cases of gonorrhea and 101,000 of syphilis. There was, moreover, a sharp increase in antibiotic-resistant cases of gonorrhea. In 1976 all gonorrhea infections were curable by penicillin; between 1987 and 1994 the proportion of resistant infections rose from 2 to 30 percent.[63]

After 1970 there was a sharp increase in the identification of other STDs. Between 1980 and 1995 eight new sexually transmitted pathogens were identified. It became clear, in addition, that sexual contacts were the major route of adult transmission of some previously described pathogens, notably the hepatitis B virus and cytomegalovirus. The Centers for Disease Control and Prevention (more popularly known as the CDC) estimated in 1993 that more than 12 million Americans (3 million of whom were teenagers) were infected with STDs each year. They accounted for about 87 percent of all cases reported among the top ten most frequently reported infectious diseases in 1995.[64]

The significance of many STDs and their relationship to chronic conditions later in life were often overlooked. Some STDs were asymptomatic and therefore remained undetected. Others led to chronic diseases years after the initial infection. They resulted in a variety of clinical syndromes that had serious health consequences, including cancers, infertility, neurologic damage, pelvic inflammatory disease, low-birthweight infants, urethritis, and even death. Human papillomavirus is associated with cervical and other genital and anal cancers; herpes simplex results in genital ulcers; hepatitis B can lead to chronic hepatitis, cirrhosis, and liver carcinoma; chlamydial genital infection can result in pelvic inflammatory disease. The consequences for fetuses and the newborn were even more severe.[65]

However significant their role in creating morbidity, most STDs–unlike cancer–aroused relatively little public concern or anxiety.[66] AIDS, which made a spectacular appearance in the early 1980s, was an exception. In 1981 cases of *Pneumocystis carinii* pneumonia and Kaposi's sarcoma were reported in previously healthy gay men, accompanied by an extraordinarily high death rate. Both were generally found in humans with compromised immune systems. The following year the disease had been named AIDS (acquired immunodeficiency syndrome). Subsequently a retrovirus–human immunodeficiency virus (HIV-1)–provided the link between AIDS and HIV-1; the retrovirus compromises the T-cells, a critical component of the immune system. The disease is transmitted not only by sexual contact but by blood from a pregnant mother to her fetus, by contaminated needles used by intravenous drug users, and by transfusions. In the symptomatic phase, an impaired immune system renders individuals susceptible to a host of opportunistic infections and diseases that often prove fatal.

The AIDS pandemic initially escaped detection because of its relatively long incubation period, sometimes as long as a decade from the initial infection to the appearance of clinical symptoms. By 1996 estimates of the number of reported cases in the United States exceeded 500,000, with nearly 340,000 fatalities. In the aggregate it was not among the ten leading causes of death. Among males aged 35 to 44, however, HIV-1 infection in 1995 was the leading cause of death, and the third leading cause among women in the same age group, accounting for 23 and 11 percent of total mortality, respectively. Indeed, by the early 1990s it was clear that AIDS was a pandemic; according to some estimates nearly 30 million people worldwide had been infected by 1997.[67]

The origin of AIDS remains uncertain, but whatever its origins, it is clear that social factors played a key role in the pandemic. In the second half of the twentieth century the intermingling of populations, the use of intravenous drugs, and novel techniques of blood transfusion combined to create conditions conducive to the spread of AIDS and other STDs. Equally important were changes in sexual behavioral standards that increased promiscuity among both homosexual and heterosexual groups. Novel cultural and behavioral norms combined with the belief that antibiotic drugs and more-effective birth-control techniques had reduced the risk of disease and pregnancy to facilitate sexual behavioral change. Indeed, there was evidence that behavioral change among gay males had created health problems that antedated the appearance of AIDS in this population subgroup. Between 1958 and 1978, for example, there was a sharp increase in amebiasis cases in New York City among homosexual males. An intestinal disorder, amebiasis is normally found in tropical areas with poor sanitation. In New York City, however, it was spread by oral-anal practices of sexually active persons. Had poor sanitation played a role, the disease would have been distributed equally throughout the population. In New York City, however, amebiasis was concentrated among male homosexuals living in well-defined neighborhoods.[68]

But social factors, however important, do not by themselves explain the AIDS pandemic. Complex biological mechanisms are also involved. The AIDS virus, for example, is extremely variable and mutates rapidly. It is entirely possible that in the past highly virulent strains were eliminated because the death of an infected individual broke the chain of transmissibility. Diseases that resulted from compromised immune systems, therefore, were relatively rare. Social, medical, and behavioral changes after 1950, however, fostered rapid transmissibility among virgin populations, thus permitting viral strains with high virulence levels to maintain themselves.[69] Moreover, there is evidence that a variety of STDs (including chancroid, syphilis, genital herpes, gonorrhea, chlamydia, and trichomoniasis) among the heterosexual population increased the risk of HIV-1 infection.[70]

STDs remain a persistent problem because their causative pathogens survive in human hosts and are transmitted by intimate human contact. There is a synergistic relationship between STDs and other infectious diseases that exacerbates morbidity. Moreover, the traditional belief that the host-pathogen relationship evolves toward benignity is not always accurate. Natural selection does not necessarily lead toward equilibrium. Variations in host susceptibility and pathogen virulence, Paul W. Ewald has observed, "is a race between our resistance to pathogens and pathogens resistance to us . . . As resistant humans become more numerous, pathogens that are not controlled by the human defenses are favored and they begin to prosper. In turn, new resistance mechanisms emerge in hosts." In short, the race is neverending; adaptation and change proceed simultaneously.[71]

The startling emergence of the AIDS epidemic led to more-widespread concern about "emerging infections." The fear was that pathogens–both known and unknown–could spread quickly throughout the world. In the case of AIDS, behavioral elements played critical roles in the dissemination of a disease that was–unlike plague and influenza–largely preventable. The concept of emerging infections also reflected a subordinate concern with resistant strains. Biomedical and scientific leaders called for better international surveillance systems, accelerated research for vaccine and drug development, the maintenance of a strong public health infrastructure, more careful deployment of antibiotic drugs, and greater attention to the ways in which human beings interacted and transformed their environment. The evidence, according to a report prepared by the Institute of Medicine, indicated "that humankind is beset by a greater variety of microbial pathogens than ever before . . . Clearly, despite a great deal of progress in detecting, preventing, and treating infectious diseases, we are a long way from eliminating the human health threats posed by bacteria, viruses, protozoans, helminths, and fungi."[72]

Prepared by a group of distinguished scientists, the report hinted that the prevention, control, and even elimination of infectious agents was a distinct possibility, given the will and appropriate resources. Such beliefs, as René Dubos once observed, reflect the age-old illusion that a disease-free world is possible. All efforts to create a "self-chosen pattern of life," he wrote in a classic and influential book, "involves many unknown consequences . . . The multiplicity of determinants which affect biological systems limits the power of the experimental method to predict their trends and behaviors." That the risks posed by pathogens can be partially limited is probable; that they can be eliminated is dubious.[73]

This book's focus on long-duration and infectious diseases, whether of unknown or known etiology, provides a necessarily incomplete portrait of the evolution of health patterns in late twentieth-century America. Morbidity and mortality indicators are also shaped by a variety of human activities that result in injury, disability, and death. Curiously enough, the unavoidable and avoidable risks to health and life, precisely because of their predictability, generally aroused less public apprehension, whereas relatively isolated and statistically insignificant events were often transformed into public health crises.

Consider, for example, the extent of trauma caused by intentional and unintentional injuries. In 1998 unintentional injuries killed nearly 98,000 people and accounted for 4 percent of total mortality. Indeed, unintentional injuries were the leading cause of death of individuals between ages 1 and 44. Within this category motor vehicle accidents accounted for about 45 percent of deaths and was the leading cause of death among those aged 1 to 34. To be sure, motor vehicle death rates, after rising dramatically in the early twentieth century, fell from 23.3 per 100,000 in 1950 to 15.6 in 1998, but the number of deaths remained high. Equally significant, such accidents resulted in serious injuries. Some population-based regional studies in the late 1970s and early 1980s estimated that 10 percent of emergency room admissions were the result of motor vehicle accidents, which also accounted for about 44 percent of brain and 56 percent of acute spinal cord injuries. Yet motor vehicle accidents aroused relatively little public concern or apprehension.[74]

The death rate from all unintentional injuries was highest among the elderly, largely because of falls. In 1998 accidents were the seventh leading cause of death among those 65 and older. Falls accounted for nearly half of the 1 million visits to hospital emergency departments by the elderly. Not only were they more likely to fall, but when they did they were more apt to sustain a fracture, especially of the hip.[75]

A comprehensive history of health patterns would also have to take into account a variety of other diseases, as well as suicide, homicide, violence, substance abuse, and specific and *proven* environmental and occupational risks. Though accounting for considerable morbidity, they play a much smaller role in mortality. The limitations of space, however, preclude detailed analyses of these and other topics.

▼ ▼ ▼

At the beginning of the twenty-first century life expectancy stood at an all-time high. Indeed, the fastest-growing group in the population was the very old (currently defined as those over age 85). In 1900 this group was not enumerated separately, but was included in the 65-and-older category. In 1997, by contrast, the very old included more than 3.8 million persons, and the Bureau of the Census projected that by 2050 this group could be as large as 31 million.[76] To be sure, the gains in longevity were not equally distributed. Yet virtually all groups were better off than their predecessors at the beginning of the twentieth century.

To many Americans the gains in longevity and health appeared to be the consequences of medical progress since World War II. Predictions about future progress seemed to suggest that Ponce de León's fountain of youth might somehow become a reality. "If developments in research maintain their current pace," according to William B. Schwartz, "it seems likely that a combination of improved attention to dietary and environmental factors along with advances in gene therapy and protein-targeted drugs will have virtually eliminated most major classes of disease." Moreover, a molecular understanding of the process of aging could result in ways of controlling its progress. Conceivably, "by 2050, aging may in fact prove to be simply another disease to be treated."[77]

Schwartz's optimism was by no means idiosyncratic; many shared a faith in the redemptive authority of medicine. Indeed, the presence of numerous groups that lobbied for greater funding for research and treatment of specific diseases suggested that many Americans believed that the very conquest of disease was a possibility, given will and adequate resources. The war on disease required the same judicious mix of people, resources, and technology that enabled the United States to emerge the victor in World War II and meet the challenges of a new space age.

In the last edition of his classic work on infectious disease in 1972, Sir Macfarlane Burnet, the distinguished Australian virologist and recipient of the Nobel Prize in medicine, observed that "young people today have had almost no experience of serious infectious disease." What about the future, he asked?

> If for the present we retain a basic optimism and assume no major catastrophes occur and that any wars are kept at the "brush fire" level, the most likely forecast about the future of infectious disease is that it will be very dull. There may be some wholly unexpected emergence of a new and dangerous infectious disease, but nothing of the sort has marked the last fifty years. There have been isolated outbreaks of fatal infections derived from exotic animals as in the instance of the laboratory workers struck down with the Marburg virus from African monkeys and the cases of severe haemorrhagic fever due to Lassa virus infection in Nigeria. Similar episodes will doubtless occur in the future but they will presumably be safely contained.

Burnet conceded that ecological changes could lead once again to the emergence of infectious diseases with the potential to "play havoc in our crowded world."[78] Nevertheless, he and his collaborator looked forward to a better future.

Burnet, of course, was both right and wrong. His prediction of the emergence of "a new and dangerous infectious disease" was accurate, but his belief that it could be "safely contained" was erroneous. Writing in 1972, he could not have predicted the extent of the AIDS pandemic. According to data compiled by the Joint United Nations Programme on HIV/AIDS, nearly 22 million people worldwide had died from the disease by 2000 (3 million in the year 2000 alone). As many as 36 million people were infected with the virus by the beginning of the twenty-first century. Although the rate of new infections may have stabilized, there were over 5 million newly infected persons in 2000. Even with allowances for inflated prevalence and mortality data, there was no doubt that the HIV virus represented a threat to life of global proportions.

How realistic is the faith that diseases can be conquered? The history of predictions—medical and others—offers relatively little support for such an optimistic view of the future. For several centuries numerous individuals have provided estimates of the maximum number of people that the Earth can support; all such estimates have proven wrong.[79] The same is true of population estimates by such agencies as the Bureau of the Census. The census of 1940 reported a population of 131 million. The bureau then estimated that by 1980 population would reach 153 million. In fact the actual number for 1980 was nearly 227 million.[80] Such an error was not due to incompetence; it simply reflected an inability to predict both the increase in the birthrate after World War II and the number of immigrants to the United States. Most predictions, after all, are based on an extension of linear trends into the future; they cannot take into account unforeseen developments.

In recent years the advances in molecular biology and genetics have led to claims that in the near future it will become possible, in the words of Leroy Hood, "to take DNA from newborns and analyze fifty or more genes for the allelic forms that can predispose the infant to many common diseases—cardiovascular, cancer, autoimmune, or metabolic. For each defective gene there will be therapeutic regimes that will circumvent the limitations of the defective gene." Medicine, therefore, would move from a merely reactive to a preventive mode. "This is truly the golden age of biology," Hood concluded. "I believe that we will learn more about human development and pathology in the next twenty-five years than we have in the past two thousand."[81]

The historical record offers little to sustain such sanguine predictions. Most contemporary diseases, as David Weatherall has noted in a work critical of Hood and others, do not have a single cause; they have "complex and multiple pathologies that reflect the effects of both nature and nurture together with the damage that our tissues sustain as we age." Human systems are complex, interactive, and involve large numbers of genes; there are multiple routes to a given disease. Thus the search for a single "magic bullet" to prevent or cure a specific disease is likely to be futile.[82]

"Complete and lasting freedom from disease is but a dream remembered from imaginings of a Garden of Eden designed for the welfare of man."[83] So wrote René Dubos more than forty years ago, and his words remain as compelling as ever. Diseases may appear and disappear; some may be amenable to human control, and others perhaps not. Moreover, the disappearance of one category of disease invariably sets the stage for the emergence of others. The faith that disease can be completely conquered is at best a harmless and at worst a dangerous utopian illusion.

In our modern Western culture we have grown accustomed to the belief that all things are possible and that humans can completely control their destiny. History, however, suggests that we cannot always predict the unanticipated consequences of our actions. Confidence in our ability to control the world should be tempered by a wise skepticism and a recognition of our limitations. This is not in any way to suggest that we are powerless. Biomedical science, for example, has much to offer in controlling and alleviating many diseases. Yet we must be aware that the complexity of reality far exceeds our very real abilities to understand and shape our world.

"And at the end [of life], what?" George H. Bigelow and Herbert L. Lombard asked more than seventy years ago in an important study of chronic disease. Their answer remains as relevant today as when it was written.

> Is it not that we would have, after a span of years passed in reasonable serenity, a reduction to a minimum of the span of crippling and terminal illness, and then a humane departure, which can certainly be faced with more assurance than could an irrevocable guarantee

of immortality here. If anything like the above can be accepted generally, we see that the complete elimination of sickness and death may not be even theoretically desirable, but rather some conscious and rational control of sickness and death . . . [The goal is not to] entirely eliminate disease and death but . . . delay them and make them more humane.[84]

Notes

PROLOGUE

1. René Dubos, *The Dreams of Reason: Science and Utopias* (New York: Columbia University Press, 1961), p. 71.
2. Paul B. Beeson, "Changes in Medical Therapy during the Past Half Century," *Medicine,* 59 (1980): 79–85.
3. James Le Fanu, *The Rise and Fall of Modern Medicine* (New York: Carroll & Graf, 1999), especially pp. xv–xvii and 22–23.
4. William B. Schwartz, *Life without Disease: The Pursuit of Medical Utopia* (Berkeley: University of California Press, 1998), p. 149.
5. Susan Sontag, *Illness as Metaphor* (New York: Farrar, Straus and Giroux, 1978), pp. 64–66.
6. Dubos, *Dreams of Reason,* pp. 84–85. See also his classic and influential *Mirage of Health: Utopias, Progress, and Biological Change* (New York: Harper & Brothers, 1959).
7. David J. Weatherall, *Science and the Quiet Art: The Role of Medical Research in Health Care* (New York: W. W. Norton, 1995), pp. 223–224.
8. Ibid., pp. 63, 167–173.
9. See especially Renée C. Fox and Judith P. Swazy, *Spare Parts: Organ Replacement in American Society* (New York: Oxford University Press, 1992), pp. 3–10, 204–210.
10. See Linda T. Cohen, Janet M. Corrigan, and Molla S. Donaldson, eds., *To Err Is Human: Building a Safer Health System* (Washington, D.C.: National Academy Press, 2000), pp. 26–48.
11. The traditional distinction between acute infectious and chronic degenerative diseases is somewhat spurious. Miliary tuberculosis, for example, can

kill quickly, whereas pulmonary and other forms of tuberculosis tend to be chronic. Similarly, malaria can kill infants but be chronic and episodic in adults. Until the development of antibiotic drugs, many forms of tuberculosis and syphilis more properly belonged in the chronic category; the same is currently true for HIV infections. A more accurate conceptualization distinguishes between long- and short-duration illnesses. In general, chronic illnesses are of long duration; they gradually impair organs, a result that in turn leads to health problems and disability. The causes of such illnesses are complex, and can include pathogens, environmental factors, injuries, and a variety of unknown elements related to aging.

1. THE PRE-COLUMBIANS

1. Ilza Veith, ed. and trans., *Huang Ti Nei Ching Su Wên: The Yellow Emperor's Classic of Internal Medicine,* 2d ed. (Berkeley: University of California Press, 1966), pp. 97–98.

2. Charles L. Redman, *Human Impact on Ancient Environments* (Tucson: University of Arizona Press, 1999), pp. 199–207.

3. The distinction between epidemic and endemic diseases is somewhat artificial. Cholera and yellow fever represent one model; they are either present or absent at given times. Smallpox, by contrast, may be present in most years even though in certain years mortality rises precipitously. In many respects the distinction between the two types of infections was a construct designed by public health officials in order to introduce some element of clarity into data gathering and to assist in policy formulation.

4. This and preceding paragraphs are based largely on Mark N. Cohen, *Health and the Rise of Civilization* (New Haven: Yale University Press, 1989), pp. 32–38.

5. William H. McNeill, *Plagues and Peoples* (Garden City, N.Y.: Doubleday/ Anchor, 1976), pp. 27–32; Jared Diamond, *Guns, Germs, and Steel: The Fates of Human Societies* (New York: W. W. Norton, 1997), pp. 212–213.

6. Paul A. Janssens, *Paleopathology: Diseases and Injuries of Prehistoric Man* (London: John Baker, 1970), pp. 60–63.

7. For elaborations see Cohen, *Health and the Rise of Civilization;* and McNeill, *Plagues and Peoples.*

8. A. T. Sandison and Edmund Trapp, "Disease in Ancient Egypt," in *Mummies, Disease, and Ancient Cultures,* ed. Aidan Cockburn, Eve Cockburn, and Theodore A. Reyman, 2d ed. (New York: Cambridge University Press, 1998), pp. 38–44; J. Thompson Rowling, "Respiratory Disease in Egypt," in *Diseases in Antiquity: A Survey of the Diseases, Injuries, and Surgery of Early Populations,* ed. Don Brothwell and A. T. Sandison (Springfield, Ill.: Charles C. Thomas, 1967), pp. 489–497 (quotation p. 492).

9. James B. Pritchard, ed., *Ancient Near Eastern Texts Relating to the Old Testament,* 3d ed. (Princeton: Princeton University Press, 1969), pp. 394–395. Other texts contain similar passages. See ibid., pp. 346–347, 393–394.

10. Exodus 12:30, 1 Samuel 6:17, 2 Samuel 24:15, Isaiah 37:36, in *The Holy Scriptures According to the Masoretic Text* (Philadelphia: Jewish Publication Society of America, 1955).

11. *Thucydides History II,* trans. P. J. Rhodes (Warminster: Aris & Phillips, 1988), pp. 95–101; Diodorus Siculus, *History,* quoted in Adam Patrick, "Disease in Antiquity: Ancient Greece and Rome," in Brothwell and Sandison, *Disease in Antiquity,* pp. 239–240; *Hippocrates, Volume I,* trans. W. H. S. Jones (Cambridge: Harvard University Press, 1923), pp. 83–89, 147, 155–157, 253–257.

12. McNeill, *Plagues and Peoples,* pp. 77–149.

13. David Grigg, *Population Growth and Agrarian Change: An Historical Perspective* (Cambridge: Cambridge University Press, 1980), pp. 281–283; David Herlihy, *The Black Death and the Transformation of the West* (Cambridge: Harvard University Press, 1997), pp. 31–32; Ann G. Carmichael and Arthur M. Silverstein, "Smallpox in Europe before the Seventeenth Century: Virulent Killer or Benign Disease?" *Journal of the History of Medicine and Allied Sciences* 42 (1987): 147–168.

14. Walter G. Bell, *The Great Plague in London in 1665,* rev. ed. (London: Bodley Head, 1951), pp. x–xi, 12–13, 176–177 (quote), 325; Roy Porter, *London: A Social History* (Cambridge: Harvard University Press, 1995), pp. 80–84.

15. The debate concerning the origin of New World peoples can be followed in the *Chronicle of Higher Education,* March 13, 1998, pp. A22–23; *New York Times,* November 9, 1999, sec. F, pp. 1, 4; *Science* 275 (1997): 1256–57 and 286 (1999): 657, 659; and Thomas D. Dillehay, *The Settlement of the Americas: A New Prehistory* (New York: Basic Books, 2000). See also Russell Thornton, *American Indian Holocaust and Survival: A Population History since 1492* (Norman: University of Oklahoma Press, 1987), pp. 3–11.

16. Alfred W. Crosby, *The Columbian Exchange: Biological and Cultural Consequences of 1492* (Westport, Conn.: Greenwood Press, 1972), pp. 21–31; Francis L. Black, "Why Did They Die?" *Science* 258 (1992): 1739–40; idem, "An Explanation of High Death Rates among New World Peoples When in Contact with Old World Diseases," *Perspectives in Biology and Medicine* 37 (1994): 292–307.

17. Marshall T. Newman, "Aboriginal New World Epidemiology and Medical Care, and the Impact of Old World Disease Imports," *American Journal of Physical Anthropology* 45 (1976): 667–672.

18. Diamond, *Guns, Germs, and Steel,* pp. 212–214, 354–358.

19. For a discussion of methodological problems, see Clark S. Larsen and

George R. Milner, eds., *In the Wake of Contact: Biological Responses to Conquest* (New York: Wiley-Liss, 1993), especially chap. 1.

20. John W. Verano and Douglas B. Ubelaker, eds., *Disease and Demography in the Americas* (Washington, D.C.: Smithsonian Institution Press, 1992), pp. 5–6. See also Saul Jarcho, "Some Observations on Disease in Prehistoric America," *Bulletin of the History of Medicine* 38 (1964): 1–19; and Donald Journal Ortner and Walter G. Journal Putschar, *Identification of Pathological Conditions in Human Skeletal Remains* (Washington, D.C.: Smithsonian Institution Press, 1981).

21. George R. Milner, "Disease and Sociopolitical Systems in Late Prehistoric Illinois," in Verano and Ubelaker, *Disease and Demography,* pp. 103–112.

22. Newman, "Aboriginal New World Epidemiology," pp. 667–672.

23. Charles F. Merbs, "A New World of Infectious Disease," *Yearbook of Physical Anthropology* 35 (1992): 3–42.

24. Mary L. Powell, "Health and Disease in the Late Prehistoric Southeast," in Verano and Ubelaker, *Disease and Demography,* pp. 41–46; Jane E. Buikstra, ed., *Prehistoric Tuberculosis in the Americas* (Evanston: Northwestern University Archeological Program, 1981), pp. 1–14.

25. Powell, "Health and Disease in Late Prehistoric Southeast," pp. 41–50.

26. This and the preceding paragraph are based on Merbs, "New World of Infectious Disease," pp. 26–28; Victoria A. Harden, *Rocky Mountain Spotted Fever: History of a Twentieth-Century Disease* (Baltimore: Johns Hopkins University Press, 1990), pp. 1–8; James R. Busvine, *Disease Transmission by Insects: Its Discovery and Ninety Years of Efforts to Prevent It* (New York: Springer Verlag, 1993), pp. 38–39, 82–85, 93.

27. Merbs, "New World of Infectious Disease," p. 35; Ernest C. Faust, "History of Human Parasitic Infections," *Public Health Reports* 70 (1955): 958.

28. Merbs, "New World of Infectious Disease," pp. 30–32.

29. Charles F. Merbs, "Patterns of Health and Sickness in the Precontact Southwest," and Phillip L. Walker, Patricia Lambert, and Michael Journal DeNiro, "The Effects of European Contact on the Health of Alta California Indians," in *Columbian Consequences,* ed. David H. Thomas, 3 vols. (Washington, D.C.: Smithsonian Institution Press, 1989–1991), 1: 41–55, 349–364.

30. *The Book of Chilam Balam of Chumayel,* ed. Ralph L. Roys (Washington, D.C.: Carnegie Institution of Washington, 1933), p. 83. See also Virgil J. Vogel, *American Indian Medicine* (Norman: University of Oklahoma Press, 1970), pp. 148–161.

31. Marcus S. Goldstein, "Some Vital Statistics Based on Skeletal Material," *Human Biology* 25 (1953): 3–12; Christopher B. Ruff, "Reassessment of Demographic Estimates for Pecos Pueblo," *American Journal of Physical Anthropology* 54 (1981): 147–151; Douglas H. Ubelaker, *Reconstruction of*

Demographic Profiles from Ossuary Skeletal Samples: A Case Study from the Tidewater Potomac (Washington, D.C.: Smithsonian Institution Press, 1974), pp. 63–64.

32. John W. Lallo and Jerome C. Rose, "Patterns of Stress, Disease, and Mortality in Two Prehistoric Populations from North America," *Journal of Human Evolution* 8 (1979): 323–335; Rebecca Storey, "An Estimate of Mortality in a Pre-Columbian Urban Population," *American Anthropologist* 87 (1985): 519–535.

33. Richard H. Steckel, Paul W. Sciulli, and Jerome C. Rose, "Skeletal Remains, Health, and History: A Project on Long Term Trends in the Western Hemisphere," in *The Biological Standard of Living in Comparative Perspective,* ed. John Komlos and Joerg Baten (Stuttgart: Franz Steiner Verlag, 1998), pp. 139–154; Claire M. Cassidy, "Skeletal Evidence for Prehistoric Subsistence Adaptation in the Central Ohio River Valley," in *Paleopathology at the Origins of Agriculture,* ed. Mark N. Cohen and George Journal Armelagos (Orlando: Academic Press, 1984), pp. 307–345. Other essays in the latter collection offer corroborating data.

34. Storey, "Mortality in a Pre-Columbian Urban Population," pp. 520–522; Mary J. Dobson, *Contours of Death and Disease in Early Modern England* (Cambridge: Cambridge University Press, 1997), p. 185. London data can be found in Roger Finlay, *Population and Metropolis: The Demography of London, 1580–1650* (Cambridge: Cambridge University Press, 1981).

35. Approximately eleven methods have been used to derive population estimates; none has been demonstrated to have significant reliability. A survey of methodologies and estimates can be found in John D. Daniels, "The Indian Population of North America in 1492," *William and Mary Quarterly* 49 (1992): 298–320; Ubelaker, *Reconstruction of Demographic Profiles,* pp. 1–7; and William M. Denevan, ed., *The Native Population of the Americas in 1492,* 2d ed. (Madison: University of Wisconsin Press, 1992), pp. xvii–xxix, 235–292. For a devastating (if exaggerated) attack on population estimates for the Americas by the "High Counters" see David Henige, *Numbers from Nowhere: The American Indian Contact Population Debate* (Norman: University of Oklahoma Press, 1998).

2. NEW DISEASES IN THE AMERICAS

1. Adrián Recinos and Delia Goetz, eds., *The Annals of the Cakchiquels* (Norman: University of Oklahoma Press, 1953), p. 116.

2. Adam Smith, *An Inquiry into the Nature and Causes of the Wealth of Nations* (1776; reprint, New York: Random House, 1937), p. 590.

3. These themes are imaginatively developed in the writings of Alfred W. Crosby. See especially *The Columbian Exchange: Biological and Cultural*

Consequences of 1492 (Westport, Conn.: Greenwood Press, 1972), *Ecological Imperialism: The Biological Expansion of Europe, 900–1900* (New York: Cambridge University Press, 1986), and *Germs, Seeds, and Animals: Studies in Ecological History* (Armonk, N.Y.: M. E. Sharpe, 1994).

4. Richard H. Steckel, Paul W. Sciulli, and Jerome C. Rose, "Skeletal Remains, Health, and History: A Project on Long-Term Trends in the Western Hemisphere," in *The Biological Standard of Living in Comparative Perspective*, ed. John Komlos and Joerg Baten (Stuttgart: Franz Steiner Verlag, 1998), p. 151.

5. William M. Denevan, "The Pristine Myth: The Landscape of the Americas in 1492," *Annals of the Association of American Geographers* 82 (1992): 370.

6. Noble D. Cook, "Disease and Depopulation of Hispaniola, 1492–1518," *Colonial Latin American Review* 2 (1993): 213–245; idem, *Born to Die: Disease and New World Conquest, 1492–1650* (New York: Cambridge University Press, 1998), pp. 23–24.

7. Contemporary interpretations of disease can be found in *The Merck Manual of Diagnosis and Therapy*, 17th ed. (Rahway, N.J.: Merck Research Laboratories, 1999); and *The Cambridge World History of Human Disease*, ed. Kenneth F. Kiple (New York: Cambridge University Press, 1993).

8. Francisco Guerra, "The Earliest American Epidemic: The Influenza of 1493," *Social Science History* 12 (1988): 305–325; Cook, *Born to Die*, pp. 28–45.

9. Cyril W. Dixon, *Smallpox* (London: J. & A. Churchill, 1962), pp. 6–7. An overview of the history of smallpox can be found in Donald R. Hopkins, *Princes and Peasants: Smallpox in History* (Chicago: University of Chicago Press, 1983).

10. Ann G. Carmichael and Arthur M. Silverstein, "Smallpox in Europe before the Seventeenth Century: Virulent Killer or Benign Disease?" *Journal of the History of Medicine and Allied Sciences* 42 (1987): 146–168.

11. *Motolinía's History of the Indians of New Spain*, ed. and trans. Elizabeth A. Foster (Berkeley: Cortés Society, 1950), p. 38.

12. W. George Lovell, "'Heavy Shadows and Black Night': Disease and Depopulation in Colonial Spanish America," *Annals of the Association of American Geographers* 82 (1992): 429; Sherburne F. Cook and Woodrow Borah, *Essays in Population History: Mexico and the Caribbean*, 3 vols. (Berkeley: University of California Press, 1971–1979), 1: viii; Noble D. Cook, *Demographic Collapse: Indian Peru, 1520–1620* (New York: Cambridge University Press 1981); *Motolinía's History*, p. 38. For analysis of the exaggerated population estimates for the New World see Shepard Krech III, *The Ecological Indian: Myth and History* (New York: W. W. Norton, 1999), pp. 73–99; and David Henige, *Numbers from Nowhere: The American Indian Population Debate* (Norman: University of Oklahoma Press, 1998).

13. *Motolinía's History*, p. 38. See especially Noble D. Cook and W. George Lovell, eds., *"Secret Judgments of God": Old World Disease in Colonial Spanish America* (Norman: University of Oklahoma Press, 1991); and Cook, *Demographic Collapse.*

14. Cook's *Born to Die* provides a synthesis of the literature dealing with the impact of disease on Spanish America (quote from p. 13). For yellow fever in Yucatán, see Richard M. Taylor, "Epidemiology," in *Yellow Fever*, ed. George K. Strode (New York: McGraw-Hill, 1951), pp. 529–530.

15. Clark Spencer Larsen et al., "Beyond Demographic Collapse: Biological Adaptation and Change in the Native Populations of La Florida," in *Columbian Consequences*, ed. David H. Thomas, 3 vols. (Washington, D.C.: Smithsonian Institution Press, 1989–1991), 2: 409–428.

16. Henry F. Dobyns, *Their Number Become Thinned: Native American Population Dynamics in Eastern North America* (Knoxville: University of Tennessee Press, 1983), pp. 254–289. Dobyns' work has come under criticism. See, for example, David Henige, "Primary Source by Primary Source? On the Role of Epidemics in New World Depopulation," *Ethnohistory* 33 (1986): 293–312, and especially *Numbers from Nowhere*. A more supportive critique is Ann F. Ramenofsky, *Vectors of Death: The Archeology of European Contact* (Albuquerque: University of New Mexico Press, 1987).

17. Jerald T. Milanich, "The European Entrada in La Florida: An Overview," in Thomas, *Columbian Consequences*, 2: 9; idem, *Florida Indians and the Invasion from Europe* (Gainesville: University Press of Florida, 1995), pp. 221–222.

18. George R. Milner, "Epidemic Disease in the Postcontact Southeast: A Reappraisal," *Mid-Continental Journal of Archeology* 5 (1980): 39–56; Robert L. Blakely and Bettina Detweiler-Blakely, "The Impact of European Diseases in the Sixteenth-Century Southeast: A Case Study," ibid., 14 (1989): 62–89. David E. Stannard's *American Holocaust: Columbus and the Conquest of the New World* (New York: Oxford University Press, 1992), while conceding the significance of disease, emphasizes instead the brutality of Europeans in the destruction of the inhabitants of the Americas. His thesis is both grossly exaggerated and hardly supported by empirical data.

19. See John C. Ewers, "The Influence of Epidemics on the Indian Populations and Cultures of Texas," *Plains Anthropologist* 18 (1973): 104–115.

20. Robert H. Jackson, *Indian Population Decline: The Missions of Northwestern New Spain, 1687–1840* (Albuquerque: University of New Mexico Press, 1994), p. 4 and passim.

21. Ibid., pp. 116–123, 141.

22. Ibid., pp. 117–143. The classic works by Sherburne F. Cook, *The Population of the California Indians, 1769–1970* (Berkeley: University of California Press, 1976), and Cook and Borah, *Essays in Population History*, vol. 3,

confirm most of Jackson's findings even though based on less sophisticated data. See also the essays in Thomas, *Columbian Consequences,* 1: 303–449.

23. Material in this and the previous two paragraphs is drawn from James Mooney, "The Powhatan Confederacy, Past and Present," *American Anthropologist,* n.s. 9 (1907): 129–152; Russell Thornton, *American Indian Holocaust and Survival: A Population History since 1492* (Norman: University of Oklahoma Press, 1987), pp. 67–70; John Duffy, *Epidemics in Colonial America* (Baton Rouge: Louisiana State University Press, 1953), p. 69; idem, "Smallpox and the Indians in the American Colonies," *Bulletin of the History of Medicine* 25 (1951): 330; Peter C. Mancall, *Deadly Medicine: Indians and Alcohol in Early America* (Ithaca: Cornell University Press, 1995), p. 92.

24. Timothy L. Bratton, "The Identity of the New England Indian Epidemic of 1616–19," *Bulletin of the History of Medicine* 62 (1988): 351–383; Sherburne F. Cook, "The Significance of Disease in the Extinction of the New England Indians," *Human Biology* 45 (1973): 485–508; Crosby, *Germs, Seeds, and Animals,* pp. 109–119. Scholarly disagreements persist. Arthur E. and Bruce D. Spiess, for example, have argued in favor of hepatitis in their article "New England Pandemic of 1616–1622: Cause and Archaeological Implication," *Man in the Northeast* 34 (1987): 71–83.

25. Duffy, "Smallpox and the Indians," pp. 327–328.

26. Dean R. Snow and Kim M. Lanphear, "European Contact and Indian Depopulation in the Northeast: The Timing of the First Epidemics," *Ethnohistory* 35 (1988): 23–24; E. Wagner Stearn and Allen E. Stearn, *The Effect of Smallpox on the Destiny of the Amerindian* (Boston: Bruce Humphries, 1945), chap. 2; Thornton, *American Indian Holocaust,* pp. 72–74.

27. Cook, "Significance of Disease," pp. 485–508. For estimates of the New England Indian population both before and after the first contacts, see Dean R. Snow, *The Archaeology of New England* (New York: Academic Press, 1980), pp. 33–42.

28. Thornton, *American Indian Holocaust,* pp. 78 ff.; Duffy, "Smallpox and the Indians," pp. 332–341; Laurence M. Hauptman, "Smallpox and the American Indian: Depopulation in Colonial New York," *New York State Journal of Medicine* 79 (1979): 1945–49; Peter H. Wood, "The Impact of Smallpox on the Native Population of the 18th Century South," ibid., 87 (1987): 30–36; Stearn and Stearn, *Effect of Smallpox,* pp. 34–52.

29. Calvin Martin, "Wildlife Diseases as a Factor in the Depopulation of the North American Indian," *Western Historical Quarterly* 7 (1976): 47–62; idem, *Keepers of the Game: Indian-Animal Relationships and the Fur Trade* (Berkeley: University of California Press, 1978), pp. 40–65, 130–149.

30. Russell Thornton, "Cherokee Population Losses during the 'Trail of Tears':

A New Perspective and a New Estimate," *Ethnohistory* 31 (1984): 289–300; idem, *American Indian Holocaust*, pp. 113–131; James Mooney, *Historical Sketch of the Cherokee* (1900; reprint, Chicago: Aldine, 1975), pp. 124–130.

31. Robert Boyd, *The Coming of the Spirit of Pestilence: Introduced Infectious Diseases and Population Decline among Northwest Coast Indians, 1774–1874* (Seattle: University of Washington Press, 1999), pp. 22, 88–89, 231–261.

32. Virginia R. Allen, "The White Man's Road: The Physical and Psychological Impact of Relocation on the Southern Plains Indians," *Journal of the History of Medicine and Allied Sciences* 30 (1975): 148–163. In line with post-World War II intellectual trends, Allen emphasized the psychological impact of stress and the inability of the Plains Indians to adapt to their new circumstances, which in turn magnified the importance of disease. Although stress played a role, the material circumstances of life of the Southern Plains Indians were largely responsible for high morbidity and mortality rates.

33. Paul Stuart, *Nations within a Nation: Historical Statistics of American Indians* (New York: Greenwood Press, 1987), p. 52; Thornton, *American Indian Holocaust*, pp. 91–133; Dobyns, *Their Number Become Thinned*, pp. 15–26. For more specific examples of decline see Clyde D. Dollar, "The High Plains Smallpox Epidemic of 1837–38," *Western Historical Quarterly* 8 (1977): 15–38; John C. Ewers, "The Influence of Epidemics on the Indian Populations and Cultures of Texas," *Plains Anthropologist* 18 (1973): 104–115; Jody F. Decker, "Depopulation of the Northern Plains Natives," *Social Science and Medicine* 33 (1991): 381–393; Herbert C. Taylor Jr. and Lester L. Hoaglin Jr., "The 'Intermittent Fever' Epidemic of the 1830's on the Lower Columbia River," *Ethnohistory* 9 (1962): 160–178; Richard White, *The Organic Machine* (New York: Hill and Wang, 1995), pp. 24 ff.

34. Population data are taken from U.S. Bureau of the Census, *Statistical Abstract of the United States, 1996* (Washington, D.C.: Government Printing Office, 1996), p. 21. Internal analysis of the age distribution data suggests that the increase in population in this fifteen-year period is overstated, and may result from the fact that more individuals identified themselves in this category.

35. Alfred W. Crosby, "Virgin Soil Epidemics as a Factor in the Aboriginal Depopulation in America," *William and Mary Quarterly* 33 (1976): 289–299.

36. The contemporary study of "genetic markers" is of individuals who survived the epidemics that killed their ancestors. In virtually every population, there are "natural" immunes. Peter L. Panum's classic study of measles in the Faroe Islands in 1846 suggested as much. Measles had been absent on the islands since 1781. In the epidemic of 1846 there were 6,000 cases of measles in a population of 7,782. Panum, *Observations Made during the Epidemic*

of Measles on the Faroe Islands in the Year 1846 (New York: Delta Omega Society, 1940), p. 49. The essay was first published in the *Bibliothek for Laeger* in 1847.

37. This and the preceding two paragraphs are based on Francis L. Black, "Why Did They Die?" *Science* 258 (1992): 1739–40 and "An Explanation of High Death Rates among New World Peoples When in Contact with Old World Diseases," *Perspectives in Biology and Medicine* 37 (1994): 292–307. Peter Aaby's work can be followed in Aaby et al., "Overcrowding and Intensive Exposure as Determinants of Measles Mortality," *American Journal of Epidemiology* 120 (1984): 49–63; Aaby, "Malnutrition and Overcrowding/Intensive Exposure in Severe Measles Infection: Review of Community Studies," *Reviews of Infectious Diseases* 10 (1988): 478–491; idem, "Determinants of Measles Mortality: Host or Transmission Factors?" in *Medical Virology 10: Proceedings of the 1990 Symposium on Medical Virology . . . 1990,* ed. Luis M. De la Maza and Ellena M. Peterson (New York: Plenum, 1991), pp. 83–116.

38. William Bradford, *Of Plymouth Plantation, 1620–1647,* ed. Samuel E. Morison (New York: Alfred A. Knopf, 1975), pp. 270–271.

39. Richard White, *The Roots of Dependency: Subsistence, Environment, and Social Change among the Choctaws, Pawnees, and Navajos* (Lincoln: University of Nebraska Press, 1983); Stephen J. Kunitz, *Disease and Social Diversity: The European Impact on the Health of Non-Europeans* (New York: Oxford University Press, 1994); idem, *Disease Change and the Role of Medicine: The Navajo Experience* (Berkeley: University of California Press, 1983). See also Richard White, *The Middle Ground: Indians, Empires, and Republics in the Great Lakes Region, 1650–1815* (New York: Cambridge University Press, 1991).

40. White, *Roots of Dependency;* Mancall, *Deadly Medicine.* For a discussion of the use of alcohol by Navajos and other Southwestern native Americans since the 1970s, see Stephen J. Kunitz and Jerrold E. Levy, "Changes in Alcohol Use among Navajos and Other Indians of the American Southwest," in *Drugs and Narcotics in History,* ed. Roy Porter and Mikulas Teich (New York: Cambridge University Press, 1995), pp. 133–155.

41. Martin, *Keepers of the Game.*

42. René Dubos and Jean Dubos, *The White Plague: Tuberculosis, Man, and Society* (Boston: Little, Brown, 1952), pp. 190–191; Jane E. Buikstra, *Prehistoric Tuberculosis in the Americas* (Evanston: Northwestern University Archeological Program, 1981), pp. 1–14.

3. COLONIES OF SICKNESS

1. William Wood, *New England's Prospect* (1635), ed. Alden T. Vaughan, 2d ed. (Amherst: University of Massachusetts Press, 1977), pp. 110–111.

2. Karen O. Kupperman, "The Puzzle of the American Climate in the Early Colonial Period," *American Historical Review* 87 (1982): 1262–89.

3. Thomas Hariot, *A Brief and True Report of the New Found Land of Virginia* (London: n.p., 1588), fol. 3; David W. Stahle et al., "The Lost Colony and Jamestown Droughts," *Science* 280 (1998): 564–567; Gordon W. Jones, "The First Epidemic in English America," *Virginia Magazine of History and Biography* 71 (1963): 3–10; Kupperman, "Puzzle of the American Climate," p. 1272.

4. Carville Earle, "Environment, Disease, and Mortality in Early Virginia," *Journal of Historical Geography* 5 (1979): 365–366.

5. Joyce E. Chaplin, "Natural Philosophy and an Early Racial Idiom in North America: Comparing English and Indian Bodies," *William and Mary Quarterly* 44 (1997): 241.

6. George Percy, "Discourse," in *The Genesis of the United States,* ed. Alexander Brown, 2 vols. (Boston: Houghton, Mifflin, 1890), 1: 167–168; Earle, "Environment, Disease, and Mortality in Early Virginia," p. 367; Dana P. Arneman, "Mortality in the Early Colonies of Jamestown, Plymouth, and Massachusetts Bay Colony: A New Interpretation" (M.A. thesis, University of South Carolina, 1990), pp. 9–10.

7. Earle, "Environment, Disease, and Mortality in Early Virginia," pp. 373–383; John Duffy, *Epidemics in Colonial America* (Baton Rouge: Louisiana State University Press, 1953), p. 13.

8. Karen O. Kupperman, using analogies from World War II and the Korean War, suggests that malnutrition and nutritional deficiency diseases led to a form of apathy. Apathy, in turn, led to neglect of agriculture and other vital tasks necessary to the survival of the colony. The interaction of psychological and physical causes resulted in high rates of mortality in Jamestown from 1607 to 1624, just as it did among American prisoners of war during the Korean conflict. See Kupperman, "Apathy and Death in Early Jamestown," *Journal of American History* 66 (1979): 24–40.

   Malnutrition clearly played a role in high mortality rates among American prisoners of war in the Korean conflict. Yet other factors shaped mortality patterns: the length of time an individual was a prisoner, the ability of the enemy to break down structures of loyalty and command, as well as respiratory illnesses and diarrhea. Physicians found that anger often was a means of surviving. See Albert E. Cowdrey, *The Medics' War* (Washington, D.C.: U.S. Army Center of Military History, 1987), pp. 300–306.

9. Earle, "Environment, Disease, and Mortality in Early Virginia," pp. 370–371; Arneman, "Mortality in the Early Colonies," pp. 20–23.

10. See Adelia M. Beeuwkes, "The Prevalence of Scurvy among Voyageurs to America—1493–1600," *Journal of the American Dietetic Association* 24 (1948): 300–303.

11. Arneman, "Mortality in the Early Colonies," pp. 33–54; William Bradford, *Of Plymouth Plantation, 1620–1647*, ed. Samuel E. Morison (New York: Alfred A. Knopf, 1975), pp. 77–78.

12. Arneman, "Mortality in the Early Colonies," pp. 60–70; John Smith, "Advertisements for the Unexperienced Planters of New England, or Any Where" (1631), in *The Complete Works of Captain John Smith*, ed. Philip L. Barbour, 3 vols. (Chapel Hill: University of North Carolina Press, 1986), 3: 292.

13. Arneman, "Mortality in the Early Colonies," pp. 70–86; Edward Johnson, *Wonder-Working Providence of Sions Saviour in New England* (1654; reprint, Andover, Mass.: Warren F. Draper, 1867), pp. 38–39. For Boston's early history see Darrett B. Rutman, *Winthrop's Boston: Portrait of a Puritan Town, 1630–1649* (Chapel Hill: University of North Carolina Press, 1965).

14. John Duffy, *A History of Public Health in New York City, 1625–1866* (New York: Russell Sage Foundation, 1968), pp. 5–7.

15. Dana P. Arneman, "The Medical History of Colonial South Carolina" (Ph.D. diss., University of South Carolina, 1996), pp. 32–41.

16. Gerald L. Cates, "'THE SEASONING': Disease and Death among the First Colonists of Georgia," *Georgia Historical Quarterly* 64 (1980): 146–158.

17. Farley Grubb, "Morbidity and Mortality on the North Atlantic Passage: Eighteenth-Century German Immigration," *Journal of Interdisciplinary History* 17 (1987): 565–585.

    Mortality rates for the seventeenth through the end of the nineteenth century were generally reported as deaths per thousand. Since 1900 rates have usually been expressed as deaths per 100,000.

18. This and the preceding paragraph are based on Susan E. Klepp's "Seasoning and Society: Racial Differences in Mortality in Eighteenth-Century Philadelphia," *William and Mary Quarterly* 51 (1994): 473–506, and *"The Swift Progress of Population": A Documentary and Bibliographic Study of Philadelphia's Growth, 1642–1859* (Philadelphia: American Philosophical Society, 1991).

19. The most important sources of colonial population data are Evarts B. Greene and Virginia D. Harrington, *American Population before the Federal Census of 1790* (New York: Columbia University Press, 1932); and Robert V. Wells, *The Population of the British Colonies in America before 1776* (Princeton: Princeton University Press, 1975).

20. See especially Mary J. Dobson, *Contours of Death and Disease in Early Modern England* (Cambridge: Cambridge University Press, 1997).

21. John Demos, "Notes on Life in Plymouth Colony," *William and Mary Quarterly* 22 (1965): 269–272.

22. Kenneth A. Lockridge, "The Population of Dedham, Massachusetts, 1636–

1736," *Economic History Review* 19 (1966): 318–344, and *A New England Town: The First Hundred Years, Dedham, Massachusetts, 1636–1736* (New York: W. W. Norton, 1970), pp. 66–68.

23. This and the preceding paragraph are based on Susan L. Norton, "Population Growth in Colonial America: A Study of Ipswich, Massachusetts," *Population Studies* 25 (1971): 433–452; Philip J. Greven Jr., *Four Generations: Population, Land, and Family in Colonial Andover, Massachusetts* (Ithaca: Cornell University Press, 1970), pp. 22–30; Richard Archer, "New England Mosaic: A Demographic Analysis for the Seventeenth Century," *William and Mary Quarterly* 47 (1990): 477–502.

24. Duffy, *Public Health in New York City,* pp. 27–29, 34–36; John B. Blake, *Public Health in the Town of Boston, 1630–1822* (Cambridge: Harvard University Press, 1959), pp. 23–29, 34–36; Darrett B. Rutman and Anita H. Rutman, "Of Agues and Fevers: Malaria in the Early Chesapeake," *William and Mary Quarterly* 33 (1976): 48. See also Maris A. Vinovskis, "Angels' Heads and Weeping Willows: Death in Early America," *American Antiquarian Society Proceedings,* n.s. 86 (1976): 278–279; idem, "Mortality Rates and Trends in Massachusetts before 1860," *Journal of Economic History* 32 (1972): 195–201; and Mary J. Dobson, "Mortality Gradients and Disease Exchanges: Comparisons from Old England and Colonial America," *Social History of Medicine* 2 (1989): 259–297.

25. Edmund S. Morgan, *American Slavery American Freedom: The Ordeal of Colonial Virginia* (New York: W. W. Norton, 1975), pp. 158–162, 180–185, 395–405. Wyndham B. Blanton attributes the slow growth of Virginia's population to the sex imbalance; "Epidemics, Real and Imaginary, and Other Factors Influencing Seventeenth-Century Virginia's Population," *Bulletin of the History of Medicine* 31 (1957): 454–462.

26. Daniel B. Smith, "Mortality and Family in the Chesapeake," *Journal of Interdisciplinary History* 8 (1978): 403–427.

27. Lorena S. Walsh and Russell R. Menard, "Death in the Chesapeake: Two Life Tables for Men in Early Colonial Maryland," *Maryland Historical Magazine* 69 (1974): 211–227; Daniel S. Levy, "The Life Expectancies of Colonial Maryland Legislators," *Historical Methods* 20 (1987): 17–27. See also Lorena S. Walsh, "'Till Death Us Do Part': Marriage and Family in Seventeenth-Century Maryland," in *The Chesapeake in the Seventeenth Century: Essays on Anglo-American Society and Politics,* ed. Thad W. Tate and David L. Ammerman (Chapel Hill: University of North Carolina Press, 1979), pp. 126–152.

28. See especially Dobson, *Contours of Death and Disease,* pp. 287–367.

29. Ibid., pp. 157–159, 339.

30. Charles F. Merbs, "A New World of Infectious Disease," *Yearbook of Physical Anthropology* 35 (1992): 10–13; Frederick L. Dunn, "On the Antiquity

of Malaria in the Western Hemisphere," *Human Biology* 37 (1965): 385–393.

31. Rutman and Rutman, "Of Agues and Fevers," pp. 42–54; Jon Kukla, "Kentish Agues and American Distempers: The Transmission of Malaria from England to Virginia in the Seventeenth Century," *Southern Studies* 25 (1986): 135–147; Duffy, *Epidemics in Colonial America,* pp. 204–214.

32. Rutman and Rutman, "Of Agues and Fevers," pp. 47–51; D. J. Bradley, "Malaria: Old Infections, Changing Epidemiology," *Health Transition Review,* suppl. to vol. 2 (1992): 145.

33. Rutman and Rutman, "Of Agues and Fevers," pp. 49–52. See also Guy P. Youmans, Philip Y. Paterson, and Herbert M. Sommers, *The Biologic and Clinical Basis of Infectious Diseases,* 3d ed. (Philadelphia: W. B. Saunders, 1985), p. 709.

34. H. Roy Merrens and George D. Terry, "Dying in Paradise: Malaria, Mortality, and the Perceptual Environment in Colonial South Carolina," *Journal of Southern History* 50 (1984): 533–537; Peter H. Wood, *Black Majority: Negroes in Colonial South Carolina from 1670 through the Stono Rebellion* (New York: Alfred A. Knopf, 1974), pp. 63–64 (quotation).

35. St. Julien R. Childs, *Malaria and Colonization in the Carolina Low Country, 1526–1696* (Baltimore: Johns Hopkins Press, 1940), pp. 88–110.

36. Ibid., pp. 221–226; Wood, *Black Majority,* pp. 64–65, 87–88.

37. See Peter A. Coclanis, *The Shadow of a Dream: Economic Life and Death in the South Carolina Low Country, 1670–1920* (New York: Oxford University Press, 1989).

38. Wood, *Black Majority,* pp. 71–72; Merrens and Terry, "Dying in Paradise," pp. 541–547.

4. THE PROMISE OF ENLIGHTENED HEALTH

1. A completed marriage is one in which the woman has lived to an age when she is no longer able to bear children (generally in the mid-forties).

2. Population data drawn from U.S. Bureau of the Census, *Historical Statistics of the United States: Colonial Times to 1970,* 2 vols. (Washington, D.C.: Government Printing Office, 1975), 1: 1168–72; Robert V. Wells, *The Population of the British Colonies in America before 1776* (Princeton: Princeton University Press, 1975), pp. 259–284; Evarts B. Greene and Virginia D. Harrington, *American Population before the Federal Census of 1790* (New York: Columbia University Press, 1932), pp. 3–8. See also Russell R. Menard, "Whatever Happened to Early American Population History?" *William and Mary Quarterly* 50 (1993): 356–366.

3. Descriptions of colonial urban life can be found in Carl Bridenbaugh's *Cities in the Wilderness: The First Century of Urban Growth in America, 1625–*

1742 (New York: Ronald Press, 1938), and *Cities in Revolt: Urban Life in America, 1743–1776* (New York: Alfred A. Knopf, 1955), as well as John Duffy's *A History of Public Health in New York City, 1625–1866* (New York: Russell Sage Foundation, 1968).

4. John Duffy, *Epidemics in Colonial America* (Baton Rouge: Louisiana State University Press, 1953), pp. 43–50.

5. Cotton Mather to John Cotton, November 1678, quoted in David E. Stannard, "Death and the Puritan Child," *American Quarterly* 26 (1974): 464.

6. Ann G. Carmichael and Arthur M. Silverstein, "Smallpox in Europe before the Seventeenth Century: Virulent Killer or Benign Disease?" *Journal of the History of Medicine and Allied Sciences* 42 (1987): 147–168; Duffy, *Epidemics in Colonial America,* pp. 21–22. For a chronology of epidemic disease and mortality in seventeenth- and eighteenth-century England see Mary J. Dobson, *Contours of Death and Disease in Early Modern England* (New York: Cambridge University Press, 1997), pp. 383–449.

7. John B. Blake, *Public Health in the Town of Boston, 1630–1822* (Cambridge: Harvard University Press, 1959), pp. 52–98.

8. Duffy, *Epidemics in Colonial America,* pp. 55–69.

9. Ibid., pp. 69–82; Duffy, *Public Health in New York City,* pp. 54–56; Billy G. Smith, *The "Lower Sort": Philadelphia's Laboring People, 1750–1800* (Ithaca: Cornell University Press, 1990), p. 48.

   There has been a long and heated debate over what is now referred to as biological warfare–particularly the use of smallpox as a military weapon–in the eighteenth century. "Biological warfare," according to Elizabeth Fenn, "was therefore a reality in eighteenth-century North America, not a distant, abstract threat as it is today." That it was used by all participants seems likely. Nevertheless, from a demographic perspective biological warfare played no role in the reduction of the Indian population. See Fenn, "Biological Warfare in Eighteenth-Century America: Beyond Jeffery Amherst," *Journal of American History* 86 (2000): 1552–80.

10. Duffy, *Epidemics in Colonial America,* pp. 7, 82–83, 92–95, 99–100; Dana P. Arneman, "The Medical History of Colonial South Carolina" (Ph.D. diss., University of South Carolina, 1996), pp. 141–148, 163–168.

11. Absalom Jones and Richard Allen, *A Narrative of the Proceedings of the Black People, during the Late Awful Calamity in Philadelphia, in the Year 1793* (Philadelphia: William W. Woodward, 1794), p. 16.

12. The classic work on the origins of yellow fever is Henry R. Carter's *Yellow Fever: An Epidemiological and Historical Study of Its Place of Origin* (Baltimore: Williams & Wilkins, 1931). See also George K. Strode, ed., *Yellow Fever* (New York: McGraw-Hill, 1951).

13. Duffy, *Epidemics in Colonial America,* pp. 141–146; idem, *Public Health in*

New York City, pp. 35–36; Arneman, "Medical History of Colonial South Carolina," pp. 194–195.

14. K. David Patterson, "Yellow Fever Epidemics and Mortality in the United States, 1693–1905," *Social Science and Medicine* 34 (1992): 856–857; Duffy, *Epidemics in Colonial America,* pp. 146–163.

15. Ernest Caulfield, "Early Measles Epidemics in America," *Yale Journal of Biology and Medicine* 15 (1943): 531–538; Duffy, *Epidemics in Colonial America,* pp. 164–169.

16. Caulfield, "Early Measles Epidemics," pp. 538–545; Noah Webster, *A Brief History of Epidemic and Pestilential Diseases,* 2 vols. (Hartford: Hudson & Goodwin, 1799), 1: 259–260.

17. Caulfield, "Early Measles Epidemics," pp. 550–555.

18. *The Diary of Ebenezer Parkman 1703–1782,* ed. Francis G. Walett (Worcester, Mass.: American Antiquarian Society, 1974), p. 1.

19. My discussion of diphtheria is based upon Ernest Caulfield's classic *A True History of the Terrible Epidemic Vulgarly Called the Throat Distemper* (New Haven: Yale Journal of Biology and Medicine, 1939). A different but unsupported interpretation can be found in Mary K. Matossian, "The Throat Distemper Reappraised" (with a critique by Robert P. Hudson), *Bulletin of the History of Medicine* 54 (1980): 529–543.

20. Caulfield, *True History,* pp. 14–23.

21. Ibid., pp. 32–34, 49.

22. Ibid., p. 5; H. Louis Settler, "The New England Throat Distemper and Family Size," in *Empirical Studies in Health Economics: Proceedings of the Second Conference in the Economics of Health,* ed. Herbert E. Klarman (Baltimore: Johns Hopkins Press, 1970), p. 19.

23. Caulfield, *True History,* p. 101.

24. Ibid., pp. 99–113; Ernest Caulfield, "Some Common Diseases of Colonial Children," *Publications of the Colonial Society of Massachusetts* 35 (1951): 15–24; Duffy, *Epidemics in Colonial America,* pp. 123–129.

25. Caulfield, "Some Common Diseases," pp. 24–36; Duffy, *Epidemics in Colonial America,* pp. 129–135.

26. Caulfield, "Some Common Diseases," pp. 36–42; Duffy, *Epidemics in Colonial America,* pp. 179–183.

27. Gottlieb Mittelberger, *Journey to Pennsylvania* (1756), ed. and trans. Oscar Handlin and John Clive (Cambridge: Harvard University Press, 1960), pp. 15–16.

28. Waldemar Westergaard, ed., "Two Germantown Letters of 1738," *Pennsylvania Magazine of History and Biography* 56 (1932): 12.

29. Webster, *Brief History,* 1: 239; Caulfield, "Some Common Diseases," pp. 43–65; Duffy, *Epidemics in Colonial America,* pp. 214–222.

30. Duffy, *Epidemics in Colonial America,* pp. 204–214; Paul F. Russell, "The

United States and Malaria: Debits and Credits," *Bulletin of the New York Academy of Medicine* 44 (1968): 623–625; Pascal James Imperato, Howard B. Shookhoff, and Robert P. Harvey, "Malaria in New York City," *New York State Journal of Medicine* 73 (1973): 2372–81.

31. See Arneman, "Medical History of Colonial South Carolina," pp. 90–124; and Peter A. Coclanis, *The Shadow of a Dream: Life and Death in the South Carolina Low Country, 1670–1920* (New York: Oxford University Press, 1989), pp. 42–47.

32. Peter H. Wood, *Black Majority: Negroes in Colonial South Carolina from 1670 through the Stono Rebellion* (New York: Alfred A. Knopf, 1974), pp. 70–76, 85–91.

33. [Alexander Hewat,] *An Historical Account of the Rise and Progress of the Colonies of South Carolina and Georgia,* 2 vols. (London, 1779), 1: 120, quoted in Winthrop D. Jordan, *White over Black: American Attitudes toward the Negro, 1550–1812* (Chapel Hill: University of North Carolina Press, 1968), p. 262.

34. John Tennent, *An Essay on the Pleurisy* (Williamsburg and New York, 1742), p. 3, quoted in Duffy, *Epidemics in Colonial America,* p. 200.

35. K. David Patterson, *Pandemic Influenza, 1700–1900: A Study in Historical Epidemiology* (Totowa, N.J.: Rowman & Littlefield, 1986), pp. 11–28. See especially Ernest Caulfield, "The Pursuit of a Pestilence," *Proceedings of the American Antiquarian Society,* n.s. 60 (1950): 21–52.

36. Scott D. Holmberg, "The Rise of Tuberculosis in America before 1820," *American Review of Respiratory Diseases* 142 (1990): 1228–32; Journal P. Brissot de Warville, *New Travels in the United States of America, 1788* (1791; reprint, Cambridge: Harvard University Press, 1964), pp. 279–280. See also E. R. N. Grigg, "The Arcana of Tuberculosis," *American Review of Tuberculosis and Pulmonary Diseases* 78 (1958): 426–432.

37. Holmberg, "Rise of Tuberculosis," pp. 1228–32; Michael Wigglesworth, "God's Controversy with New-England," *Massachusetts Historical Society Proceedings* 12 (1871–1873): 91.

38. Peter Kalm, *Travels into North America* (1772; reprint, Barre, Mass.: Imprint Society, 1972), p. 37; Holmberg, "Rise of Tuberculosis," pp. 1229–30.

39. Holmberg, "Rise of Tuberculosis," pp. 1228–32; Webster, *Brief History,* 2: 209.

40. U.S. Bureau of the Census, *Historical Statistics,* 1: 16, 19.

41. Howard H. Peckham, ed., *The Toll of Independence: Engagements and Battle Casualties of the American Revolution* (Chicago: University of Chicago Press, 1974), pp. xi–xiv, 130–133.

42. Mary C. Gillett, *The Army Medical Department, 1775–1818* (Washington, D.C.: Government Printing Office, 1981), pp. 3–6, 10–11, 77, 84–85, 94–97; Stanhope Bayne-Jones, *The Evolution of Preventive Medicine in the*

United States Army, 1607–1939 (Washington, D.C.: Department of the Army Office of the Surgeon General, 1968), pp. 45, 51–59. See also James E. Gibson, "The Role of Disease in the 70,000 Casualties in the American Revolutionary Army," *Transactions and Studies of the College of Physicians of Philadelphia* 17 (1949): 121–127; and Reuben Friedman, *The Story of Scabies* (New York: Froben Press, 1947).

43. De Warville, *New Travels*, p. 294.

44. Blake, *Public Health in the Town of Boston*, pp. 247–250.

45. Maris A. Vinovskis, "Mortality Rates and Trends in Massachusetts before 1860," *Journal of Economic History* 32 (1972): 184–213; R. S. Meindl and A. C. Swedlund, "Secular Trends in Mortality in the Connecticut Valley, 1700–1850," *Human Biology* 49 (1977): 389–414; Susan L. Norton, "Population Growth in Colonial America: A Study of Ipswich, Massachusetts," *Population Studies* 25 (1971): 433–452; Philip Greven Jr., *Four Generations: Population, Land, and Family in Colonial Andover, Massachusetts* (Ithaca: Cornell University Press, 1970), pp. 175–210; John W. Florin, *Death in New England: Regional Variations in Mortality* (Chapel Hill: University of North Carolina, Department of Geography, 1971), pp. 40–72.

46. Mary J. Dobson, "Mortality Gradients and Disease Exchanges: Comparisons from Old England and Colonial America," *Social History of Medicine* 2 (1989): 259–297; Maris A. Vinovskis, "Angels Heads and Weeping Willows: Death in Early America," *Proceedings of the American Antiquarian Society* 86 (1976): 273–302; Stannard, "Death and the Puritan Child," pp. 456–476; Rose Lockwood, "Birth, Illness, and Death in 18th-Century New England," *Journal of Social History* 12 (1978): 11–28.

47. This and the preceding paragraph are based on Susan E. Klepp, "Fragmented Knowledge: Questions in Regional Demographic History," *Proceedings of the American Philosophical Society* 133 (1989): 223–233; idem, *"The Swift Progress of Population": A Documentary and Bibliographic Study of Philadelphia's Growth, 1600–1859* (Philadelphia: American Philosophical Society, 1989); Billy G. Smith, "Death and Life in a Colonial Immigrant City: A Demographic Analysis of Philadelphia," *Journal of Economic History* 37 (1977): 863–889; idem, *The "Lower Sort,"* pp. 204–212; Louise Kantrow, "Life Expectancy of the Gentry in Eighteenth- and Nineteenth-Century Philadelphia," *Proceedings of the American Philosophical Society* 133 (1989): 312–327; and James T. Lemon, *The Best Poor Man's Country: A Geographical Study of Early Southeastern Pennsylvania* (Baltimore: Johns Hopkins Press, 1972).

48. Dobson, "Mortality Gradients and Disease Exchanges," pp. 271–274, 283.

49. Arneman, "Medical History of Colonial South Carolina," pp. 364–372, 377–393; Coclanis, *Shadow of a Dream*, pp. 42–47, 161–174; H. Roy Merrens and George D. Terry, "Dying in Paradise: Malaria, Mortality, and

the Perceptual Environment in Colonial South Carolina," *Journal of Southern History* 50 (1984): 533–550; James M. Gallman, "Mortality among White Males: Colonial North Carolina," *Social Science History* 4 (1980): 295–316; Daniel S. Levy, "The Life Expectancies of Colonial Maryland Legislators," *Historical Methods* 20 (1987): 17–27.

5. THREATS TO URBAN HEALTH

1. *New York Times,* March 13, 1865, reprinted in Stephen Smith, *The City That Was* (New York: Frank Allaban, 1911), pp. 100–101.
2. Adna F. Weber, *The Growth of Cities in the Nineteenth Century* (New York: Macmillan, 1899), p. 22.
3. Joel A. Tarr, *The Search for the Ultimate Sink: Urban Pollution in Historical Perspective* (Akron: University of Akron Press, 1996), pp. 10, 114.
4. Joel A. Tarr, "The Evolution of the Urban Infrastructure in the Nineteenth and Twentieth Centuries," in *Perspectives on Urban Infrastructure,* ed. Royce Hanson (Washington, D.C.: National Academy Press, 1984), pp. 4–21; Nelson M. Blake, *Water for the Cities: A History of the Urban Water Supply in the United States* (Syracuse: Syracuse University Press, 1956); Joanne A. Goldman, *Building New York's Sewers: Developing Mechanisms of Urban Management* (West Lafayette, Ind.: Purdue University Press, 1997), pp. 22–23; Theodore Steinberg, *Nature Incorporated: Industrialization and the Waters of New England* (New York: Cambridge University Press, 1991), pp. 205–239 (quote from p. 210).
5. See Tarr's essay "The Horse–Polluter of the City," in his *Search for the Ultimate Sink,* pp. 323–333.
6. John H. Griscom, *The Sanitary Condition of the Laboring Population of New York* (New York: Harper and Bros., 1845), pp. 6–12, 46–52; idem, *The Uses and Abuses of Air* (New York: J. S. Redfield, 1850), pp. 248–249.
7. *Report of the Council of Hygiene and Public Health of the Citizens' Association of New York, upon the Sanitary Condition of the City* (New York: D. Appleton, 1866), pp. xv, lxxxiii.
8. Massachusetts Sanitary Commission [Lemuel Shattuck], *Report of a General Plan for the Promotion of Public and Personal Health, Devised, Prepared and Recommended by the Commissioners Appointed under a Resolve of the Legislature of Massachusetts, Relating to a Sanitary Survey of the State* (Boston: Dutton & Wentworth, 1850); Isaac D. Rawlings, *The Rise and Fall of Disease in Illinois,* 2 vols. (Springfield: Illinois Department of Public Health, 1927), 1: 101–112. See also Oscar Handlin, *Boston's Immigrants: A Study in Acculturation,* rev. ed. (Cambridge: Harvard University Press, 1959); and Stuart Galishoff, *Newark: The Nation's Unhealthiest City, 1832–1895* (New Brunswick, N.J.: Rutgers University Press, 1988).

9. Quoted in J. Worth Estes and Billy G. Smith, eds., *A Melancholy Scene of Devastation: The Public Response to the 1793 Philadelphia Yellow Fever Epidemic* (Canton, Mass.: Science History Publications, 1997), p. 35.

10. Data on the epidemic of 1793 are found in Estes and Smith, *A Melancholy Scene of Devastation;* and J. H. Powell, *Bring Out Your Dead: The Great Plague of Yellow Fever in Philadelphia in 1793* (Philadelphia: University of Pennsylvania Press, 1949). See also Martin S. Pernick, "Politics, Parties, and Pestilence: Epidemic Yellow Fever in Philadelphia and the Rise of the First Party System," *William and Mary Quarterly* 29 (1972): 559–586; and Kenneth F. and Virginia H. Kiple, "Black Yellow Fever Immunities, Innate and Acquired, as Revealed in the American South," *Social Science History* 1 (1977): 419–436.

11. For a contemporary account see Ashbel Smith, *Yellow Fever in Galveston, Republic of Texas, 1839* (1839; reprint, Austin: University of Texas Press, 1951).

12. John Duffy, "Yellow Fever in the Continental United States during the Nineteenth Century," *Bulletin of the New York Academy of Medicine* 44 (1968): 687–701; Jo Ann Carrigan, *The Saffron Scourge: A History of Yellow Fever in Louisiana* (Lafayette: Center for Louisiana Studies, 1994), pp. 20–57 (quote from p. 32).

13. *Daily Crescent,* August 9, 1853, quoted in Jo Ann Carrigan, "Impact of Epidemic Yellow Fever on Life in Louisiana," *Louisiana History* 4 (1963): 30.

14. Statistical data in this and the previous paragraph are taken from John Duffy, *Sword of Pestilence: The New Orleans Yellow Fever Epidemic of 1853* (Baton Rouge: Louisiana State University Press, 1966), pp. 39, 115–119, 167–172; and Carrigan, *Saffron Scourge,* pp. 58–81.

15. K. David Patterson, "Yellow Fever Epidemics and Mortality in the United States, 1693–1905," *Social Science and Medicine* 34 (1992): 855–865; Duffy, "Yellow Fever," pp. 693–696. See also Margaret Humphries, *Yellow Fever and the South* (New Brunswick, N.J.: Rutgers University Press, 1992); John H. Ellis, *Yellow Fever and Public Health in the New South* (Lexington: University Press of Kentucky, 1992); Khaled J. Bloom, *The Mississippi Valley's Great Yellow Fever Epidemic of 1878* (Baton Rouge: Louisiana State University Press, 1993).

16. See especially W. E. van Heyningen and John R. Seal, *Cholera: The American Scientific Experience, 1947–1980* (Boulder: Westview Press, 1983).

17. See L. A. McNicol and R. N. Doetsch, "A Hypothesis Accounting for the Origin of Pandemic Cholera: A Retrograde Analysis," *Perspectives in Biology and Medicine* 26 (1983): 547–552.

18. See the exhaustive study by Robert Pollitzer, *Cholera* (Geneva: World Health Organization, 1959).

19. Ibid., pp. 11–50; van Heyningen and Seal, *Cholera,* pp. 4–10; G. F. Pyle,

"The Diffusion of Cholera in the United States in the Nineteenth Century," *Geographical Analysis* 1 (1969): 59–75. The classic study of the American reaction to the epidemics is Charles E. Rosenberg, *The Cholera Years: The United States in 1832, 1849, and 1866* (Chicago: University of Chicago Press, 1962).

20. J. S. Chambers, *The Conquest of Cholera: America's Greatest Scourge* (New York: Macmillan, 1938); U.S. Surgeon General, *The Cholera Epidemic of 1873* (Washington, D.C.: Government Printing Office, 1875), pp. 530–682; van Heyningen and Seal, *Cholera,* p. 8.

21. Rosenberg, *Cholera Years,* pp. 33–35, 108, 184; John Duffy, *A History of Public Health in New York City, 1625–1866* (New York: Russell Sage Foundation, 1968), p. 588.

22. John V. Cotter and Larry L. Patrick, "Disease and Ethnicity in an Urban Environment," *Annals of the Association of American Geographers* 71 (1981): 40–49. See also the description of conditions among the Boston Irish by two physicians in Massachusetts Sanitary Commission, *Report of a General Plan,* pp. 425–436.

23. John Snow, *On the Mode of Communication of Cholera,* 2d ed. (London, 1855), reprinted in *Snow on Cholera,* ed. Wade Hampton Frost (New York: Commonwealth Fund, 1936), p. 56.

24. Ibid., pp. 133–136; Rosenberg, *Cholera Years,* pp. 193–194.

25. Gretchen A. Condran, "Changing Patterns of Epidemic Disease in New York City," in *Hives of Sickness: Public Health and Epidemics in New York City,* ed. David Rosner (New Brunswick, N.J.: Rutgers University Press, 1995), p. 31; Duffy, *Public Health in New York City,* pp. 447–448; Donald R. Hopkins, *Princes and Peasants: Smallpox in History* (Chicago: University of Chicago Press, 1983), pp. 268–269; William T. Howard, *Public Health Administration and the Natural History of Disease in Baltimore, Maryland, 1797–1920* (Washington, D.C.: Carnegie Institution of Washington, 1924), pp. 282–283.

26. Patterson, "Yellow Fever Epidemics and Mortality," pp. 857–858; Chambers, *Conquest of Cholera,* pp. 285–286; van Heyningen and Seal, *Cholera,* p. 8.

27. Quoted in René Dubos and Jean Dubos, *The White Plague: Tuberculosis, Man, and Society* (Boston: Little, Brown, 1952), pp. 44–66.

28. Sheila M. Rothman, *Living in the Shadow of Death: Tuberculosis and the Social Experience of Illness in American History* (New York: Basic Books, 1994), pp. 118–127.

29. See Godias J. Drolet, "Epidemiology of Tuberculosis," in *Clinical Tuberculosis,* ed. Benjamin Goldberg, 5th ed., 2 vols. (Philadelphia: F. A. David, 1946), 1: A3 ff.; Richard H. Shryock, *National Tuberculosis Association: A Study of the Voluntary Health Movement in the United States* (New York:

National Tuberculosis Foundation, 1957), pp. 30–32; Dubos and Dubos, *White Plague.*

30. E. R. N. Grigg, "The Arcana of Tuberculosis," *American Review of Tuberculosis and Respiratory Diseases* 78 (1958): 429–430; Drolet, "Epidemiology of Tuberculosis," p. A3; Duffy, *Public Health in New York City,* p. 587.

31. Massachusetts Sanitary Commission, *Report of a General Plan,* pp. 94–99; Howard, *Public Health Administration,* p. 384.

32. Howard, *Public Health Administration,* pp. 391–392; Duffy, *Public Health in New York City,* pp. 585–587; Massachusetts Sanitary Commission, *Report of a General Plan,* p. 96.

33. Handlin, *Boston's Immigrants,* pp. 100–115, 329. Often responsibility for disease was attributed to the behavior of impoverished immigrants. For elaborations of this theme see Alan M. Kraut, *Silent Travelers: Germs, Genes, and the "Immigrant Menace"* (New York: Basic Books, 1994); and Howard Markel, *Quarantine: East European Jewish Immigrants and the New York City Epidemics of 1892* (Baltimore: Johns Hopkins University Press, 1997).

34. John E. Murray, "The White Plague in Utopia: Tuberculosis in Nineteenth-Century Shaker Communes," *Bulletin of the History of Medicine* 68 (1994): 278–306.

35. Wilson G. Smillie, *Public Health: Its Promise for the Future* (New York: Macmillan, 1955), p. 150.

36. See the classic work by Hans Zinsser, *Rats, Rice, and History* (Boston: Little, Brown, 1935).

37. *Report of the Council of Hygiene,* p. xlv; Smith, *The City That Was,* pp. 113–116; George Rosen, "Tenements and Typhus in New York City, 1840–1875," *American Journal of Public Health* 62 (1972): 590–593; Howard, *Public Health Administration,* p. 219.

38. Condran, "Changing Patterns of Epidemic Disease in New York City," p. 34.

39. Howard, *Public Health Administration,* pp. 232–237.

40. Ibid., pp. 435–468.

41. See Roger Lane, *Violent Death in the City: Suicide, Accident, and Murder in Nineteenth-Century Philadelphia* (Cambridge: Harvard University Press, 1979); and Howard, *Public Health Administration,* pp. 479–486, 554–555.

42. *Report on Insanity and Idiocy in Massachusetts, by the Commission on Lunacy, under Resolve of the Legislature of 1854,* Massachusetts *House Document No. 144* (Boston, 1855), p. 103. See also Gerald N. Grob, *Mental Institutions in America: Social Policy to 1875* (New York: Free Press, 1973); and Herbert Goldhamer and Andrew W. Marshall, *Psychosis and Civilization: Two Studies in the Frequency of Mental Disease* (Glencoe, Ill.: Free Press, 1953).

43. Richard A. Meckel, *Save the Babies: American Public Health Reform and the Prevention of Infant Mortality, 1850–1929* (Baltimore: Johns Hopkins University Press, 1990), pp. 28–29; Charles V. Chapin, "Deaths among Taxpayers and Non-Taxpayers, Income Tax Providence, 1865," *American Journal of Public Health* 14 (1924): 647–651.

44. Howard, *Public Health Administration,* pp. 507–517.

45. Ibid., p. 517; Duffy, *Public Health in New York City,* pp. 578–579; Meckel, *Saving the Babies,* p. 29.

46. Chapin, "Deaths among Taxpayers and Non-Taxpayers," pp. 648–651.

47. See W. Peter Ward, *Birth Weight and Economic Growth: Women's Living Standards in the Industrializing West* (Chicago: University of Chicago Press, 1993), pp. 10–21.

48. Claudia Goldin and Robert A. Margo, "The Poor at Birth: Birth Weights and Infant Mortality at Philadelphia's Almshouse Hospital, 1848–1873," *Explorations in Economic History* 26 (1989): 360–379; Ward, *Birth Weight,* pp. 82–97. The history of diet can be followed in Sarah F. McMahon, "Provisions Laid Up for the Family: Toward a History of Diet in New England, 1650–1850," *Historical Methods* 14 (1981): 4–21; Harvey A. Levenstein, *Revolution at the Table: The Transformation of the American Diet* (New York: Oxford University Press, 1988); and Richard O. Cummings, *The American and His Food: A History of Food Habits in the United States,* rev. ed. (Chicago: University of Chicago Press, 1941).

49. Maris Vinovskis, "Mortality Rates and Trends in Massachusetts before 1860," *Journal of Economic History* 32 (1972): 1211; A. J. Jaffe and W. I. Lourie Jr., "An Abridged Life Table for the White Population of the United States in 1830," *Human Biology* 14 (1942): 357; R. S. Meindl and A. C. Swedlund, "Secular Trends in Mortality in the Connecticut Valley, 1700–1850," ibid., 49 (1977): 403; Yasukichi Yasuba, *Birth Rates of the White Population in the United States: An Economic Study* (Baltimore: Johns Hopkins Press, 1962), p. 75; Clayne L. Pope, "Adult Mortality in America: A View from Family Histories," in *Strategic Factors in Nineteenth-Century American Economic History,* ed. Claudia Goldin and Hugh Rockoff (Chicago: University of Chicago Press, 1992), pp. 267–296.

50. Duffy, *Public Health in New York City,* pp. 532–538; Howard, *Public Health Administration,* pp. 508–509; Vinovskis, "Mortality Rates," p. 206; Stephen J. Kunitz, "Mortality Change in America, 1620–1920," *Human Biology* 56 (1984): 566–568; Mary Dalton, "Mortality in New York City a Century and a Quarter Ago," ibid., 6 (1934): 87–97.

51. Pope, "Adult Mortality," pp. 281–282. For a controversial analysis of the problem of sickness rates, see James C. Riley's *Sickness, Recovery, and Death: A History and Forecast of Ill Health* (Iowa City: University of

Iowa Press, 1989) and *Sick, Not Dead: The Health of British Workingmen During the Mortality Decline* (Baltimore: Johns Hopkins University Press, 1997).

52. Smith, *The City That Was*, pp. 18–19.

6. EXPANDING AMERICA, DECLINING HEALTH

1. Herman Melville, *Pierre; or, The Ambiguities* (1852), in *The Writings of Herman Melville*, vol. 7 (Evanston: Northwestern University Press, 1971), pp. 13, 240–241.

2. Adam Seybert, *Statistical Annals . . . of the United States of America* (Philadelphia: Thomas Dobson & Son, 1818), pp. 51–52.

3. R. S. Maindl and A. C. Swedlund, "Secular Trends in Mortality in the Connecticut Valley, 1700–1850," *Human Biology* 49 (1977): 389–414.

4. A. J. Jaffe and W. I. Lourie Jr., "An Abridged Life Table for the White Population of the United States in 1830," ibid., 14 (1942): 352–371. J. Worth Estes and David Goodman, *The Changing Humors of Portsmouth: The Medical Biography of an American Town, 1623–1983* (Boston: Francis A. Countway Library of Medicine, 1986), offer a microanalysis of a New Hampshire town.

5. Michael R. Haines, "Mortality in Nineteenth-Century America: Estimates from New York and Pennsylvania Census Data, 1865 and 1900," *Demography* 14 (1977): 326.

6. Stephen E. Ambrose and Sam Abell, *Lewis and Clark: Voyage of Discovery* (Washington, D.C.: National Geographic Society, 1998), pp. 54–55. For a description of the travails of the expedition, see Ambrose, *Undaunted Courage: Meriwether Lewis, Thomas Jefferson, and the Opening of the American West* (New York: Simon & Schuster, 1996).

7. J. Howard Beard, "The Medical Observations and Practice of Lewis and Clark," *Scientific Monthly* 20 (1925): 506–523.

8. Lillian Schlissel, *Women's Diaries of the Westward Journey*, rev. ed. (New York: Schocken, 1992), p. 129; Peter D. Olch, "Treading the Elephant's Tail: Medical Problems on the Overland Trails," *Bulletin of the History of Medicine* 59 (1985): 196–212; Thomas B. Hall, *Medicine on the Santa Fe Trail* (Dayton, Ohio: Morningside Bookshop, 1971), p. 90.

9. Olch, "Treading the Elephant's Tail," pp. 202–204; Robert T. Boyd, "Another Look at the 'Fever and Ague' of Western Oregon," *Ethnohistory* 22 (1975): 133–154; idem, *The Coming of the Spirit of Pestilence: Introduced Infectious Diseases and Population Decline among Northwest Coast Indians, 1774–1874* (Seattle: University of Washington Press, 1999); Hall, *Medicine on the Santa Fe Trail*, p. 88.

10. Olch, "Treading the Elephant's Tail," p. 203. See also Hall, *Medicine on the Santa Fe Trail*, pp. 98–101.

11. Anthony J. Lorenz, "Scurvy in the Gold Rush," *Journal of the History of Medicine and Allied Sciences* 12 (1957): 473–510. See also Georgia W. Read, "Diseases, Drugs, and Doctors on the Oregon-California Trail in the Gold-Rush Years," *Missouri Historical Review* 38 (1944): 260–276; and George W. Groh, *Gold Fever* (New York: William Morrow, 1966).

12. Olch, "Treading the Elephant's Tail," pp. 197, 205–209; Hall, *Medicine on the Santa Fe Trail*, pp. 102–111.

13. M. G. Wadsworth, "Auburn and Vicinity Forty Years Ago," in *History of Sangamon County* (Springfield, Ill., 1881), quoted in Paul M. Angle, "The Hardy Pioneer: How He Lived in the Early Middle West," in University of Illinois College of Medicine, *Essays in the History of Medicine in Honor of David J. Davis, M.D., Ph.D.* (Urbana: University of Illinois Press, 1965), pp. 132–133.

14. Madge E. Pickard and R. Carlyle Buley, *The Midwest Pioneer: His Ills, Cures, and Doctors* (Crawfordsville, Ind.: R. E. Banta, 1945), pp. 13–14.

15. Ibid., pp. 16–17; William Oliver, *Eight Months in Illinois; with Information to Emigrants* (Newcastle-upon-Tyne: W. A. Mitchell, 1843), p. 65.

16. A. D. P. Van Buren, in *Michigan Pioneer Collections* 5 (1882): 300–301, quoted in Angle, "The Hardy Pioneer," p. 134.

17. Pickard and Buley, *Midwest Pioneer*, p. 17.

18. Erwin H. Ackerknecht, *Malaria in the Upper Mississippi Valley, 1760–1900* (Baltimore: Johns Hopkins Press, 1945), pp. 6–9; Joseph J. Woodward, *Outlines of the Chief Camp Diseases of the United States Armies* (Philadelphia: J. B. Lippincot, 1863), p. 74. See also Woodward's *Typho-Malarial Fever: Is It a Special Type of Fever?* (Philadelphia: Washington, Gibson Brothers, 1876). For a detailed history of the diagnosis of typhomalarial fever see Dale C. Smith, "The Rise and Fall of Typhomalarial Fever," *Journal of the History of Medicine and Allied Sciences* 37 (1982): 182–220, 287–321.

19. Daniel Drake, *A Systematic Treatise, Historical, Etiological, and Practical, on the Principal Diseases of the Interior Valley of North America*, 2 vols. (Cincinnati: Winthrop B. Smith, 1850; Philadelphia: Lippincott, 1854), 2: 17–186.

20. My discussion draws largely on Ackerknecht's classic *Malaria in the Upper Mississippi Valley* and his "Diseases in the Middle West," in University of Illinois College of Medicine, *Essays in the History of Medicine*, pp. 168–181. See also Isaac D. Rawlings, *The Rise and Fall of Disease in Illinois*, 2 vols. (Springfield: Illinois Department of Public Health, 1927), 1: 35–43.

21. Drake, *Systematic Treatise*, 2: 186.

22. Noah Webster, *A Brief History of Epidemic and Pestilential Diseases*, 2 vols.

(Hartford: Hudson and Goodwin, 1799), 2: 229–230; Benjamin W. McCready, *On the Influence of Trades, Professions, and Occupations in the United States, in the Production of Disease* (1837; reprint, Baltimore: Johns Hopkins Press, 1943), p. 36.

23. The previous paragraphs are based on Ackerknecht, *Malaria in the Upper Mississippi Valley*, pp. 62–130. See also Peter T. Harsted, "Sickness and Disease on the Wisconsin Frontier: Malaria, 1820–1850," *Wisconsin Magazine of History* 43 (1959–60): 83–96; Mark F. Boyd, "An Historical Sketch of the Prevalence of Malaria in North America," *American Journal of Tropical Medicine* 21 (1941): 223–244; idem, *An Introduction to Malariology* (Cambridge: Harvard University Press, 1930).

24. Oliver, *Eight Months in Illinois*, p. 77.

25. For full descriptions of midwestern pioneer life see R. Caryle Buley, *The Old Northwest: Pioneer Period, 1815–1840*, 2 vols. (Bloomington: Indiana University Press, 1951).

26. Pickard and Buley, *Midwest Pioneer*, pp. 22–23; Rawlings, *Rise and Fall of Disease in Illinois*, 1: 69–83; Ackerknecht, "Diseases in the Middle West," pp. 174–175.

27. Pickard and Buley, *Midwest Pioneer*, pp. 9–34; Rawlings, *Rise and Fall of Disease in Illinois*, 1: 27–119; Peter T. Harsted, "Health in the Upper Mississippi River Valley" (Ph.D. diss., University of Wisconsin, 1963), pp. 207–222.

28. On the shortcomings of the mid-nineteenth-century federal censuses see Gerald N. Grob, *Edward Jarvis and the Medical World of Nineteenth-Century America* (Knoxville: University of Tennessee Press, 1978), pp. 137–154.

29. J. D. B. De Bow, *Mortality Statistics of the Seventh Census of the United States, 1850* (Washington, D.C.: A. O. P. Nicholson, 1855), pp. 88–89; Rawlings, *Rise and Fall of Disease in Illinois*, 1: 89.

30. Richard H. Steckel, "The Health and Mortality of Women and Children, 1850–1860," *Journal of Economic History* 48 (1988): 333–345; Lee L. Bean, Geraldine P. Mineau, and Douglas L. Anderton, "High-Risk Childbearing: Fertility and Infant Mortality on the American Frontier," *Social Science History* 16 (1992): 337–363.

31. Philip D. Jordan, "Milksickness in Kentucky and the Western Country," *Filson Club History Quarterly* 19 (1945): 29–40; Rawlings, *Rise and Fall of Disease in Illinois*, 1: 66–69; Pickard and Buley, *Midwest Pioneer*, pp. 20–21.

32. David T. Courtwright, "Disease, Death, and Disorder on the American Frontier," *Journal of the History of Medicine and Allied Sciences* 46 (1991): 457–492. See also Courtwright's *Violent Land: Single Men and Social Disorder from the Frontier to the Inner City* (Cambridge: Harvard University Press, 1996).

33. Schlissel, *Women's Diaries,* pp. 35, 171; Courtwright, "Disease Death, and Disorder on the American Frontier," p. 469. This paragraph draws heavily on Courtwright's perceptive analysis.

34. K. David Patterson, "Disease Environments of the Antebellum South," in *Science and Medicine in the Old South,* ed. Ronald L. Numbers and Todd L. Savitt (Baton Rouge: Louisiana State University Press, 1989), pp. 152–165. For a general account see Albert E. Cowdry, *This Land, This South: An Environmental History* (Lexington: University of Kentucky Press, 1983).

35. Jack E. Eblen, "New Estimates of the Vital Rates of the United States Black Population during the Nineteenth Century," *Demography* 11 (1974): 304–305; U.S. Bureau of the Census, *Historical Statistics of the United States: Colonial Times to 1970,* 2 vols. (Washington, D.C.: Government Printing Office, 1975), 1: 22.

36. Patterson, "Disease Environments," p. 157.

37. Ibid., pp. 152–165; Kenneth F. Kiple and Virginia H. King, *Another Dimension to the Black Diaspora: Diet, Disease, and Racism* (New York: Cambridge University Press, 1981), pp. 14–21, 53–55; Jill Dubisch, "Low Country Fevers: Cultural Adaptations to Malaria in Antebellum South Carolina," *Social Science and Medicine* 21 (1985): 641–649; John Duffy, "The Impact of Malaria on the South," in *Disease and Distinctiveness in the American South,* ed. Todd L. Savitt and James Harvey Young (Knoxville: University of Tennessee Press, 1988), pp. 29–54.

38. Todd L. Savitt, "Filariasis in the United States," *Journal of the History of Medicine and Allied Sciences* 32 (1977): 140–150. See also Kenneth F. Kiple, *The Caribbean Slave: A Biological History* (New York: Cambridge University Press, 1984).

39. Patterson, "Disease Environments," pp. 161–162.

40. Clayne L. Pope, "Adult Mortality in America before 1900: A View from Family Histories," in *Strategic Factors in Nineteenth-Century American Economic History,* ed. Claudia Goldin and Hugh Rockoff (Chicago: University of Chicago Press, 1992), pp. 284–296.

41. The literature on the slave trade is large. For recent findings see Herbert S. Klein, *The Middle Passage* (Princeton: Princeton University Press, 1978), pp. 228–251; Philip D. Curtin, *The Atlantic Slave Trade: A Census* (Madison: University of Wisconsin Press, 1969), pp. 275–286; Joseph C. Miller, "Mortality in the Atlantic Slave Trade: Statistical Evidence on Causality," *Journal of Interdisciplinary History* 11 (1981): 385–423; Richard H. Steckel and Richard A. Jensen, "New Evidence on the Causes of Slave and Crew Mortality in the Atlantic Slave Trade," *Journal of Economic History* 46 (1986): 57–77; David Eltis, "Mortality and Voyage Length in the Middle Passage: New Evidence from the Nineteenth Century," ibid., 44 (1984): 301–308; idem, "Fluctuations in Mortality in the Last Half Century of the

Transatlantic Slave Trade," *Social Science History* 13 (1989): 315–340; Kenneth F. Kiple and Brian T. Higgins, "Mortality Caused by Dehydration during the Middle Passage," ibid., pp. 421–437.

42. Philip D. Morgan, *Slave Counterpoint: Black Culture in the Eighteenth-Century Chesapeake and Lowcountry* (Chapel Hill: University of North Carolina Press, 1998), pp. 444–445. See also Allan Kulikoff, "A 'Prolifick' People: Black Population Growth in the Chesapeake Colonies, 1700–1790," *Southern Studies* 16 (1977): 396–398.

43. Kiple and King, *Another Dimension to the Black Diaspora*, pp. 8–10.

44. Ibid., pp. 6–11; Todd L. Savitt, *Medicine and Slavery: The Diseases and Health Care of Blacks in Antebellum Virginia* (Urbana: University of Illinois Press, 1978), pp. 35–47; Nicholas S. Cardell and Mark H. Hopkins, "The Effect of Milk Intolerance on the Consumption of Milk by Slaves in 1860," *Journal of Interdisciplinary History* 8 (1978): 507–513.

45. Savitt, *Medicine and Slavery*, pp. 49–81. See also Jeffrey R. Young, "Ideology and Death on a Savannah River Rice Plantation, 1833–1867: Paternalism amidst 'a Good Supply of Disease and Pain,'" *Journal of Southern History* 59 (1993): 673–706; and the older account of William D. Postell, *The Health of Slaves on Southern Plantations* (Baton Rouge: Louisiana State University Press, 1951).

46. Savitt, *Medicine and Slavery*, pp. 83–109; Young, "Ideology and Death," pp. 689–691.

47. For a description of the southern diet see Sam B. Hilliard, *Hog Meat and Hoecake: Food Supply in the Old South, 1840–1860* (Carbondale: Southern Illinois University Press, 1972).

48. Kiple and King, *Another Dimension to the Black Diaspora*, pp. 96–116; Richard H. Steckel, "A Dreadful Childhood: The Excess Mortality of American Slaves," *Social Science History* 4 (1986): 427–465; idem, "A Peculiar Population: The Nutrition, Health, and Mortality of American Slaves from Childhood to Maturity," *Journal of Economic History* 46 (1986): 721–741; idem, "Birth Weights and Infant Mortality among American Slaves," *Explorations in Economic History* 23 (1986): 173–198; idem, "Slave Mortality: Analysis of Evidence from Plantation Records" and "Work, Disease, and Diet in the Health and Mortality of American Slaves," in *Without Consent or Contract: The Rise and Fall of American Slavery*, vol. 2: *Conditions of Slave Life and the Transition to Freedom: Technical Papers*, ed. Robert W. Fogel and Stanley L. Engerman (New York: W. W. Norton, 1992), pp. 393–412, 489–507; John Komlos, "Toward an Anthropometric History of African Americans: The Case of the Free Blacks in Antebellum Maryland," in Goldin and Rockoff, *Strategic Factors*, p. 299; John Campbell, "Work, Pregnancy, and Infant Mortality among Southern Slaves," *Journal of Interdisciplinary History* 14 (1984): 793–812.

49. Richard H. Steckel, "Slave Height Profiles from Coastwise Manifests," *Explorations in Economic History* 16 (1979): 363–380; Robert A. Margo and Richard H. Steckel, "The Height of American Slaves: New Evidence on Slave Nutrition and Health," *Social Science History* 6 (1982): 516–538; Richard H. Steckel, "Growth Depression and Recovery: The Remarkable Case of American Slaves," *Annals of Human Biology* 14 (1987): 111–132; Robert A. Margo and Richard H. Steckel, "The Nutrition and Health of Slaves and Antebellum Southern Whites," in Fogel and Engerman, *Without Consent or Contract,* 2: 508–521; Steckel, "A Peculiar Population," p. 733; Charles S. Sydnor, "Life Span of Mississippi Slaves," *American Historical Review* 35 (1930): 566–574; John Komlos, "On the Biological Standard of Living of African-Americans: The Case of the Civil War Soldiers," in *The Biological Standard of Living in Comparative Perspective,* ed. Komlos and Joerg Baten (Stuttgart: Franz Steiner Verlag, 1998), pp. 236–249.

50. Steckel, "A Peculiar Population," pp. 738–741. See also Doris H. Calloway, "Functional Consequences of Malnutrition," *Reviews of Infectious Diseases* 4 (1982): 736–745.

51. Mary C. Gillett, *The Army Medical Department, 1775–1818* (Washington, D.C.: Government Printing Office, 1981), pp. 136–138; idem, *The Army Medical Department, 1818–1865* (Washington, D.C.: Government Printing Office, 1987), pp. 43–44, 38–50, 87–93, 134–150.

52. James O. Breeden, "Health of Early Texas: The Military Frontier," *Southwestern Historical Quarterly* 80 (1977): 357–398. Detailed medical data can be found in the three volumes published between 1840 and 1860 titled *Statistical Report on the Sickness and Mortality in the Army of the United States* and found in the federal document series. Volume 1 covers 1819–1839, volume 2 1839–1855, and volume 3 1855–1860.

53. Donald R. Hickey, *The War of 1812: A Forgotten Conflict* (Urbana: University of Illinois Press, 1989), pp. 78–79, 302–303; J. C. A. Stagg, "Enlisted Men in the United States Army, 1812–1815: A Preliminary Survey," *William and Mary Quarterly* 43 (1986): 624.

54. Richard H. Coolidge, *Statistical Report on the Sickness and Mortality of the Army of the United States . . . 1839 to . . . 1855,* 34th Cong., 1st sess., *Senate Executive Document* 96 (Washington, D.C.: A. P. Nicholson, 1856), p. 606; George W. Smith and Charles Judah, eds., *Chronicles of the Gringos: The U.S. Army in the Mexican War, 1846–1848: Accounts of Eyewitnesses and Combatants* (Albuquerque: University of New Mexico Press, 1968), pp. 318–350 (quote from p. 323); Stanhope Bayne-Jones, *The Evolution of Preventive Medicine in the United States Army, 1607–1939* (Washington, D.C.: Office of the Surgeon General, Department of the Army, 1968), p. 86; Gillett, *Army Medical Department 1775–1818,* pp. 157–171, 190–195; idem, *Army Medical Department 1818–1865,* pp. 95–105, 116–125;

K. Jack Bauer, *The Mexican War, 1846–1848* (New York: Macmillan, 1974), p. 397.

55. Paul E. Steiner, *Disease in the Civil War: Natural Biological Warfare in 1861–1865* (Springfield, Ill.: Charles C. Thomas, 1968), pp. 3–5. Statistical data on disease in the Union forces during the Civil War can be found in the massive compilation prepared under the direction of Joseph K. Barnes, *The Medical and Surgical History of the War of the Rebellion (1861–65*, 6 vols. (Washington, D.C.: Government Printing Office, 1870–1888), 1: parts I–III. Confederate data can be found in Thomas L. Livermore, *Numbers and Losses in the Civil War in America, 1861–65* (Boston: Houghton Mifflin, 1901), pp. 2–8.

56. See Steiner, *Disease in the Civil War;* idem, *Medical History of a Civil War Regiment: Disease in the Sixty-Fifth United States Colored Infantry* (Clayton, Mo.: Institute for Civil War Studies, 1977); George W. Adams, *Doctors in Blue: The Medical History of the Union Army in the Civil War* (New York: Henry Schuman, 1952); H. H. Cunningham, *Doctors in Gray: The Confederate Medical Service* (Baton Rouge: Louisiana State University Press, 1958); Stewart Brooks, *Civil War Medicine* (Springfield, Ill.: Charles C. Thomas, 1966).

57. See Alfred J. Bollet, "Scurvy and Chronic Diarrhea in Civil War Troops: Were They Both Nutritional Deficiency Syndromes?" *Journal of the History of Medicine and Allied Sciences* 47 (1992): 49–67.

58. Barnes, *Medical and Surgical History,* 1, pt. 1: xxxvii–xliii, 636–641, 710–712; 1, pt. 3: 1–5; Bayne-Jones, *Evolution of Preventive Medicine,* pp. 98–99; Steiner, *Disease in the Civil War,* pp. 9–11; Louis C. Duncan, "The Comparative Mortality of Disease and Battle Casualties in the Historic Wars of the World," in *The Medical Department of the United States Army in the Civil War* (Washington, D.C.: n.p., n.d.), pp. 27–28.

59. Barnes, *Medical and Surgical History,* 1: pt. II, p. 8, pt. III, pp. 1–25.

60. *The Journals and Miscellaneous Notebooks of Ralph Waldo Emerson,* ed. William H. Gilman et al., 16 vols. (Cambridge: Harvard University Press, 1960–1982), 7: 403.

61. Pope, "Adult Mortality in America before 1900," pp. 279–283; Joseph P. Ferrie, *Yankeys Now: Immigrants in the Antebellum United States, 1840–1860* (New York: Oxford University Press, 1999), pp. 200–202.

62. Kenneth L. Sokoloff and Georgia C. Villaflor, "The Early Achievement of Modern Stature in America," *Social Science History* 6 (1982): 453–481; Robert A. Margo and Richard H. Steckel, "Heights of Native-Born Whites during the Antebellum Period," *Journal of Economic History* 43 (1983): 167–174; Robert W. Fogel, Stanley L. Engerman, and James Trussell, "Exploring the Uses of Data on Heights," *Social Science History* 6 (1982): 401–421; Robert W. Fogel et al., "Secular Changes in American and British Stat-

ure," *Journal of Interdisciplinary History* 14 (1983): 445–481; John Komlos, "The Height and Weight of West Point Cadets: Dietary Change in Antebellum America," *Journal of Economic History* 47 (1987): 897–927; Dora L. Costa, "Height, Wealth, and Disease among Native-born in the Rural, Antebellum North," *Social Science History* 17 (1993): 355–383; Richard H. Steckel, "Heights and Health in the United States, 1710–1950," in *Stature, Living Standards, and Economic Development: Essays in Anthropometric History,* ed. John Komlos (Chicago: University of Chicago Press, 1994), pp. 153–170; John Komlos, *The Biological Standard of Living on Three Continents: Further Explorations in Anthropometric History* (Boulder: Westview Press, 1995), pp. 133–150; Dora L. Costa and Richard H. Steckel, "Long-Term Trends in Health, Welfare, and Economic Growth in the United States," in *Health and Welfare during Industrialization,* ed. Steckel and Roderick Floud (Chicago: University of Chicago Press, 1997), pp. 59–60; John E. Murray, "Standards of the Present for People of the Past: Height, Weight, and Mortality among Men of Amherst College, 1834–1949," *Journal of Economic History* 57 (1997): 585–606; Timothy Cuff, "The Body Mass Index Values of Mid-Nineteenth-Century West Point Cadets: A Theoretical Application of Waaler's Curves to a Historical Population," *Historical Methods* 26 (1993): 171–182; idem, "Variation and Trends in the Stature of Pennsylvanians, 1820–1860," in Komlos and Baten, *Biological Standard of Living in Comparative Perspective,* pp. 208–235.

63. Costa, "Height, Wealth, and Disease," p. 358; Michael R. Haines, "Health, Height, Nutrition, and Mortality: Evidence on the 'Antebellum Puzzle' from Union Army Recruits for New York State and the United States," in Komlos and Baten, *Biological Standard of Living in Comparative Perspective,* pp. 155–180; Lee A. Craig and Thomas Weiss, "Nutritional Status and Agricultural Surpluses in the Antebellum United States," ibid., pp. 190–207.

64. Claudia Goldin and Robert A. Margo, "Wages, Prices, and Labor Markets before the Civil War," in Goldin and Rockoff, *Strategic Factors,* pp. 67–104; Costa and Steckel, "Long-Term Trends," pp. 48–50.

65. Costa and Steckel, "Long-Term Trends," pp. 65–67; Richard H. Steckel and Roderick Floud, "Conclusions," in Steckel and Floud, *Health and Welfare during Industrialization,* p. 435; Richard H. Steckel, "The Health and Mortality of Women and Children, 1850–1860," *Journal of Economic History* 48 (1988): 333–345.

66. Costa and Steckel, "Long-Term Trends," pp. 64–65; Nevin S. Scrimshaw, "Ecological Factors in Nutritional Disease," in *Chronic Disease and Public Health,* ed. Abraham M. Lilienfeld and Alice J. Gifford (Baltimore: Johns Hopkins Press, 1966), pp. 114–125. The latter work, however suggestive, must be used with caution because of the author's occasional tendency to shade data to support his thesis. See also Robert W. Fogel, "The Conquest of

High Mortality and Hunger in Europe and America: Timing and Mechanisms," in *Favorites of Fortune: Technology, Growth, and Economic Development since the Industrial Revolution,* ed. Patrice Higonnet, David S. Landes, and Henry Rosovsky (Cambridge: Harvard University Press, 1991), pp. 33–71; Roderick Floud, "Anthropometric Measures of Nutritional Status in Industrialized Societies: Europe and North America since 1750," in *Nutrition and Poverty,* ed. S. R. Osmani (New York: Oxford University Press, 1992), pp. 219–241; Richard H. Steckel and Donald R. Haurin, "Health and Nutrition in the American Midwest: Evidence from the Height of Ohio National Guardsmen, 1850–1910," and Steckel, "Heights and Health in the United States, 1710–1950," pp. 117–128, 153–170; Massimo Livi-Bacci, *Population and Nutrition: An Essay on European Demographic History* (New York: Cambridge University Press, 1990); Roderick Floud, Kenneth Wachter, and Annabel Gregory, *Height, Health, and History: Nutritional Status in the United Kingdom, 1750–1980* (New York: Cambridge University Press, 1990).

In recent years David Parker and his followers have argued that undernutrition *in utero* and infancy plays a key role in adult health. See David J. P. Parker, ed., *Fetal and Infant Origins of Adult Disease* (London: British Medical Journal, 1992) and *Fetal Origins of Cardiovascular and Lung Disease* (New York: M. Dekker, 2001).

7. THREATS OF INDUSTRY

1. Benjamin W. McCready, *On the Influence of Trades, Professions, and Occupations in the United States, in the Production of Disease* (1837; reprint, Baltimore: Johns Hopkins Press, 1943), p. 117.
2. Bernardino Ramazzini, *Diseases of Workers,* translation of Latin text of 1713 *De Morbis Artificum* by Wilmer C. Wright (New York: Hafner, 1964).
3. Henry E. Sigerist, "Historical Background of Industrial and Occupational Diseases," *Bulletin of the New York Academy of Medicine* 12 (1936): 597–609; Charles Turner Thackrah, *The Effects of Arts, Trades, and Professions, and of Civic Service and Habits of Living, on Health and Longevity,* 2d ed. (London: Longman, 1832), pp. 4–5. The first and much shorter edition of Thackrah's work appeared in 1831. The second edition was reprinted in A. Meiklejohn, *The Life, Work and Times of Charles Turner Thackrah, Surgeon and Apothecary of Leeds (1795–1833)* (Edinburgh: E. & S. Livingstone, 1957).
4. A full discussion can be found in Robert Straus, *Medical Care for Seamen: The Origin of Public Medical Service in the United States* (New Haven: Yale University Press, 1950).
5. Richard Wedeen, *Poison in the Pot: The Legacy of Lead* (Carbondale:

Southern Illinois University Press, 1984); Jacqueline K. Corn, "Historical Perspective to a Current Controversy on the Clinical Spectrum of Plumbism," *Milbank Memorial Fund Quarterly* 53 (1975): 93–114; George Rosen, *A History of Public Health,* enl. ed. (Baltimore: Johns Hopkins University Press, 1993), p. 250.

6. McCready, *On the Influence of Trades,* pp. 61–62, 88–91.
7. Ibid., pp. 33–37.
8. Ibid., pp. 39, 46–65.
9. Ibid., pp. 67–117.
10. Ibid., pp. 117–120, 123–124.
11. Ibid., pp. 117–118, 124–129.
12. For a lengthy treatment of McCready, see Craig Donegan, "For the Good of Us All: Early Attitudes toward Occupational Health with Emphasis on the Northern United States from 1787 to 1870" (Ph.D. diss., University of Maryland, 1984), pp. 128–158.
13. Bruce Laurie, *Working People of Philadelphia, 1800–1850* (Philadelphia: Temple University Press, 1980), pp. 3–30.
14. Michael Chevalier, *Society, Manners, and Politics in the United States: Being a Series of Letters on North America* (Boston: Weeks, Jordan, 1839), pp. 125–144; Charles Dickens, *American Notes and Pictures from Italy* (1842; reprint, London: Oxford University Press, 1957), pp. 62–70. For a full description of the medical aspects of factory work see George Rosen, "The Medical Aspects of the Controversy over Factory Conditions in New England, 1840–1850," *Bulletin of the History of Medicine* 15 (1944): 483–497.
15. John R. Commons et al., *History of Labour in the United States,* 4 vols. (New York: Macmillan, 1918–1935), 1: 319–320, 428–429.
16. Josiah Quincy, "Public Hygiene of Massachusetts; but More Particularly of the Cities of Boston and Lowell," *American Medical Association Transactions* 2 (1849): 510, 513.
17. Ibid., pp. 514–519; Jacqueline K. Corn, *Response to Occupational Health Hazards: A Historical Perspective* (New York: Van Nostrand Reinhold, 1992), pp. 152–154.
18. Quincy, "Public Hygiene of Massachusetts", pp. 514–519; Corn, *Response to Occupational Health Hazards,* p. 148. See also Mark Aldrich, "Mortality from Byssinosis among New England Cotton Mill Workers, 1905–1912," *Journal of Occupational Medicine* 24 (1982): 977–980.
19. Martin V. Melosi, *Coping with Abundance: Energy and Environment in Industrial America* (Philadelphia: Temple University Press, 1985), pp. 17–23.
20. Ibid., pp. 26–32; Jacqueline K. Corn, *Environment and Health in Nineteenth-Century America: Two Case Studies* (New York: Peter Lang, 1989), pp. 16–17; U.S. Bureau of the Census, *Historical Statistics of the United*

States: Colonial Times to 1970, 2 vols. (Washington, D.C.: Government Printing Office, 1975), 1: 590–593.

21. See George Rosen, *The History of Miners' Diseases: A Medical and Social Interpretation* (New York: Schuman's, 1943).

22. For an illuminating discussion of mining technology see Anthony F. C. Wallace, *St. Clair: A Nineteenth-Century Coal Town's Experience with a Disaster-Prone Industry* (New York: Alfred A. Knopf, 1987).

23. Rosen, *History of Miners' Diseases*, pp. 200–201.

24. Alan Derickson, *Black Lung: Anatomy of a Public Health Disaster* (Ithaca: Cornell University Press, 1998), pp. 4–63; idem, "The United Mine Workers of America and the Recognition of Occupational Respiratory Diseases, 1902–1968," *American Journal of Public Health* 81 (1991): 782–790. See also Barbara E. Smith, *Digging Our Own Graves: Coal Miners and the Struggle over Black Lung Disease* (Philadelphia: Temple University Press, 1987); and Daniel M. Fox and Judith F. Stone, "Black Lung: Miners' Militancy and Medical Uncertainty, 1968–1972," *Bulletin of the History of Medicine* 54 (1980): 43–63.

25. Derickson, *Black Lung*, p. 27; Rosen, *History of Miners' Diseases*, pp. 213–225, 240–241.

26. Frederick L. Hoffman, *Mortality from Respiratory Diseases in Dusty Trades (Inorganic Dusts)*, U.S. Bureau of Labor Statistics Bulletin 231 (Washington, D.C.: Government Printing Office, 1918), pp. 323, 398, 403, 409, 443.

    The prevalence of CWP is unknown; estimates vary in the extreme. In 1969 the U.S. surgeon general estimated that 100,000 coal miners had CWP; four years later 150,000 miners received federal compensation benefits for total disability from the disease. Epidemiological estimates range from 10 to 30 percent of the workforce. Prevalence rates may vary over time, depending on the age of the workforce and length of time worked as well as dust levels. Whatever the actual numbers, there is no doubt that coal mining was one of the most dangerous occupations in the late nineteenth and early twentieth centuries. See Smith, *Digging Our Own Graves*, pp. 145–147.

27. Hoffman, *Mortality from Respiratory Diseases*, pp. 12–42.

28. Ibid., pp. 426–432. See also David Rosner and Gerald Markowitz, *Deadly Dust: Silicosis and the Politics of Occupational Disease in Twentieth-Century America* (Princeton: Princeton University Press, 1991).

29. Edward H. Beardsley, *A History of Neglect: Health Care for Blacks and Mill Workers in the Twentieth-Century South* (Knoxville: University of Tennessee Press, 1987), pp. 62–65; Carl Gersuny, *Work Hazards and Industrial Conflict* (Hanover, N.H.: University Press of New England, 1981), pp. 20–25, 36–37; Aldrich, "Mortality from Byssinosis," pp. 977–980.

30. Wallace, *St. Clair*, pp. 249–258.

31. Ibid., pp. 253, 258.
32. Ibid., pp. 296–302; Daniel J. Curran, *Dead Laws for Dead Men: The Politics of Federal Coal Mine Health and Safety Reform* (Lexington: University Press of Kentucky, 1976), pp. 2–3.
33. William Graebner, *Coal-Mining Safety in the Progressive Period: The Political Economy of Reform* (Lexington: University Press of Kentucky, 1976), pp. 2–3.
34. Curran, *Dead Laws for Dead Men,* pp. 50–52. See also Alan Derickson, *Workers' Health Workers' Democracy: The Western Miners' Struggle, 1891–1925* (Ithaca: Cornell University Press, 1988); James Whiteside, *Regulating Danger: The Struggle for Mine Safety in the Rocky Mountain Coal Industry* (Lincoln: University of Nebraska Press, 1990); and Price V. Fishback, "Workplace Safety during the Progressive Era: Fatal Accidents in Bituminous Coal Mining, 1912–1923," *Explorations in Economic History* 23 (1986): 269–298.
35. U.S. Bureau of the Census, *Historical Statistics,* 2: 731, 765.
36. Walter Licht, *Working for the Railroad: The Organization of Work in the Nineteenth Century* (Princeton: Princeton University Press, 1983), pp. 181–188. See also Robert B. Shaw, *A History of Railroad Accidents, Safety Precautions and Operating Practices* (n.p.: Vail-Ballou Press, 1978).
37. Licht, *Working for the Railroad,* pp. 190–197; U. S. Bureau of the Census, *Historical Statistics,* 2: 739–740.
38. Ethelbert Stewart, "Industrial Accidents in the United States," *Annals of the American Academy of Political and Social Science* 123 (1926): 1–3.
39. U.S. Bureau of the Census, *Historical Statistics,* 1: 604; Hoffman, *Mortality from Respiratory Diseases,* pp. 274–278, 354–366; Christopher C. Sellers, *Hazards of the Job: From Industrial Disease to Environmental Health Science* (Chapel Hill: University of North Carolina Press, 1997), pp. 15–17; Christian Warren, *Brush with Death: A Social History of Lead Poisoning* (Baltimore: Johns Hopkins University Press, 2000), pp. 13–26.
40. George Rosen, "Urbanization, Occupation and Disease in the United States, 1870–1920: The Case of New York City," *Journal of the History of Medicine and Allied Sciences* 43 (1988): 396–397.
41. Alice Hamilton to Mr. Foster, May 22, 1911, in Barbara Sicherman, *Alice Hamilton: A Life in Letters* (Cambridge: Harvard University Press, 1984), pp. 159–161. See also Hamilton's *Exploring the Dangerous Trades: The Autobiography of Alice Hamilton* (Boston: Little, Brown, 1943); and the discussion in Sellers, *Hazards of the Job,* pp. 69–106.
42. U.S. Bureau of the Census, *Historical Statistics,* 1: 138; Sellers, *Hazards of the Job,* pp. 16–18.
43. Helen E. Sheehan and Richard P. Wedeen, "Hatters' Shakes," in *Toxic Cir-*

cles: Environmental Hazards from the Workplace into the Community, ed. Sheehan and Wedeen (New Brunswick: Rutgers University Press, 1993), pp. 26–54.

44. Keith Wailoo, *Drawing Blood: Technology and Disease Identity in Twentieth-Century America* (Baltimore: Johns Hopkins University Press, 1997), pp. 88–96.

45. Rosen, "Urbanization, Occupation and Disease," pp. 394–395.

46. Jacob A. Riis, *The Battle with the Slum* (New York: Macmillan, 1902), pp. 102–103; idem, *How the Other Half Lives: Studies among the Tenements of New York* (1890; reprint, New York: Sagamore Press, 1957), pp. 77–78. See also Deborah Dwork, "Health Conditions of Immigrant Jews on the Lower East Side of New York: 1880–1914," *Medical History* 25 (1981): 1–40.

47. Rosen, "Urbanization, Occupation and Disease," pp. 398–400; Riis, *How the Other Half Lives,* p. 103.

48. Dwork, "Health Conditions of Immigrant Jews," p. 3.

49. Riis, *How the Other Half Lives,* pp. 91–92; *Medical Record,* March 7, 1908, quoted in Rosen, "Urbanization, Occupation and Disease," p. 415.

50. Dwork, "Health Conditions of Immigrant Jews," pp. 20–27

51. Rosen, "Urbanization, Occupation and Disease," pp. 414, 417.

52. Sellers, *Hazards of the Job,* pp. 21–43.

53. Rosner, *Deadly Dust,* pp. 15–22; Ludwig Teleky, *History of Factory and Mine Legislation* (New York: Columbia University Press, 1948), pp. 199–200 (quote).

54. See Barbara G. Rosenkrantz, *Public Health and the State: Changing Views in Massachusetts, 1842–1936* (Cambridge: Harvard University Press, 1972); and Nancy Tomes, *The Gospel of Germs: Men, Women, and the Microbe in American Life* (Cambridge: Harvard University Press, 1998).

55. Paul Uselding, "In Dispraise of the Muckrakers: United States Occupational Mortality, 1890–1910," *Research in Economic History* 1 (1976): 334–371.

56. Ibid., pp. 348–351.

8. STOPPING THE SPREAD OF INFECTION

1. Florence Kelley, "Children in the Cities," *National Municipal Review* 4 (1915): 199, quoted in Nancy S. Dye and Daniel B. Smith, "Mother Love and Infant Death, 1750–1920," *Journal of American History* 75 (1986): 347. See also Lillian D. Wald, *The House on Henry Street* (New York: Henry Holt, 1915).

2. U.S. Bureau of the Census, *Statistical Abstract of the United States: 1996* (Washington, D.C.: Government Printing Office, 1996), pp. 14–16.

3. See Charles E. Rosenberg, *The Cholera Years: The United States in 1832,*

1849, and 1866 (Chicago: University of Chicago Press, 1962); and Howard Markel, *Quarantine! East European Jewish Immigrants and the New York City Epidemics of 1892* (Baltimore: Johns Hopkins University Press, 1997).

4. A. J. Mercer, "Smallpox and Epidemiological-Demographic Change in Europe: The Role of Vaccination," *Population Studies* 39 (1985): 287–307.

5. Gretchen A. Condran, "Changing Patterns of Epidemic Disease in New York City," in *Hives of Sickness: Public Health and Epidemics in New York City,* ed. David Rosner (New Brunswick: Rutgers University Press, 1995), p. 31; William T. Howard, *Public Health Administration and the Natural History of Disease in Baltimore, Maryland, 1797–1920* (Washington, D.C.: Carnegie Institution of Washington, 1924), pp. 277–291; Judith W. Leavitt, *The Healthiest City: Milwaukee and the Politics of Health Reform* (Princeton: Princeton University Press, 1982), p. 29; John Duffy, ed., *The Rudolph Matas History of Medicine in Louisiana,* 2 vols. (Baton Rouge: Louisiana State University Press, 1958–1962), 2: 438–443; Donald R. Hopkins, *Princes and Peasants: Smallpox in History* (Chicago: University of Chicago Press, 1983), p. 287; Mercer, "Smallpox and Epidemiological-Demographic Change," pp. 302–307.

6. Judith W. Leavitt, "Be Safe. Be Sure: New York City's Experience with Epidemic Smallpox," in Rosner, *Hives of Sickness,* pp. 104–110; Hopkins, *Princes and Peasants,* p. 282; Duffy, *Rudolph Matas History,* 2: 441.

7. Charles V. Chapin, "Changes in Type of Contagious Disease with Special Reference to Smallpox and Scarlet Fever," *Journal of Preventive Medicine* 1 (1926): 1–29; Cyril W. Dixon, *Smallpox* (London: J. & A. Churchill, 1962), pp. 204–205; Frank Fenner et al., *Smallpox and Its Eradication* (Geneva: World Health Organization, 1988), pp. 327–332; Anne Hardy, *The Epidemic Streets: Infectious Disease and the Rise of Preventive Medicine, 1856–1900* (New York: Oxford University Press, 1993), pp. 114–115.

8. K. David Patterson, "Yellow Fever Epidemics and Mortality in the United States, 1693–1905," *Social Science and Medicine* 34 (1992): 857–858.

9. Margaret Humphreys, *Yellow Fever and the South* (New Brunswick: Rutgers University Press, 1992), p. 60.

10. Patterson, "Yellow Fever Epidemics," p. 858.

11. The discussion of yellow fever is based on Humphreys, *Yellow Fever and the South;* John H. Ellis, *Yellow Fever and Public Health in the New South* (Lexington: University Press of Kentucky, 1992); Khaled J. Bloom, *The Mississippi Valley's Great Yellow Fever Epidemic of 1878* (Baton Rouge: Louisiana State University Press, 1993); Jo Ann Carrigan, *The Saffron Scourge: A History of Yellow Fever in Louisiana, 1796–1905* (Lafayette: Center for Louisiana Studies, 1994); and Francois Delaporte, *The History of Yellow Fever: An Essay on the Birth of Tropical Medicine* (Cambridge: MIT Press, 1991).

12. Ernest C. Faust, "Malaria Mortality in the Southern United States for the Year 1937," *American Journal of Tropical Medicine* 19 (1939): 447–455; idem, "The Distribution of Malaria in North America, Mexico, Central America and the West Indies," in American Association for the Advancement of Science, *A Symposium on Human Malaria with Special Reference to North America and the Caribbean Region* (Washington, D.C., 1941), pp. 8–18; idem, "Clinical and Public Health Aspects of Malaria in the United States from an Historical Perspective," *American Journal of Tropical Medicine* 25 (1945): 185–201; idem, "The History of Malaria in the United States," *American Scientist* 39 (1951): 121–130.

13. Margaret Humphreys, *Malaria: Poverty, Race, and Public Health in the United States* (Baltimore: Johns Hopkins University Press, 2001), pp. 51–55. See also James R. Young, "Malaria in the South, 1900–1950" (Ph.D. diss., University of North Carolina, 1972).

14. Faust, "Clinical and Public Health Aspects of Malaria," p. 190.

15. Humphreys, *Malaria*, pp. 110–112. On the basis of some recent findings, Humphreys (p. 12) suggests that the weather patterns generated by El Niño might have played a role in malarial cycles (although she concedes that such a connection has yet to be proven). See also Jack T. Kirby, *Rural Worlds Lost: The American South, 1920–1960* (Baton Rouge: Louisiana State University Press, 1987).

    Oddly enough, the federal government launched an intensive antimalarial campaign after the disease had become virtually extinct in the South. In 1942 it created the Malaria Control in War Areas (MCWA) agency within the Public Health Service. Its alleged success led to larger appropriations, and in 1945 it was renamed as the Communicable Disease Center and eventually became the contemporary Centers for Disease Control (CDC). See Margaret Humphreys, "Kicking a Dying Dog: DDT and the Demise of Malaria in the American South, 1942–1950," *Isis* 87 (1996): 1–17.

16. For a brief discussion see Robert F. Breiman, "Impact of Technology on the Emergence of Infectious Diseases," *Epidemiologic Reviews* 18 (1996): 4–9.

17. U.S. Bureau of the Census, *Historical Statistics of the United States: Colonial Times to 1970*, 2 vols. (Washington, D.C.: Government Printing Office, 1975), 1: 11; Joel A. Tarr, *The Search for the Ultimate Sink: Urban Pollution in Historical Perspective* (Akron: University of Akron Press, 1996), pp. 43–44.

18. See especially Martin V. Melosi, *The Sanitary City: Urban Infrastructure in America from Colonial Times to the Present* (Baltimore: Johns Hopkins University Press, 2000).

19. Quoted in Alan D. Anderson, *The Origin and Resolution of an Urban Crisis: Baltimore, 1890–1930* (Baltimore: Johns Hopkins University Press, 1977), p. 66.

20. Tarr, *Search for the Ultimate Sink*, pp. 111–190.

21. Ibid., p. 188; Howard, *Public Health Administration,* pp. 260–265; Louis I. Dublin, Alfred J. Lotka, and Mortimer Spiegelman, *Length of Life: A Study of the Life Table,* rev. ed. (New York: Ronald Press, 1949), pp. 158–159; Robert Higgs and David Booth, "Mortality Differentials within Large American Cities in 1890," *Human Ecology* 7 (1979): 353–370; Melosi, *Sanitary City,* p. 138.

    Quantitative data on typhoid fever are unavailable before the 1870s, largely because of the confusion with other infectious diseases. The typhoid bacillus was not identified until 1880, although medical thinkers had begun to differentiate typhoid from other fevers during the previous three decades.

22. Tarr, *Search for the Ultimate Sink,* p. 356.

23. Ibid., pp. 179–217. See also Robert V. Wells, *Facing the "King of Terrors": Death and Society in an American Community, 1750–1900* (New York: Cambridge University Press, 2000), p. 180.

24. John R. Paul, "Historical and Geographical Aspects of the Epidemiology of Poliomyelitis," *Yale Journal of Biology and Medicine* 27 (1954): 101–113.

25. Much of my discussion of polio is based on John R. Paul, *A History of Poliomyelitis* (New Haven: Yale University Press, 1971).

26. This and the previous paragraph are based on C. Lavinder, A. W. Freeman, and W. H. Frost, *Epidemiologic Studies of Poliomyelitis in New York City and the North-Eastern United States during the Year 1916, Public Health Bulletin* 91 (Washington, D.C.: Government Printing Office, 1918), p. 109; Robert E. Serfling and Ida L. Sherman, "Poliomyelitis Distribution in the United States," *Public Health Reports* 68 (1953): 453–466; John R. Paul, "The Peripheral Spread of Poliomyelitis through Rural and Urban Areas: Observations from a Recent Epidemic," *Yale Journal of Biology and Medicine* 19 (1947): 521–536. See also Paul, "A Review of Recent Studies on the Epidemiology of Poliomyelitis in the United States," ibid., 10 (1938): 577–590; Herbert A. Wenner, "An Ecologic Study of Poliomyelitis in Connecticut," ibid., 15 (1943): 707–722; idem, "Poliomyelitis in Alabama: Epidemiological Considerations," ibid., 18 (1946): 281–306; idem, "Comparative Statistical Studies of Epidemics of Poliomyelitis in and about the City of New Haven, 1916–1943," ibid., 19 (1947): 331–343; Julien I. Pichel, "The Age Incidence of Poliomyelitis in Connecticut, 1921–1947," ibid., 22 (1950): 327–340; Alexander G. Gilliam, "Changes in Age Selection of Fatal Poliomyelitis," *Public Health Reports* 63 (1948): 1334–39; and W. J. Hall, N. Nathanson, and A. D. Langmuir, "The Age Distribution of Poliomyelitis in the United States in 1955," *American Journal of Hygiene* 66 (1957): 214–234.

27. Tony Gould, *A Summer Plague: Polio and Its Survivors* (New Haven: Yale University Press, 1995), p. 6. See also Naomi Rogers, *Dirt and Disease: Polio before FDR* (New Brunswick, N.J.: Rutgers University Press, 1992).

28. Lavinder, Freeman, and Frost, *Epidemiologic Studies,* p. 214. See also New

York City Department of Health, *A Monograph on the Epidemic of Polio-myelitis in New York City in 1916* (New York: Department of Health, 1917), which was largely the work of Haven Emerson.

29. John R. Paul, "Poliomyelitis Attack Rates in American Troops (1940–1948)," *American Journal of Hygiene* 50 (1949): 57–62.

30. Carl L. Erhardt and Joyce E. Berlin, eds., *Mortality and Morbidity in the United States* (Cambridge: Harvard University Press, 1974), pp. 24–26. More complete data can be found in Forrest E. Linder and Robert D. Grove, *Vital Statistics Rates in the United States, 1900–1940* (Washington, D.C.: Government Printing Office, 1940).

31. Richard A. Meckel, *Save the Babies: American Public Health Reform and the Prevention of Infant Mortality, 1850–1929* (Baltimore: Johns Hopkins University Press, 1990), p. 29; U. S. Bureau of the Census, *Historical Statistics,* 1: 58. For a community study of Schenectady, New York, see Wells, *Facing the "King of Terrors,"* pp. 172–178.

32. Erhardt and Berlin, *Mortality and Morbidity,* pp. 4–5.

    In 1900 the Death Registration Area included only Maine, New Hampshire, Vermont, Massachusetts, New York, New Jersey, Indiana, Michigan, and the District of Columbia and covered only about a quarter of the population; complete national coverage took several more decades. Data from 1900 are therefore biased because urban areas were overrepresented and rural areas underrepresented. As a result, the differentials between the white and nonwhite (largely African-American) population were overstated; urban African Americans probably had higher death rates than their rural brethren in the South (where the majority lived).

33. Samuel H. Preston and Michael R. Haines, *Fatal Years: Child Mortality in Late Nineteenth-Century America* (Princeton: Princeton University Press, 1991), pp. 3–6.

34. Ibid., pp. 186–187, 209.

35. See ibid., pp. 3–48; and Nancy Tomes, *The Gospel of Germs: Men, Women, and the Microbe in American Life* (Cambridge: Harvard University Press, 1998).

36. The discussion of the Spanish-American War is based on Vincent J. Cirillo, "The Spanish-American War and Military Medicine" (Ph.D. diss., Rutgers University, 1999), chaps. 1–2; and Mary C. Gillett, *The Army Medical Department, 1865–1917* (Washington, D.C.: Government Printing Office, 1995), pp. 148–155, 173–199.

    The devastating nature of epidemics in military camps led to the appointment of a Typhoid Board headed by Walter Reed and including two others. Their report at the beginning of 1899 emphasized that polluted water played only a minor role in the epidemic. More important was the movement of flies from latrines to kitchens, which contaminated the food supply, as well as person-to-person transmission from infected to healthy persons by hand contact. Reed also recognized the role of the typhoid carrier–an individual who acted as a host for the bacillus but did not develop the disease. Walter Reed, Victor C. Vaughan, and E. O. Shakespeare, "Preliminary Report on Typhoid Fever in Military Camps of the United States, 1898" (January 25, 1899), reprinted in *Army Medical Bulletin* 53 (1940): 73–102.

37. This discussion is based upon John Ettling, *The Germ of Laziness: Rockefeller Philanthropy and Public Health in the New South* (Cambridge: Harvard University Press, 1981). See also Stephen J. Kunitz, "Hookworm and Pellagra: Exemplary Diseases in the New South," *Journal of Health and Social Behavior* 29 (1988): 139–148.

38. See Henry F. Dowling, *Fighting Infection: Conquests of the Twentieth Century* (Cambridge: Harvard University Press, 1977), pp. 82–104; and Allan M. Brandt, *No Magic Bullet: A Social History of Venereal Disease in the United States since 1880,* enl. ed. (New York: Oxford University Press, 1987).

39. Lawrence R. Murphy, "The Enemy among Us: Venereal Disease among Union Soldiers in the Far West, 1861–1865," *Civil War History* 31 (1985): 257–269; Brandt, *No Magic Bullet,* pp. 12–13; Gerald N. Grob, *Mental Illness and American Society, 1875–1940* (Princeton: Princeton University Press, 1983), pp. 188–189. See also James F. Donohue and Quentin R. Remein, "Long-Term Trend and Economic Factors of Paresis in the United States," *Public Health Reports* 69 (1954): 758–765.

40. E. E. Southard and H. C. Solomon, *Neurosyphilis: Modern Systematic Diagnosis and Treatment Presented in One Hundred and Thirty-Seven Case Histories* (Boston: W. M. Leonard, 1917), pp. 133–134.

41. Metropolitan Life Insurance data are illustrative. See Louis I. Dublin and Alfred J. Lotka, *Twenty-five Years of Health Progress: A Study of the Experience among the Industrial Policyholders of the Metropolitan Life Insurance Company, 1911 to 1935* (New York: Metropolitan Life Insurance Company, 1937).

42. The discussion of pellagra is based upon Milton Terris, ed., *Goldberger on Pellagra* (Baton Rouge: Louisiana State University Press, 1964); Richard V. Kasius, ed., *The Challenge of Facts: Selected Public Health Papers of Edgar Sydenstricker* (New York: Prodist, 1974); Elmer V. McCollum, *A History of Nutrition: The Sequence of Ideas in Nutrition Investigations* (Boston: Houghton Mifflin, 1957), pp. 302–318; and especially Elizabeth W. Etheridge, *The Butterfly Caste: A Social History of Pellagra in the South* (Westport, Conn.: Greenwood, 1972). The quote is from Goldberger's "Pellagra: Its Nature and Prevention," *Public Health Reports* 42 (1927): 2193–2200.

43. Etheridge, *Butterfly Caste,* pp. 206–217.

44. Selwyn D. Collins, Katherine S. Trantham, and Josephine L. Lehmann, "Illness and Mortality among Infants during the First Year of Life," *Public Health Monograph* No. 31 (Washington, D.C.: Government Printing Office, 1955), pp. 1–4, 19; Linder and Grove, *Vital Statistics Rates,* p. 161; U.S. Bureau of the Census, *Historical Statistics,* 1: 56; Samuel H. Preston, Douglas Ewbank, and Mark Hereward, "Child Mortality Differences by Ethnicity and Race in the United States, 1900–1910," in *After Ellis Island: Newcomers and Natives in the 1910 Census,* ed. Susan C. Watkins (New York: Russell Sage Foundation, 1994), pp. 41–47.

45. See Louis I. Dublin and Alfred J. Lotka, "The History of Longevity in the United States," *Human Biology* 6 (1934): 43–86; and Albert J. Mayer, "Life Expectancy in the City of Chicago, 1880–1950," ibid., 27 (1955): 202–210.

46. The literature on the epidemiological or health transition is enormous. For a very small sampling of a very large literature see Thomas McKeown, *The Role of Medicine: Dream, Mirage, or Nemesis?* (Princeton: Princeton University Press, 1979); Abdel R. Omran, "The Epidemiologic Transition: A Theory of the Epidemiology of Population Change," *Milbank Memorial Fund Quarterly* 49 (1971): 509–538; idem, "A Century of Epidemiologic Transition in the United States," *Preventive Medicine* 6 (1977): 30–51; idem, "The Epidemiologic Transition Theory: A Preliminary Update," *Journal of Tropical Pediatrics* 29 (1983): 305–316; David Coleman and Roger Schofield, eds., *The State of Population Theory: Forward from Malthus* (Oxford: Basil Blackwell, 1986); John Landers, ed., "Historical Epidemiology and the Health Transition," *Health Transition Review,* suppl. to vol. 2 (1992); Robert W. Fogel, *Nutrition and the Decline in Mortality since 1700: Some Preliminary Findings,* National Bureau of Economic Research Working Paper No. 1402 (Washington, D.C., 1984); idem, "Economic Growth, Population Theory, and Physiology: The Bearing of Long-Term Processes on the Making of Economic Policy," *American Economic Review* 84 (1994): 369–395; Alex Mercer, *Mortality and Population in Transition: Epidemiological-Demographic Change in England since the Eighteenth Century as Part of a Global Phenomenon* (Leicester: Leicester University Press, 1990); Patrice Higonnet, David S. Landes, and Henry Rosovsky, eds., *Favorites of Fortune: Technology, Growth, and Economic Development since the Industrial Revolution* (Cambridge: Harvard University Press, 1991); Richard H. Steckel and Roderick Floud, eds., *Health and Welfare during Industrialization* (Chicago: University of Chicago Press, 1997); S. Ryan Johansson, "Food for Thought: Rhetoric and Reality in Modern Mortality History," *Historical Methods* 27 (1994): 101–125. For a comprehensive global survey that examines the manner in which health risks were reduced, see James C. Riley, *Rising Life Expectancy: A Global History* (New York: Cambridge University Press, 2001).

47. Paul B. Beeson, "Changes in Medical Therapy during the Past Half Cen-

tury," *Medicine* 59 (1980): 79–85; John B. McKinlay and Sonja M. McKin-
lay, "The Questionable Contribution of Medical Measures to the Decline of
Mortality in the United States in the Twentieth Century," *Milbank Memorial
Fund Quarterly* 55 (1977): 405–428.

48. See Simon Szreter, "The McKeown Thesis," *Journal of Health Services Research and Policy* 5 (2000): 119–121.

49. Gretchen A. Condran and Rose A. Cheyney, "Mortality Trends in Philadelphia: Age- and Cause-Specific Death Rates, 1870–1930," *Demography* 19
(1982): 103; Eileen M. Crimmins and Gretchen A. Condran, "Mortality
Variation in U.S. Cities in 1900," *Social Science History* 7 (1983): 36;
Meckel, *Save the Babies*, pp. 37, 95; Robert M. Woodbury, *Infant Mortality
and Its Causes* (Baltimore: Williams & Wilkins, 1926), pp. 39, 75–101.

50. Condran and Cheyney, "Mortality Trends in Philadelphia," p. 103;
Gretchen A. Condran, Henry Williams, and Rose A. Cheyney, "The Decline
of Mortality in Philadelphia from 1870 to 1930: The Role of Municipal Services," *Pennsylvania Magazine of History and Biography* 108 (1984): 159–
161. See the data in Linder and Grove, *Vital Statistics Rates;* and Sam
Shapiro, Edward R. Schlesinger, and Robert E. L. Nesbitt Jr., *Infant,
Perinatal, Maternal, and Childhood Mortality in the United States* (Cambridge: Harvard University Press, 1968).

51. L. Emmett Holt, *The Diseases of Infancy and Childhood* (New York:
D. Appleton, 1897), p. 41; Meckel, *Save the Babies,* p. 61.

52. Jane E. Sewell, *Medicine in Maryland: The Practice and Profession, 1799–
1999* (Baltimore: Johns Hopkins University Press, 1999), p. 140.

53. The generalizations in this and the previous paragraphs are based on Preston
and Haines, *Fatal Years;* Gretcen A. Condran and Michael R. Haines,
"Child Mortality Differences, Personal Health Care Practices, and Medical
Technology: The United States, 1900–1930," in *Health and Change in Inter-
national Perspective,* ed. Lincoln C. Chen, Arthur Kleinman, and Norma C.
Ware (Boston: Harvard School of Public Health, 1993), pp. 171–224;
Woodbury, *Infant Mortality;* Preston, Ewbank, and Hereward, "Child Mor-
tality Differences," pp. 35–82; Meckel, *Save the Babies;* Wells, *Facing the
"King of Terrors,"* p. 181; Rima D. Apple, *Mothers and Medicine: A Social
History of Infant Feeding, 1890–1950* (Madison: University of Wisconsin
Press, 1987), chaps. 1–2.

54. Woodbury, *Infant Mortality,* pp. 107–122; Preston, Ewbank, and Hereward,
"Child Mortality Differences," pp. 64–69; Condran and Preston, "Child
Mortality Differences," pp. 173–177; Maurice Fishberg, *The Jews: A Study
of Race and Environment* (New York: Charles Scribner's Sons, 1911),
pp. 255–269; Gretchen A. Condran and Ellen A. Kramarow, "Child Mortality among Jewish Immigrants to the United States," *Journal of Interdisciplinary History* 22 (1991): 223–254.

55. Shapiro, Schlesinger, and Nesbitt, *Infant, Perinatal, Maternal, and Child-*

hood Mortality, pp. 336–339; Linder and Grove, *Vital Statistics Rates,* pp. 210, 216, 222, 228, 238.

56. Arthur Newsholme, *Epidemic Diphtheria: A Research on the Origin and Spread of the Disease from an International Standpoint* (London: Swann Sonnenschein, 1898), pp. 9–22; Howard, *Public Health Administration,* p. 344; Haven Emerson and Harriet E. Hughes, *Population, Births, Notifiable Diseases, and Deaths, Assembled for New York City, New York, 1866–1938, from Official Records* (New York: DeLamar Institute of Public Health, Columbia University, 1941), unpaginated; Condran and Cheney, "Mortality Trends in Philadelphia," pp. 102–111.

57. See Peter C. English, "Diphtheria and Theories of Infectious Disease: Centennial Appreciation of the Critical Role of Diphtheria in the History of Medicine," *Pediatrics* 76 (1985): 1–9; and Evelynn M. Hammonds, *Childhood's Deadly Scourge: The Campaign to Control Diphtheria in New York City, 1880–1930* (Baltimore: Johns Hopkins University Press, 1999).

58. Selwyn D. Collins, "Diphtheria Incidence and Trends in Relation to Artificial Immunization, with some Comparative Data for Scarlet Fever," *Public Health Reports* 61 (1946): 203–240; Elizabeth Fee and Evelynn M. Hammonds, "Science, Politics, and the Art of Persuasion: Promoting the New Scientific Medicine in New York City," in Rosner, *Hives of Sickness,* pp. 165–175; Hardy, *Epidemic Streets,* pp. 82–109; Hammonds, *Childhood's Deadly Scourge.*

59. Charles V. Chapin, "Measles in Providence, R.I., 1858–1923," *American Journal of Hygiene* 5 (1925): 635–655; A. W. Hedrich, "The Corrected Average Attack Rate from Measles among City Children," ibid., 11 (1930): 576–600; Howard, *Public Health Administration,* pp. 314–322; Andrew Cliff, Peter Haggett, and Matthew Smallman-Raynor, *Measles: An Historical Geography of a Major Human Viral Disease from Global Expansion to Local Retreat, 1840–1990* (Oxford: Blackwell, 1993), pp. 98–101.

60. David Morley, "Severe Measles," in *Changing Disease Patterns and Human Behaviour,* ed. N. F. Stanley and R. A. Joske (New York: Academic Press, 1980), pp. 116–128; Peter Aaby et al., "Overcrowding and Intensive Exposure as Determinants of Measles Mortality," *American Journal of Epidemiology* 120 (1984): 49–63; Aaby, "Malnutrition and Overcrowding/Intensive Exposure in Severe Measles Infection: Review of Community Studies," *Reviews of Infectious Diseases* 10 (1988): 478–491; idem, "Determinants of Measles Mortality: Host or Transmission Factors?" in *Medical Virology 10: Proceedings of the 1990 Symposium on Medical Virology . . . 1990,* ed. Luis M. De la Maza and Ellena M. Peterson (New York: Plenum Press, 1991), pp. 83–116; Hardy, *Epidemic Streets,* pp. 28–55; Dublin and Lotka, *Twenty-five Years of Health Progress,* p. 61.

61. Dublin and Lotka, *Twenty-five Years of Health Progress,* pp. 73–75; Hardy,

Epidemic Streets, pp. 9–27. See also Joseph H. Lapin, *Whooping Cough* (Springfield, Ill.: Charles C. Thomas, 1943).

62. Dublin and Lotka, *Twenty-five Years of Health Progress,* pp. 67–72; Condran and Cheyney, "Mortality Trends in Philadelphia," p. 109; Chapin, "Changes in Type of Contagious Disease," pp. 20–29.

63. Peter C. English, *Rheumatic Fever in America and Britain: A Biological, Epidemiological, and Medical History* (New Brunswick, N.J.: Rutgers University Press, 1999), pp. 1–14, 113–114; May G. Wilson, *Rheumatic Fever: Studies of the Epidemiology, Manifestations, Diagnosis, and Treatment of the Disease during the First Three Decades* (New York: Commonwealth Fund, 1940), p. 11.

64. English, *Rheumatic Fever;* Benedict E. Massell, *Rheumatic Fever and Streptococcal Infection: Unraveling the Mysteries of a Dread Disease* (Boston: Francis A. Countway Library of Medicine, 1997), p. 271.

65. Edward H. Kass, "Infectious Diseases and Social Change," *Journal of Infectious Diseases* 123 (1971): 112–113.

66. See Irvine Loudon, *Death in Childbirth: An International Study of Maternal Care and Maternal Mortality, 1800–1950* (New York: Oxford University Press, 1992); idem, *The Tragedy of Childhood Fever* (New York: Oxford University Press, 2000); and Judith W. Leavitt, *Brought to Bed: Childbearing in America, 1750–1950* (New York: Oxford University Press, 1986).

The decline in maternal mortality that began in the late 1930s was due to a variety of factors, including better obstetrical care, the introduction of drugs (including the sulfonamides and penicillin), and blood transfusion.

67. Ernest Poole, "The Plague in its Stronghold: Tuberculosis in the New York Tenement," in *A Handbook on the Prevention of Tuberculosis* (New York: Charity Organization Society of the City of New York, 1903), p. 307.

68. Howard, *Public Health Administration,* p. 384; Barron H. Lerner, "New York City's Tuberculosis Control Efforts: The Historical Limitations of the 'War on Consumption,'" *American Journal of Public Health* 83 (1993): 759; Anthony M. Lowell, Lydia B. Edwards, and Carroll E. Palmer, *Tuberculosis* (Cambridge: Harvard University Press, 1969), p. 68; Albert P. Iskrant and Eugene Rogot, "Trends in Tuberculosis Mortality in Continental United States," *Public Health Reports* 68 (1953): 911.

69. Iskrant and Rogot, "Trends in Tuberculosis Mortality," pp. 912–913; Louis I. Dublin, "The Course of Tuberculosis Mortality and Morbidity in the United States," *American Journal of Public Health* 48 (1958): 1439–48; Theodore C. Doege, "Tuberculosis Mortality in the United States, 1900 to 1960," *JAMA* 192 (1965): 103–106; Lowell, Edwards, and Palmer, *Tuberculosis,* p. 69.

70. See Georgina D. Feldberg, *Disease and Class: Tuberculosis and the Shaping of Modern North American Society* (New Brunswick, N.J.: Rutgers Univer-

sity Press, 1995); and Barbara Bates, *Bargaining for Life: A Social History of Tuberculosis, 1876–1938* (Philadelphia: University of Pennsylvania Press, 1992).

71. Edgar Sydenstricker, *Health and Environment* (New York: McGraw-Hill, 1933), p. 120; idem, "The Declining Death Rate from Tuberculosis," in *National Tuberculosis Association Transactions, 1927,* reprinted in Kasius, *Challenge of Facts,* pp. 345–369.

72. Leonard G. Wilson, "The Historical Decline of Tuberculosis in Europe and America: Its Causes and Significance," *Journal of the History of Medicine and Allied Sciences* 45 (1990): 366–396. See also idem, "The Rise and Fall of Tuberculosis in Minnesota: The Role of Infection," *Bulletin of the History of Medicine* 66 (1992): 16–52.

73. Wilson, "Historical Decline of Tuberculosis"; Arthur Newsholme, *The Prevention of Tuberculosis* (London: Methuen, 1908).

74. Bates, *Bargaining for Life,* pp. 313–327; Wilson, "Historical Decline of Tuberculosis," pp. 393–395; U.S. Bureau of the Census, *Historical Statistics,* 1: 78; Godias J. Drolet, "Epidemiology of Tuberculosis," in *Clinical Tuberculosis,* ed. Benjamin Goldberg, 2 vols., 5th ed. (Philadelphia: F. A. Davis, 1946), 1: 71.

75. Louis I. Dublin, *A 40 Year Campaign against Tuberculosis* (New York: Metropolitan Life Insurance Company, 1952), pp. 1–2, 37–52.

76. Ibid., pp. 80–95.

77. Charles Edward-Amory Winslow, *The City Set on a Hill: The Significance of the Health Demonstration at Syracuse, New York* (New York: Doubleday, Doran, 1934), pp. 133–167. For a discussion of the Framingham and Syracuse projects, see Mark Caldwell, *The Last Crusade: The War on Consumption, 1862–1954* (New York: Atheneum, 1988), pp. 196–205.

78. Wade Hampton Frost, "How Much Control of Tuberculosis?" *American Journal of Public Health* 27 (1937): 759–766 and "The Age Selection of Mortality from Tuberculosis in Successive Decades," *American Journal of Hygiene* 30 (1939): 91–96, both reprinted in Barbara G. Rosenkrantz, ed., *From Consumption to Tuberculosis: A Documentary History* (New York: Garland, 1994), pp. 562–579.

79. Arnold R. Rich, *The Pathogenesis of Tuberculosis,* 2d ed. (Springfield, Ill.: Charles C. Thomas, 1951), pp. 897–914; Lowell, Edwards, and Palmer, *Tuberculosis,* pp. 84–93. See also E. R. N. Grigg, "The Arcana of Tuberculosis," *American Review of Tuberculosis and Pulmonary Diseases* 78 (1958): 151–172, 426–453, 583–603; Caldwell, *Last Crusade,* pp. 276–278; René Dubos and Jean Dubos, *The White Plague: Tuberculosis, Man, and Society* (Boston: Little, Brown, 1952); Richard H. Shryock, *National Tuberculosis Association, 1904–1954: A Study of the Voluntary Health Movement in the United States* (New York: National Tuberculosis Association, 1957); Selman

A. Waksman, *The Conquest of Tuberculosis* (Berkeley: University of California Press, 1966); and Frank Ryan, *The Forgotten Plague: How the Battle against Tuberculosis was Won–and Lost* (Boston: Little, Brown, 1993).

80. U.S. Army Medical Department, *The Medical Department of the United States Army in the World War,* 15 vols. (Washington, D.C.: Government Printing Office, 1921–1929), 15: 576–579; Stanhope Bayne-Jones, *The Evolution of Preventive Medicine in the United States Army, 1607–1939* (Washington, D.C.: Department of the Army, 1968), pp. 151–152.

81. Robert W. Fogel, "The Conquest of High Mortality and Hunger in Europe and America: Timing and Mechanisms," in Higonnet and Rosovsky, *Favorites of Fortune,* p. 34.

9. THE DISCOVERY OF CHRONIC ILLNESS

1. George H. Bigelow and Herbert L. Lombard, *Cancer and Other Chronic Diseases in Massachusetts* (Boston: Houghton Mifflin, 1933), pp. 1, 3–4, 10.

2. U.S. Census Office, *Compendium of the Tenth Census (June 1, 1880)* (Washington, D.C.: Government Printing Office 1883), pp. 1729–31.

3. U.S. Census Office, *Report on the Defective, Dependent, and Delinquent Classes of the Population of the United States, as Returned at the Tenth Census (June 1, 1880)* (Washington, D.C.: Government Printing Office, 1880), pp. vii, 39–42.

4. Herbert Goldhamer and Andrew W. Marshall, *Psychosis and Civilization: Two Studies in the Frequency of Mental Disease* (Glencoe, Ill.: Free Press, 1953); U.S. Census Office, *Report on the Defective, Dependent, and Delinquent Classes,* pp. 39–42, 215; Morton Kramer, *Psychiatric Services and the Changing Institutional Scene, 1950–1985,* DHEW Publication No. (ADM)77–433 (Washington, D.C.: Government Printing Office, 1977), p. 78.

5. Cheryl Elman and George C. Myers, "Geographic Morbidity Differentials in the Late Nineteenth-Century United States," *Demography* 36 (1999): 429–443. See also Edward Meeker, "The Improving Health of the United States, 1850–1915," *Explorations in Economic History* 9 (1972): 353–373.

6. Dora L. Costa, *The Evolution of Retirement: An American Economic History, 1880–1980* (Chicago: University of Chicago Press, 1998), pp. 160, 184–185.

7. Dora L. Costa, "Understanding the Twentieth-Century Decline in Chronic Conditions among Older Men," *Demography* 37 (2000): 53–72; idem, "Health and Labor Force Participation of Older Men, 1900–1991," *Journal of Economic History* 56 (1996): 62–89; idem, *Evolution of Retirement,* p. 62.

8. On the origins and evolution of the modern American hospital system, see

Charles E. Rosenberg, *The Care of Strangers: The Rise of America's Hospital System* (New York: Basic Books, 1987); Morris Vogel, *The Invention of the Modern Hospital: Boston, 1870–1930* (Chicago: University of Chicago Press, 1980); and Rosemary Stevens, *In Sickness and in Wealth: American Hospitals in the Twentieth Century* (New York: Basic Books, 1989).

9. Ulysses S. Grant to Dr. John Hancock Douglas, June 17, 1885, quoted in James T. Patterson, *The Dread Disease: Cancer and Modern American Culture* (Cambridge: Harvard University Press, 1987), p. 10.

10. Forrest E. Linder and Robert D. Grove, *Vital Statistics Rates in the United States, 1900–1940* (Washington, D.C.: Government Printing Office, 1943), p. 150; Alfred E. Cohn and Claire Lingg, *The Burden of Diseases in the United States* (New York: Oxford University Press, 1950), p. 27; I. S. Falk, C. Rufus Rorem, and Martha D. Ring, *The Costs of Medical Care* (Chicago: University of Chicago Press, 1933), p. 25.

11. Selwyn D. Collins, *A Review and Study of Illness and Medical Care with Special Reference to Long-Time Trends,* U.S. Public Health Service Monograph No. 48 (Washington, D.C.: Government Printing Office, 1957), pp. 1–3; Louis I. Dublin and Alfred J. Lotka, *Twenty-five Years of Health Progress: A Study of the Mortality Experience among the Industrial Policyholders of the Metropolitan Life Insurance Company, 1911 to 1935* (New York: Metropolitan Life Insurance Company, 1937); Alden B. Mills, *The Extent of Illness and of Physical and Mental Defects Prevailing in the United States* (New York: Committee on the Costs of Medical Care, 1929), pp. 19–48; Charles Edward-Amory Winslow, *The City Set on a Hill: The Significance of the Health Demonstration at Syracuse, New York* (New York: Doubleday, Doran, 1934). The Hagerstown study was covered in eleven papers written by Edgar Sydenstricker and published in *Public Health Reports* for 1926–1929.

12. Margaret L. Stecker, *Some Recent Morbidity Data* (n.p., 1919), p. 3; George S. J. Perrott and Selwyn D. Collins, "Relation of Sickness to Income and Income Change in Ten Surveyed Communities," *Public Health Reports* 50 (1935): 595.

13. On the history of influenza see K. David Patterson, *Pandemic Influenza, 1700–1900: A Study in Historical Epidemiology* (Totowa, N.J.: Rowman & Littlefield, 1986); Gerald F. Pyle, *The Diffusion of Influenza: Patterns and Paradigms* (Totowa, N.J.: Rowman & Littlefield, 1986); and Eugene P. Campbell, "The Epidemiology of Influenza Illustrated by Historical Accounts," *Bulletin of the History of Medicine* 13 (1943): 389–403.

14. The best general account is Alfred W. Crosby's *America's Forgotten Pandemic: The Influenza of 1918* (1976; reprint, New York: Cambridge University Press, 1989). See also Pyle, *Diffusion of Influenza,* pp. 54–56.

15. Crosby, *America's Forgotten Pandemic,* pp. 205–216; Charles Edward-

Amory Winslow and J. F. Rogers, "Statistics of the 1918 Epidemic of Influenza in Connecticut," *Journal of Infectious Diseases* 20 (1920): 195; Selwyn D. Collins, "Influenza and Pneumonia Excess Mortality at Specific Ages in the Epidemic of 1943–44, with Comparative Data for Preceding Epidemics," *Public Health Reports* 60 (1945): 854. Military statistics can be found in United States Army Medical Department, *The Medical Department of the United States Army in the World War,* 15 vols. (Washington, D.C.: Government Printing Office, 1921–1929), vol. 15.

16. Crosby, *America's Forgotten Pandemic,* pp. 91–120; *Chicago Tribune,* October 19, 1918, quoted in Fred R. van Hartesdeldt, ed., *The 1918–1919 Pandemic of Influenza: The Urban Impact in the Western World* (Lewiston, N.Y.: Edwin Mellen Press, 1992), p. 142.

17. See Selwyn D. Collins and Josephine Lehmann, "Trends and Epidemics of Influenza and Pneumonia, 1918–1951," *Public Health Reports* 66 (1951): 1487–1516, and *Excess Deaths from Influenza and Pneumonia and from Important Chronic Diseases during Epidemic Periods, 1918–51,* U.S. Public Health Service Monograph No. 10 (Washington, D.C.: Government Printing Office, 1953).

18. See Ann H. Reid, Thomas G. Fanning, Johan V. Hultin, and Jeffery K. Taubenberger, "Origin and Evolution of the 1918 'Spanish' Influenza Virus Hemagglutinin Gene," *Proceedings of the National Academy of Sciences* 96 (1999): 1651–56; and Robert G. Webster, "1918 Spanish Influenza: The Secrets Remain Elusive," ibid., pp. 1164–66. Gina Kolata's *Flu: The Story of the Great Influenza Pandemic of 1918 and the Search for the Virus That Caused It* (New York: Farrar, Straus and Giroux, 1999) provides a readable account for a general audience.

19. Stecker, *Some Recent Morbidity Data,* pp. 1–27.

20. Albert G. Love and Charles D. Davenport, *Defects Found in Drafted Men* (Washington D.C.: Government Printing Office, 1919), pp. 28–50.

21. Bigelow and Lombard, *Cancer and Other Chronic Diseases,* pp. 1–4, 20–26.

22. Ibid., pp. 4, 17.

23. Ibid., pp. 10–11, 18–19, 258.

24. Ibid., pp. 18, 29, 35–36, 261.

25. Mary C. Jarrett, *Chronic Illness in New York City,* 2 vols. (New York, Columbia University Press, 1933), 1: 1.

26. Ibid., pp. 23–30, 69.

27. Ibid., pp. 5–7.

28. Falk, Rorem, and Ring, *Costs of Medical Care,* pp. ix, 25–58; Mills, *Extent of Illness.* See also Daniel M. Fox, *Power and Illness: The Failure and Future of American Health Policy* (Berkeley: University of California Press, 1993).

29. For a description of the National Health Survey see George St. J. Perrott, Clark Tibbitts, and Rollo H. Britten, "The National Health Survey," *Public*

Health Reports 54 (1939): 1663–87. A bibliography of the many studies that followed can be found in *The National Health Survey 1935–1936*, U.S. Public Health Service Publication No. 85 (Washington, D.C.: Government Printing Office, 1951), pp. 25–65. See also Daniel M. Fox, "Policy and Epidemiology: Financing Health Services for the Chronically Ill and Disabled, 1930–1990," *Milbank Quarterly* 67, suppl. 2, pt. 2 (1989): 257–287.

30. Rollo H. Britten, Selwyn D. Collins, and James S. Fitzgerald, "The National Health Survey: Some General Findings as to Disease, Accidents, and Impairments in Urban Areas," *Public Health Reports* 55 (1940): 444–470; Ernst P. Boas, *The Unseen Plague: Chronic Disease* (New York: J. J. Augustin, 1940), pp. 7–14; Cohn and Lingg, *Burden of Diseases*, pp. 93 ff.

31. This term was used by Howard A. Rusk and Eugene J. Taylor in their article "Physical Disability: A National Problem," *American Journal of Public Health* 38 (1948): 1381–86.

32. David E. Hailman, "Health Status of Adults in the Productive Ages," *Public Health Reports* 56 (1941): 2071–87.

33. Britten, Collins, and Fitzgerald, "The National Health Survey: Disease, Accidents, and Impairments in Urban Areas," pp. 444–470; Boas, *Unseen Plague*, p. 13.

34. Joel A. Tarr and Mark Tebeau, "Housewives as Home Safety Managers: The Changing Perception of the Home as a Place of Hazard and Risk, 1870–1940," in *Accidents in History: Injuries, Fatalities, and Social Relations*, ed. Roger Cooter and Bill Luckin (Amsterdam: Rodopi, 1997), pp. 196–233.

35. Joan Klebba, "Public Accidents among the Urban Population as Recorded in the National Health Survey," *Public Health Reports* 56 (1941): 1419–20.

36. Ibid., pp. 1419–39; Rollo H. Britten, Joan Klebba, and David E. Hailman, "Accidents in the Urban Home as Recorded in the National Health Survey," ibid., 55 (1940): 2061–2086. See also Selwyn D. Collins, F. Ruth Phillips, and Dorothy S. Oliver, *Accident Frequency, Place of Occurrence, and Relation to Chronic Disease: Sample of White Families Canvassed on Monthly Intervals, Eastern District of Baltimore, 1938–43*, U.S. Public Health Service Monograph No. 14 (Washington, D.C.: Government Printing Office, 1953).

37. Rollo H. Britten, "Blindness as Recorded in the National Health Survey—Amount, Causes, and Relation to Certain Social Factors," *Public Health Reports* 56 (1941): 2191–2215.

38. Christopher C. Sellers, *Hazards of the Job: From Industrial Disease to Environmental Science* (Chapel Hill: University of North Carolina Press, 1997), pp. 106–110, 121–140.

39. See Hugh P. Brinton, "Disabling Sickness and Nonindustrial Injuries among Drivers and other Employees of Certain Bus and Cab Companies, 1930–34, Inclusive," *Public Health Reports* 54 (1939): 459–468; Brinton and Harry E. Seifert, "Disabling Morbidity among Employees in the Soap Industry,

1930–34, Inclusive," ibid., pp. 1301–16; Brinton, "Disabling Morbidity and Mortality among White and Negro Male Employees in the Slaughter and Meat Packing Industry, 1930–34, Inclusive," ibid., pp. 1965–77; Brinton, Seifert, and Elizabeth S. Frasier, "Disabling Morbidity among Employees in the Slaughter and Meat Packing Industry, 1930–34, Inclusive," ibid., pp. 2196–2219; Brinton and Frasier, "Disabling Morbidity among Male and Female Employees in Mail Order Stores, 1930–34, Inclusive," ibid., 55 (1940): 1163–78; and Joan Klebba, "Industrial Injuries among the Urban Population as Recorded in the National Health Survey," ibid., 56 (1941): 2375–92.

40. Hailman, "Health Status of Adults," pp. 2082–84; Rusk and Taylor, "Physical Disability," p. 1381. On the shortcomings of morbidity data from household surveys see Barkev S. Sanders, "Have Morbidity Surveys Been Oversold?" *American Journal of Public Health* 52 (1962): 1648–59.

41. Rusk and Taylor, "Physical Disability," pp. 1381–86.

42. Fox, *Power and Illness,* pp. 30–38; idem, "Policy and Epidemiology: Financing Health Services for the Chronically Ill and Disabled"; Beatrix Hoffman, *The Wages of Sickness: The Politics of Health Insurance in Progressive America* (Chapel Hill: University of North Carolina Press, 2001).

43. Bigelow and Lombard, *Cancer and Other Chronic Diseases,* p. viii; Fox, *Power and Illness,* pp. 42–47.

44. Boas, *Unseen Plague,* pp. v, 4, 17–18, 121, and passim. See also Boas' *Treatment of the Patient Past Fifty* (Chicago: Year Book Publishers, 1941).

45. Dublin and Lotka, *Twenty-five Years of Health Progress,* pp. 4, 119–142.

46. Louis I. Dublin and Richard J. Vane, "Longevity of Industrial Workers," *Statistical Bulletin of the Metropolitan Life Insurance Company* 31 (1950): 6–7.

47. See, for example, William M. Gafafer, "The Measurement of Sickness among Industrial Workers," *Medical Clinics of North America* 26 (1942): 1105–20. Gafafer was a senior statistician at the Public Health Service and chief of the Statistical Unit in the Division of Industrial Hygiene of the National Institute of Health.

48. James Whiteside, *Regulating Danger: The Struggle for Mine Safety in the Rocky Mountain Coal Industry* (Lincoln: University of Nebraska Press, 1990), pp. 132–133; Daniel J. Curran, *Dead Laws for Dead Men: The Politics of Federal Coal Mine Health and Safety Legislation* (Pittsburgh: University of Pittsburgh Press, 1993), p. 71; Barbara E. Smith, *Digging Our Own Graves: Coal Miners and the Struggle over Black Lung Disease* (Philadelphia: Temple University Press, 1987), pp. 145–147; Alan Derickson, *Black Lung: Anatomy of a Public Health Disaster* (Ithaca: Cornell University Press, 1998).

49. Material in this and the preceding paragraph is drawn from W. C. Hueper,

Environmental and Occupational Cancer, Public Health Reports, suppl. 209 (1948): 20–21; David Ozonoff, "Failed Warnings: Asbestos-Related Disease and Industrial Medicine," in *The Health and Safety of Workers: Case Studies in the Politics of Professional Responsibility,* ed. Ronald Bayer (New York: Oxford University Press, 1988), pp. 139–219; David E. Lilienfeld, "The Silence: The Asbestos Industry and Early Occupational Cancer Research–A Case Study," *American Journal of Public Health* 81 (1991): 791–800; Irving J. Selikoff and Douglas H. K. Lee, *Asbestos and Disease* (New York: Academic Press, 1978); Brooke T. Mossman and J. Bernard L. Gee, "Asbestos-Related Diseases," *New England Journal of Medicine* 320 (1989): 1721–30; and David Kotelchuck, "Asbestos: 'The Funeral Dress of Kings'–and Others," in *Dying for Work: Workers' Safety and Health in Twentieth-Century America,* ed. David Rosner and Gerald Markowitz (Bloomington: Indiana University Press, 1987), pp. 192–207.

50. The saga of the radium dial painters can be followed in Claudia Clark, *Radium Girls: Women and Industrial Health Reform, 1910–1935* (Chapel Hill: University of North Carolina Press, 1997); Angela Nugent, "The Power to Define a New Disease: Epidemiological Politics and Radium Poisoning," in Rosner and Markowitz, *Dying for Work,* pp. 177–191; and William D. Sharpe, "The New Jersey Radium Dial Workers: Seventy-Five Years Later," in *Toxic Circles: Environmental Hazards from the Workplace into the Community,* ed. Helen E. Sheehan and Richard H. Wedeen (New Brunswick: Rutgers University Press, 1993), pp. 138–163.

51. Martin Cherniack, *The Hawk's Nest Incident: America's Worst Industrial Disaster* (New Haven: Yale University Press, 1986); Jacqueline K. Corn, *Response to Occupational Health Hazards: A Historical Perspective* (New York: Van Nostrand Reinhold, 1992), pp. 118–120.

52. Sholem Asch, *East River: A Novel* (New York: G. P. Putnam's Sons, 1946), p. 151.

53. See Louis I. Dublin and Alfred J. Lotka, "The History of Longevity in the United States," *Human Biology* 6 (1934): 43–86.

54. In some controversial books, James C. Riley has argued that the decline in mortality among British workingmen in the late nineteenth and early twentieth centuries was accompanied by an increase in morbidity. See *Sick, Not Dead: The Health of British Workingmen during the Mortality Decline* (Baltimore: Johns Hopkins University Press, 1997), pp. 153–187, and *Sickness, Recovery, and Death: A History and Forecast of Ill Health* (Iowa City: University of Iowa Press, 1989), pp. 115–127.

55. Peter C. English, *Rheumatic Fever in America and Britain: A Biological, Epidemiological, and Medical History* (New Brunswick: Rutgers University Press, 1999), pp. 7–8; Benedict E. Massell, *Rheumatic Fever and Streptococcal Infection: Unraveling the Mysteries of a Dread Disease* (Boston: Francis A. Countway Library of Medicine, 1997), pp. 267–271.

56. Riley, *Sickness, Recovery, and Death,* pp. 119–121; William Ophüls, "Arteriosclerosis, Cardiovascular Disease: Their Relation to Infectious Diseases," Stanford University, *Publications. University Series. Medical Sciences,* I (1921): 95, and "A Statistical Survey of Three Thousand Autopsies from the Department of Pathology of the Stanford University Medical School," ibid., I (1926): 131–370.

57. See Sandeep Gupta, "Chronic Infection in the Aetiology of Atherosclerosis–Focus on *Chlamydia pneumoniae,*" *Atherosclerosis* 143 (1999): 1–6; "The Potential Etiologic Role of *Chlamydia pneumoniae* in Atherosclerosis: A Multidisciplinary Meeting to Promote Collaborative Research . . . 1999," *Journal of Infectious Diseases* 181, suppl. 3 (2000): s393–s86; and Joseph B. Muhlestein, "Chronic Infection and Coronary Artery Disease," *Medical Clinics of North America* 84 (2000): 123–148.

10. NO FINAL VICTORY

1. Robert W. Fogel, *The Fourth Great Awakening and the Future of Egalitarianism* (Chicago: University of Chicago Press, 2000), pp. 236–237; William B. Schwartz, *Life without Disease: The Pursuit of Medical Utopia* (Berkeley: University of California Press, 1998), p. 3.

2. Julius B. Richmond, *Currents in American Medicine: A Developmental View of Medical Care and Education* (Cambridge: Harvard University Press, 1969), p. 27.

3. President's Scientific Research Board, *Science and Public Policy,* 5 vols. (Washington, D.C.: Government Printing Office, 1947), I: 3, 115–118.

4. U.S. Bureau of the Census, *Historical Statistics of the United States: Colonial Times to 1970,* 2 vols. (Washington, D.C.: Government Printing Office, 1975), I: 74; National Center for Health Statistics, *Health, United States, 2000* (Washington, D.C.: Government Printing Office, 2000), pp. 321–322.

5. See James Le Fanu, *The Rise and Fall of Modern Medicine* (New York: Carroll & Graff, 2000); and Schwartz, *Life without Disease.*

6. U.S. Bureau of the Census, *Historical Statistics,* I: 57; National Center for Health Statistics, *Health,* pp. 152, 157.

7. Sam Shapiro, Edward R. Schlesinger, and Robert E. L. Nesbitt Jr., *Infant, Perinatal, Maternal, and Childhood Mortality in the United States* (Cambridge: Harvard University Press, 1968), pp. 3–139, 271–328; Richard A. Meckel, *Saving the Babies: American Public Health Reform and the Prevention of Infant Mortality, 1850–1929* (Baltimore: Johns Hopkins University Press, 1990), p. 227; Herbert J. Summers, "Infant Mortality in Rural and Urban Areas," *Public Health Reports* 57 (1942): 1494–1501.

8. Meckel, *Saving the Babies,* pp. 233–236; National Center for Health Statistics, *Health,* p. 151. For an analysis of infant and child mortality patterns at the turn of the century see also Samuel H. Preston and Michael R. Haines,

Fatal Years: Child Mortality in Late Nineteenth-Century America (Princeton: Princeton University Press, 1991).

9. U.S. Bureau of the Census, *Historical Statistics,* 1: 55; National Center for Health Statistics, *Health,* pp. 160–161; Eileen M. Crimmins, "The Changing Pattern of American Mortality Decline, 1940–77, and Its Implications for the Future," *Population and Development Review* 7 (1981): 229–230; Richard Cooper, Robert Cohen, and Abas Amiry, "Is the Period of Rapidly Declining Adult Mortality Coming to an End?" *American Journal of Public Health* 73 (1983): 1091–93.

10. The failure of the federal government to collect health data by socioeconomic class grew out of a curious set of circumstances. Between the two world wars officials at the Public Health Service began to call attention to the importance of occupation and income as determinants of health. But in 1946 the collection of vital statistics was transferred from the Bureau of the Census to the Public Health Service, breaking the link between vital statistics and the decennial census of death certificates. Equally important, the growing conservatism engendered during World War II and the advent of the Cold War discouraged discussion of social inequalities in health because it allegedly gave sustenance to Communist ideology. See Nancy Krieger and Elizabeth Fee, "Measuring Social Inequalities in Health in the United States: A Historical Review," *International Journal of Health Services* 26 (1996): 391–418.

11. National Center for Health Statistics, *Health,* p. 152; Gregory Pappas, Susan Queen, Wilbur Hadden, and Gail Fisher, "The Increasing Disparity in Mortality between Socioeconomic Groups in the United States, 1960 and 1986," *New England Journal of Medicine* 329 (1993): 107; Howard P. Greenwald, *Who Survives Cancer?* (Berkeley: University of California Press, 1992), pp. 161–162; Hari H. Dayal, Lincoln Polissar, and Steven Dahlberg, "Race, Socioeconomic Status, and Other Prognostic Factors for Survival from Prostate Cancer," *Journal of the National Cancer Institute* 74 (1985): 1001–06; Mary T. Bassett and Nancy Krieger, "Social Class and Black-White Differences in Breast Cancer Survival," *American Journal of Public Health* 76 (1986): 1400–03; Jing Fang, Shantha Madhavan, and Michael H. Alderman, "The Association between Birthplace and Mortality from Cardiovascular Causes among Black and White Residents of New York City," *New England Journal of Medicine* 335 (1996): 1545–51; Arlene T. Geronimus et al., "Excess Mortality among Blacks and Whites in the United States," ibid., pp. 1552–58. See also Evelyn M. Kitagawa and Philip M. Hauser, *Differential Mortality in the United States: A Study in Socioeconomic Epidemiology* (Cambridge: Harvard University Press, 1973); Stephen Marcella and Jane E. Miller, "Racial Differences in Colorectal Cancer Mortality: The Importance of Stage and Socioeconomic Status," *Journal of Clinical Epidemiology* 54

(2001): 359–366; Jane E. Miller, "The Effects of Race/Ethnicity and Income on Early Childhood Asthma Prevalence and Health Care Use," *American Journal of Public Health* 90 (2000): 428–430; Felicia B. LeClere, Richard G. Rogers, and Kimberly D. Peters, "Ethnicity and Mortality in the United States: Individual and Community Correlates," *Social Forces* 76 (1997): 169–198.

12. Gretchen A. Condran, Henry Williams, and Rose A. Cheyney, "The Decline in Mortality in Philadelphia from 1870 to 1930: The Role of Municipal Services," *Pennsylvania Magazine of History and Biography* 108 (1984): 153; Evelynn M. Hammonds, *Childhood's Deadly Scourge: The Campaign to Control Diphtheria in New York City, 1880–1930* (Baltimore: Johns Hopkins University Press, 1999), p. 29.

13. Sherry L. Murphy, "Deaths: Final Data for 1998," *National Vital Statistics Reports* 48 (July 24, 2000): 18.

14. Ibid., p. 5.

15. Ibid., p. 23.

16. In the twentieth century there have been several changes in terminology. In the early part of the century "diseases of the heart" was the diagnostic category. Subsequently "heart disease" came to include such categories as ischemic heart disease, coronary heart disease, and arteriosclerotic heart disease, all of which are basically the same. All denote the clinical symptoms of atherosclerosis, which is the obstruction of the flow of blood through the arterial network and specifically the coronary arteries.

17. Reuel A. Stallones, "The Rise and Fall of Ischemic Heart Disease," *Scientific American* 243 (1980): 53–54; National Center for Health Statistics, *Health,* pp. 163, 185.

18. William B. Kannel and Thomas J. Thom, "Declining Cardiovascular Mortality," *Circulation* 70 (1984): 331.

19. Robert A. Aronowitz, *Making Sense of Illness: Science, Society, and Disease* (New York: Cambridge University Press, 1998), p. 114; Commission on Chronic Illness, *Chronic Illness in the United States,* 4 vols. (Cambridge: Harvard University Press, 1957–1959), 1: 144, 154.

20. Aronowitz, *Making Sense of Illness,* pp. 111–144; Lester Breslow, "Occupational and Other Social Factors in the Causation of Chronic Disease," *Journal of Hygiene, Epidemiology, Microbiology and Immunology* 4 (1960): 269–270. See also Ancel Keys et al., *Seven Countries: A Multivariate Analysis of Death and Coronary Heart Disease* (Cambridge: Harvard University Press, 1980); Thomas R. Dawber, *The Framingham Study: The Epidemiology of Atherosclerosis Disease* (Cambridge: Harvard University Press, 1980); Lisa F. Berkman and Lester Breslow, *Health and Ways of Living: The Alameda County Study* (New York: Oxford University Press, 1983); and M. G. Marmot and J. F. Mustard, "Coronary Heart Disease from a Popula-

tion Perspective," in *Why Are Some People Healthy and Others Not? The Determinants of Health of Populations,* ed. Robert G. Evans, Morris L. Barer, and Theodore R. Marmor (New York: Aldine de Gruyter, 1994), pp. 189–214.

21. Berkman and Breslow, *Health and Ways of Living,* pp. 211, 219. See also Lester Breslow, "Risk Factor Intervention for Health Maintenance," *Science* 200 (1978): 908–912; and Lester Breslow and Norman Breslow, "Health Practices and Disability: Some Evidence from Alameda County," *Preventive Medicine* 22 (1993): 86–95.

22. The claim that there is a link between fat intake and atherosclerosis is hardly supported by scientific data. For a review see Gary Taubes, "The Soft Science of Dietary Fat," *Science* 291 (2001): 2536–45.

23. Stallones, "Rise and Fall of Ischemic Heart Disease," p. 59.

24. Quoted in Taubes, "The Soft Science of Dietary Fat," pp. 2544–45.

25. William C. Black and H. Gilbert Welch, "Advances in Diagnostic Imaging and Overestimation of Disease Prevalence and the Benefits of Therapy," *New England Journal of Medicine* 328 (1993): 1237–43; Elliot S. Fisher and H. Gilbert Welch, "Avoiding the Unintended Consequences of the Growth in Medical Care," *JAMA* 281 (1999): 446–453.

26. Alvan R. Feinstein, "Scientific Standards in Epidemiologic Studies of the Menace of Daily Life," *Science* 242 (1988): 1257–63. See also Le Fanu, *Rise and Fall of Modern Medicine,* pp. 289–317.

27. Kannel and Thoms, "Declining Cardiovascular Mortality," pp. 331, 335.

28. The literature on the Barker hypothesis is enormous; much of it deals with the problem of low birthweight in developing nations. See David J. P. Barker, ed., *Fetal and Infant Origins of Adult Disease* (London: British Medical Journal, 1992), quote from p. 334; and Barker, ed., *Fetal Origins of Cardiovascular and Lung Disease* (New York: M. Dekker, 2001).

29. For a summary of recent findings, see Joseph B. Muhlestein, "Chronic Infection and Coronary Artery Disease," *Medical Clinics of North America* 84 (2000): 123–148. Paul W. Ewald, an evolutionary biologist, has argued that many so-called chronic degenerative diseases have infectious origins. See his *Plague Time: How Stealth Infections Cause Cancers, Heart Disease, and Other Deadly Ailments* (New York: Free Press, 2000).

30. Paul Fremont-Smith, letter printed in the *Atlantic Monthly* 283 (May 1999): 12; Ewald, *Plague Time,* pp. 107–126; Le Fanu, *Rise and Fall of Modern Medicine,* pp. 147–156. There is considerable confusion and disagreement in explaining CHD mortality trends. See, for example, Daniel Levy and Thomas J. Thom, "Death Rates from Coronary Disease–Progress and a Puzzling Paradox," *New England Journal of Medicine* 339 (1998): 915–916; Wayne D. Rosamond et al., "Trends in the Incidence of Myocardial Infarction and in Mortality Due to Coronary Heart Disease, 1987 to 1994," ibid.,

pp. 861–867; and Stephen Klaidman, *Saving the Heart: The Battle to Conquer Coronary Disease* (New York: Oxford University Press, 2000).

31. Lewis Thomas, "Science and Health–Possibilities, Probabilities, and Limitations," *Social Research* 55 (1988): 384–385.

32. Abraham M. Lilienfeld, Morton L. Levin, and Irving I. Kessler, *Cancer in the United States* (Cambridge: Harvard University Press, 1972), p. 3; National Center for Health Statistics, *Health*, p. 172.

33. National Center for Health Statistics, *Health*, p. 191.

34. See James T. Patterson, *The Dread Disease: Cancer and Modern American Culture* (Cambridge: Harvard University Press, 1987); and Richard A. Rettig, *Cancer Crusade: The Story of the National Cancer Act of 1971* (Princeton: Princeton University Press, 1977).

35. For a sampling of the literature see Lester Breslow et al., *A History of Cancer Control in the United States, 1946–1971,* DHEW Publication Nos. (NIH) 79-1516–1519 (Washington, D.C.: U.S. Department of Health, Education and Welfare, 1979); Richard Doll and Richard Peto, *The Causes of Cancer: Quantitative Estimates of Avoidable Risks in the United States Today* (New York: Oxford University Press, 1981); Edward J. Sondik, "Progress in Cancer Prevention and Control," in *Unnatural Causes: The Three Leading Killer Diseases in America,* ed. Russell C. Maulitz (New Brunswick, N.J.: Rutgers University Press, 1988), pp. 111–131.

36. F. J. Ingelfinger, editorial in the *New England Journal of Medicine* 293 (1975): 1319–20, quoted in Patterson, *Dread Disease,* p. 255.

37. For a discussion of recent work on the biology of cancer see Harold Varmus and Robert A. Weinberg, *Genes and the Biology of Cancer* (New York: Scientific American Library, 1993); and Robert A. Weinberg, *Racing to the Beginning of the Road: The Search for the Origin of Cancer* (New York: Harmony Books, 1996).

38. Weinberg, *Racing to the Beginning of the Road,* pp. 245–250.

39. Data dealing with the epidemiology of cancer are not always accurate, depending on the period involved. Data before 1930 are often unavailable or unreliable, partly because of an inability to identify a particular neoplasm, and partly because of procedures for assigning cause of death on the death certificate. Changes in diagnostic categories throughout the twentieth century complicate the problem of identifying trends. Nevertheless, the data that have survived do not indicate sharp changes in age-adjusted mortality from this disease.

40. Interestingly, geographic differences in cancer mortality have been diminishing. See Michael R. Greenberg, *Urbanization and Cancer Mortality: The United States Experience, 1950–1975* (New York: Oxford University Press, 1983).

41. Lilienfeld, Levin, and Kessler, *Cancer in the United States,* pp. 8–48; David

Schottenfeld, "The Magnitude of the Cancer Problem," in *Chronic Disease and Public Health,* ed. Abraham M. Lilienfeld and Alice J. Gifford (Baltimore: Johns Hopkins Press, 1966), pp. 324–333.

42. American Cancer Society, *Cancer Facts and Figures–1996* (Atlanta, 1996), pp. 3–6.

43. William Haenszel, Michael B. Shimkin, and Herman P. Miller, *Tobacco Smoking Patterns in the United States,* Public Health Monograph No. 45 (1956) (Washington, D.C.: Government Printing Office, 1956), pp. 107–111; U.S. Bureau of the Census, *Statistical Abstract of the United States: 1998* (Washington, D.C.: Government Printing Office, 1998), p. 152.

44. On the history of tobacco and cancer research see John C. Burnham, "American Physicians and Tobacco Use: Two Surgeons General, 1929 and 1964," *Bulletin of the History of Medicine* 63 (1989): 1–31; Ernst L. Wynder, "Tobacco and Health: A Review of the History and Suggestions for Public Policy," *Public Health Reports* 103 (1988): 8–18; idem, "Tobacco as a Cause of Lung Cancer: Some Reflections," *American Journal of Epidemiology* 146 (1997): 687–694; Le Fanu, *Rise and Fall of Modern Medicine,* pp. 39–51; and the essays in S. Lock, L. A. Reynolds, and E. M. Tansey, eds., *Ashes to Ashes: The History of Smoking and Health* (Amsterdam: Radopi, 1998).

45. Christopher P. Howson, Tomohiko Hiyama, and Ernst L. Wynder, "The Decline in Gastric Cancer: Epidemiology of an Unplanned Triumph," *Epidemiologic Reviews* 8 (1986): 1–27; American Cancer Society, *Cancer Facts,* pp. 3–4, 6.

46. Howson, Hiyama, and Wynder, "Decline in Gastric Cancer," pp. 12–20; Schottenfeld, "Magnitude of the Cancer Problem," pp. 329–330.

47. Doll and Peto, *Causes of Cancer,* pp. 1196–97, 1256, 1258; Graham A. Colditz, "Cancer Culture: Epidemics, Human Behavior, and the Dubious Search for New Risk Factors," *American Journal of Public Health* 91 (2001): 357. This issue of the *American Journal of Public Health* includes four articles discussing risk factors (pp. 355–368).

48. For a superb analysis of the flaws of many epidemiological studies, see Feinstein, "Scientific Standards in Epidemiologic Studies." Alan I. Marcus's *Cancer from Beef: DES, Federal Food Regulation, and Consumer Confidence* (Baltimore: Johns Hopkins University Press, 1994) provides a case study of the manner in which cancer etiology becomes simplified and politicized.

49. Robert N. Proctor, *Cancer Wars: How Politics Shapes What We Know and Don't Know about Cancer* (New York: Basic Books, 1995), p. 265.

50. Screening for breast cancer in women and for prostate cancer in men has played a much smaller role in reducing mortality rates for these diseases than is commonly believed. For discussions see Barron H. Lerner, "Great Expectations: Historical Perspectives on Genetic Breast Cancer Testing," *American*

Journal of Public Health 89 (1999): 938–944; idem, "Fighting the War on Breast Cancer: Debates over Early Detection, 1945 to the Present," *Annals of Internal Medicine* 129 (1998): 74–78; and Louise B. Russell, *Educated Guesses: Making Policy about Medical Screening Tests* (Berkeley: University of California Press, 1994), pp. 25–44.

For a fascinating study of the difficulties of generating definitive data on breast cancer and the uncertainties of therapy see Barron H. Lerner, *The Breast Cancer Wars: Hope, Fear, and the Pursuit of a Cure in Twentieth-Century America* (New York: Oxford University Press, 2001).

51. John C. Bailer III and Elaine M. Smith, "Progress against Cancer," *New England Journal of Medicine* 314 (1986): 1226–32; Bailer and Heather L. Gornik, "Cancer Undefeated," ibid., 336 (1997): 1569–74. The differences between Bailer's mortality data from 1982 to 1994 and those of the National Center for Health Statistics, shown in the figure in the text, stem from the fact that the former used the age distribution of the American population for 1990, whereas the latter used 1940 as the base year. See National Center for Health Statistics, *Health*, p. 194.

52. The data and generalizations for this and the preceding paragraph come from C. Ronald Kahn and Gordon C. Weir, eds., *Joslin's Diabetes Mellitus*, 13th ed. (Philadelphia: Lea & Febiger, 1994), pp. 201–215; and Bernard N. Brodoff and Sheldon J. Bleicher, eds., *Diabetes Mellitus and Obesity* (Baltimore: Williams and Wilkins, 1982), pp. 387–397. See also James W. Presley, "A History of Diabetes Mellitus in the United States, 1880–1890" (Ph.D. diss., University of Texas, 1991); and Chris Feudtner, "A Disease in Motion: Diabetes History and the New Paradigm of Transmuted Disease," *Perspectives in Biology and Medicine* 39 (1996): 158–170.

53. Jennie J. Joe and Robert S. Young, eds., *Diabetes as a Disease of Civilization: The Impact of Cultural Change on Indigenous Peoples* (Berlin: Mouton de Gruyter, 1994), pp. 435–449 and passim; David Weatherall, *Science and the Quiet Art: The Role of Medical Research in Health Care* (New York: W. W. Norton, 1995), p. 63. See also Stephen J. Kunitz, *Disease Change and the Role of Medicine: The Navajo Experience* (Berkeley: University of California Press, 1983).

54. Center for Mental Health Services, *Mental Health, United States, 1998,* ed. Ronald W. Manderscheid and Marilyn J. Henderson (Washington, D.C.: Government Printing Office, 1998), pp. 104, 113; David Mechanic, *Mental Health and Social Policy: The Emergence of Managed Care,* 4th ed. (Boston: Allyn and Bacon, 1999), pp. 47–64.

55. Institute of Medicine, *Disability in America: Toward a National Agenda for Prevention* (Washington, D.C.: National Academy Press, 1991), pp. 1, 32.

56. Dora L. Costa, an economic historian, argues that the shift from manual to white-collar occupations and reduced exposure to infectious disease were

important determinants of a 66 percent decline in chronic respiratory problems, valvular heart disease, arteriosclerosis, and joint and back problems among men. Occupational shifts, she concludes, accounted for 29 percent of the decline, the decreased prevalence of infectious diseases for 18 percent, and the remainder is unexplained. But the causal links to support such a hypothesis are largely absent. See Costa, "Understanding the Twentieth-Century Decline in Chronic Conditions among Older Men," *Demography* 37 (2000): 53–72, and *The Evolution of Retirement: An American Economic History, 1880–1980* (Chicago: University of Chicago Press, 1998).

57. Barry R. Bloom and Christopher J. L. Murray, "Tuberculosis: Commentary on a Reemergent Killer," *Science* 257 (1992): 1055–63; Mitchell L. Cohen, "Epidemiology of Drug Resistance: Implications for a Post-Antimicrobial Era," ibid., pp. 1050–55.

58. W. Paul Glezen, "Emerging Infections: Pandemic Influenza," *Epidemiologic Reviews* 18 (1996): 64–76. Data on excess mortality in earlier epidemics appear in Selwyn D. Collins and Josephine Lehmann, *Excess Deaths from Influenza and Pneumonia and from Important Chronic Diseases during Epidemic Periods, 1918–51,* Public Health Monograph No. 10 (1953) (Washington, D.C.: Government Printing Office, 1953).

59. Arthur J. Viseltear, "A Short Political History of the 1976 Swine Influenza Legislation," in *History, Science, and Politics: Influenza in America, 1918–1976,* ed. June E. Osborn (New York: Prodist, 1977), pp. 29–58; Arthur M. Silverstein, *Pure Politics and Impure Science: The Swine Flu Affair* (Baltimore: Johns Hopkins University Press, 1981).

60. Cedric Mims, "The Emergence of New Infectious Diseases," in *Changing Disease Patterns and Human Behaviour,* ed. N. F. Stanley and R. A. Joske (New York: Academic Press, 1980), pp. 232–250; Robert G. Webster, "Influenza: An Emerging Microbial Pathogen," in *Emerging Infections: Biomedical Research Reports,* ed. Richard M. Krause (New York: Academic Press, 1998), p. 275.

61. For an elaboration see Ewald, *Plague Time,* pp. 9–31.

62. David W. Fraser et al., "Legionnaires' Disease: Description of an Epidemic of Pneumonia," *New England Journal of Medicine* 297 (1977): 1189–97; Joseph E. McDade et al., "Legionnaires' Disease: Isolation of a Bacterium and Demonstration of Its Role in Other Respiratory Disease," ibid., pp. 1197–1203; Robert P. Hudson, "Lessons from Legionnaires' Disease," *Annals of Internal Medicine* 90 (1979): 704–707.

63. William J. Brown et al., *Syphilis and Other Venereal Diseases* (Cambridge: Harvard University Press, 1970), pp. 66–67; Institute of Medicine, *The Hidden Epidemic: Confronting Sexually Transmitted Diseases* (Washington, D.C.: National Academy Press, 1997), pp. 34–35. Allan M. Brandt has traced the medical and public responses to venereal diseases in his *No Magic*

Bullet: A Social History of Venereal Disease in the United States since 1880, rev. ed. (New York: Oxford University Press, 1987).

64. Institute of Medicine, *Hidden Epidemic,* pp. 28–39.

65. Ibid., pp. 41–49, 312–315.

66. See especially William Muraskin, "The Silent Epidemic: The Social, Ethical, and Medical Problems Surrounding the Fight against Hepatitis B," *Journal of Social History* 22 (1988): 277–298, and his book *The War against Hepatitis B: A History of the International Task Force on Hepatitis B Immunization* (Philadelphia: University of Philadelphia Press, 1995).

67. Thomas C. Quinn and Anthony S. Fauci, "The AIDS Epidemic: Demographic Aspects, Population Biology, and Virus Evolution," in Krause, *Emerging Infections,* pp. 327–337; U.S. Bureau of the Census, *Statistical Abstract . . . 1998,* p. 103.

68. Barry M. Pomerantz, John S. Marr, and William D. Goldman, "Amebiasis in New York City, 1958–1978: Identification of the Male Homosexual High Risk Population," *Bulletin of the New York Academy of Medicine* 56 (1980): 232–244.

69. This thesis has been advanced by Mirko D. Grmek, "Some Unorthodox Views and a Selection Hypothesis on the Origin of the AIDS Viruses," *Journal of the History of Medicine and Allied Sciences* 50 (1995): 253–273; idem, *History of Aids: Emergence and Origin of a Modern Pandemic* (Princeton: Princeton University Press, 1990). Grmek also developed the concept of pathocoenosis, which stipulates that the frequency and overall distribution of each disease depend a great deal on the frequency and distribution of other diseases in the same population. Thus tuberculosis and a few other infectious diseases might have constituted a barrier to HIV precursors; "Some Unorthodox Views," pp. 270–272.

70. Institute of Medicine, *Hidden Epidemic,* pp. 49–51.

71. Ewald, *Plague Time,* pp. 26–27, 30, 38–40. See also Ewald's *Evolution of Infectious Disease* (New York: Oxford University Press, 1994).

72. Joshua Lederberg, Robert E. Shope, and Stanley C. Oaks Jr., eds., *Emerging Infections: Microbial Threats to Health in the United States* (Washington, D.C.: National Academy Press, 1992), pp. 26–27. See also Krause, *Emerging Infections;* and Laurie Garrett, *The Coming Plague: Newly Emerging Disease in a World Out of Balance* (New York: Farrar, Straus and Giroux, 1994).

73. René Dubos, *Mirage of Health: Utopias, Progress, and Biological Change* (New York: Harper & Brothers, 1959), p. 267.

74. National Center for Health Statistics, *Health,* pp. 172, 206; Susan P. Baker, Brian O'Neill, and Ronald S. Karpf, *The Injury Fact Book* (Lexington: D. C. Heath, 1984), p. 200. For a discussion of "self-inflicted diseases," see Howard M. Leichter, *Free to Be Foolish: Politics and Health Promotion in*

the United States and Great Britain (Princeton: Princeton University Press, 1991).

75. National Center for Health Statistics, *Health,* pp. 177, 275.

76. Ibid., p. 160; U.S. Bureau of the Census, *Statistical Abstract . . . 1998,* pp. 16–17.

77. Schwartz, *Life without Disease,* pp. 149, 153.

78. Macfarlane Burnet and David O. White, *Natural History of Infectious Disease,* 4th ed. (New York: Cambridge University Press, 1972), pp. 1, 263.

79. See especially Joel E. Cohen, *How Many People Can the Earth Support?* (New York: W. W. Norton, 1995).

80. U.S. Bureau of the Census, *Statistical Abstract of the United States: 1941* (Washington, D.C.: Government Printing Office, 1942), p. 9; idem, *Statistical Abstract . . . 1998,* p. 8.

81. Daniel Kevles and Leroy Hood, eds., *The Code of Codes: Scientific and Social Issues in the Human Genome Project* (Cambridge: Harvard University Press, 1992), pp. 157–158, 163.

82. Weatherall, *Science and the Quiet Art,* pp. 312–316. See also Evelyn Fox Keller, *The Century of the Gene* (Cambridge: Harvard University Press, 2000), pp. 68–69, 133–148.

83. Dubos, *Mirage of Health,* p. 2.

84. George H. Bigelow and Herbert L. Lombard, *Cancer and Other Chronic Diseases in Massachusetts* (Boston: Houghton Mifflin, 1933), p. 2. For a modern restatement of the theme that the postponement and compression of morbidity into as short a span of time as possible toward the end of life and the alleviation of illness are realistic goals, see James F. Fries, "The Compression of Morbidity," *Milbank Memorial Fund Quarterly* 61 (1983): 397–419.

Index

Aaby, Peter, 44
accidents, 9, 115, 137, 192, 231–233; industrial, 167–170; automobile, 248, 270–271
acquired immunodeficiency syndrome. *See* AIDS
Aedes aegypti, 75, 102, 184
African Americans: in colonies, 58–59, 60, 71; mortality, 58–59, 87, 112, 117, 193, 200, 211, 247; and slavery, 94, 140–143, 155; and yellow fever, 101–102; and tuberculosis, 111, 211; population, 138; and malaria, 139; in Civil War, 147–148; and rheumatic fever, 209; and cancer, 257–258
agricultural stage: threats to life, 11–12; and declining health, 23–24
ague, 41, 128–129
AIDS, 267–269, 273
Alameda County study, 250–251
alcoholism, 137, 144; among Indians, 37–38
Aleuts, 42
Allen, Richard, 75
amebiasis, 268–269
American Cancer Society, 256
American Medical Association, 160
American Society for the Control of Cancer, 256

Americas: origins of peoples, 15–16; biological characteristics of peoples, 16; prehistoric disease pool, 16–21; pre-Columbian population, 24–25; European transformation of, 26–28; Spanish colonization of, 28; impact of disease on indigenous peoples, 28–47; colonial misunderstanding of climate, 49–50
Anopheles mosquito, 64, 86, 126, 132, 139
Anopheles quadrimaculatis, 185
anthrax, 9, 21
anthropometric data, as measure of health, 149–150
antibiotics, 201, 244; resistance, 264; therapy, 267
Apalachee, 34
aplastic anemia, 173, 228
apoplexy, 231
Arapahoes, 42
Armed Forces Institute of Pathology, 225
army: and malaria, 126; and disease, 143–148. *See also* military, impact of disease
arteriosclerosis, 241, 250
arthritis, 208, 228, 231
asbestosis, 238